REHABILITATION IN THE AGING

Rehabilitation in the Aging

Editor
T. Franklin Williams, M.D.

Director
National Institute on Aging
National Institutes of Health
Bethesda, Maryland

Professor of Medicine
The University of Rochester
School of Medicine and Dentistry
Rochester, New York

Raven Press ■ New York

Raven Press, 1140 Avenue of the Americas, New York, New York 10036

Made in the United States of America

Library of Congress Cataloging in Publication Data
Main entry under title:

Rehabilitation in the aging.

   Includes bibliographical references and index.
   1. Geriatrics. 2. Aged—Rehabilitation. I. Williams,
T. Franklin. [DNLM: 1. Aging. 2. Geriatrics. 3. Reha-
bilitation—In old age. WT 100 R345]
RC952.5.R43   1984   615.5'47   83-42929
ISBN 0-89004-417-1

The material contained in this volume was submitted as previously unpublished material, except in the instances in which credit has been given to the source from which some of the illustrative material was derived.

Great care has been taken to maintain the accuracy of the information contained in the volume. However, Raven Press cannot be held responsible for errors or for any consequences arising from the use of the information contained herein.

Foreword

Three decades ago a great majority of the medical profession looked at rehabilitation as an extracurricular, adjunct activity of medicine. The rapid development of rehabilitation medicine was a reflection of the growing realization that to the individual patient, the capacity to function in his daily round of work, play, and family responsibilities was a matter of crucial importance. Rehabilitation medicine seeks to maximize the patient's potential through training and education and by integrating the use of his remaining abilities in the physical, social, psychological, and vocational aspects of his life.

With the significant rise in the percentage of older people, the importance of non-job-oriented rehabilitation is evident. Unfortunately, in our work-oriented culture, rehabilitation of the aging has almost inevitably received a lower priority in practice than the rehabilitation of children and adults for whom vocational possibilities were seen as realizable goals.

Preventive medicine in the form of maintenance rehabilitation for older patients is an essential approach to retard both physical and psychological deterioration. Clinical diagnoses and the usual complaints associated with the normal slope of senescence do not by themselves indicate the patient's functional capacities nor their capacity to achieve a viable living pattern. In working with older people, the overall goals may differ but the intrinsic concept of rehabilitation remains the same—to achieve and maintain the maximum degree of functional ability possible.

The editors of this book have had long experience in rendering geriatric and rehabilitative care to long-term and handicapped patients. Contributors with special expertise in the field have been selected to present a wide range of relevant topics. This material should prove invaluable to practitioners of geriatric medicine and physiatry.

Howard A. Rusk, M.D.
New York University Medical Center

Acknowledgments

In the genesis and preparation of this volume an Editorial Board was established consisting of Grady Bray, Ph.D., Clinical Psychologist, Monroe Community Hospital; Mathew H. M. Lee, M.D., M.P.H., F.A.C.P., Professor of Clinical Rehabilitation Medicine, School of Medicine, New York University; Manuel Rodstein, M.D., Director of Research, Jewish Home and Hospital; and Irving S. Wright, M.D., Emeritus Professor of Medicine, Cornell University Medical College. This Editorial Board has contributed substantially in determining the scope, selection of topics and authors, and critical review of manuscripts. The authors of the chapters have been responsive to suggestions and patient in what must have seemed to be an interminable process of assembling the wide range of contributions. Finally, Mrs. Norma G. Lee of the staff at Monroe Community Hospital, and the Editorial Staff of Raven Press, are thanked for their close, continuing attention to the preparation and editing of the material in this book.

Contents

Rehabilitation in Specific Disease Entities Commonly Presenting in Older Persons

Specific Rehabilitative Therapies

* Deceased.

Contributors

John Baum, M.D.
Director
Arthritis and Clinical Immunology Unit
Monroe Community Hospital;
Professor of Medicine University of Rochester
School of Medicine and Dentistry
Rochester, New York 14642

H. Bruce Bosmann, Ph.D.
Associate Dean and Professor of Pharmacology
University of Cincinnati College of Medicine
Cincinnati, Ohio 45267

Grady P. Bray, Ph.D.
Clinical Psychologist
Rehabilitation Unit
Monroe Community Hospital
435 E. Henrietta Rd.
Assistant Professor of Rehabilitation Medicine
University of Rochester
School of Medicine
Rochester, New York 14642

Bruce M. Caplan, M.D.
Assistant Professor
Department of Preventive, Family, and Rehabilitation Medicine
University of Rochester Medical Center
School of Medicine and Dentistry
601 Elmwood Avenue
Rochester, New York 14642

Ernesto S. Capulong, M.D.
Director
Medical Education
Nassau County Medical Center
221 Hempstead Turnpike
East Meadow, New York 11554

Gary S. Clark, M.D.
Director
Rehabilitation Unit
Monroe Community Hospital
435 E. Henrietta Rd.
Assistant Professor of Rehabilitation
University of Rochester
School of Medicine
Rochester, New York 14642

Robert S. Davis, M.D.
Associate Professor
Department of Urology
University of Rochester School of Medicine and Dentistry
601 Elmwood Avenue
Rochester, New York 14642

Carl Eisdorfer, M.D.
President
Montefoire Medical Center
111 E. 210th Street
Bronx, New York 10467

Lawrence W. Friedmann, M.D.
Chairman
Department of Physical Medicine and Rehabilitation
Nassau County Medical Center
2201 Hempstead Turnpike
East Meadow, New York 11554

Charles J. Gibson, M.D.
Associate Professor
Department of Preventive, Family, and Rehabilitation Medicine
University of Rochester Medical Center
School of Medicine and Dentistry
601 Elmwood Avenue
Rochester, New York 14642

Carl M. Harris, M.D.
Associate Professor of Orthopaedics
University of Rochester School of Medicine
and Dentistry;
Chief of Orthopaedics
The Genesee Hospital
224 Alexander Street
Rochester, New York 14607

Arthur E. Helfand, D.P.M.
Professor and Chairman
Department of Community Health
Pennsylvania College of Podiatric Medi-
cine
9 Hansen Court
Narberth, Pennsylvania 19072

Masayoshi Itoh, M.D., M.P.H.
Associate Director
Rehabilitation Medicine
Director of Rehabilitation Medicine
Goldwater Memorial Hospital
New York University Medical Center
Franklin D. Roosevelt Island
New York, New York 10044

Robert H. Jones, M.D.
Clinical Associate Professor
Family, Preventive, and Rehabilitation
Medicine
Clinical Associate Professor
Department of Medicine
Rehabilitation Consultant to the Medical
Department
University of Rochester School of Medi-
cine;
Medical Consultant to the Human Factors
Laboratory
Eastman Kodak Company
1669 Lake Avenue
Rochester, New York 14650

Harold Keltz, M.D., S.A.C.P.
Director of the Respiration Laboratory
Veterans Administration Medical Center;
Associate Clinical Professor
Albert Einstein School of Medicine
Yeshiva University
Bronx, New York 10461

Abraham L. Kornzweig, M.D. (1900–1982)
Chief and Director of Research in
Ophthalmology
The Jewish Home and Hospital for the
Aged
120 West 106 Street
New York, New York 10025

Mathew H. M. Lee, M.D., M.P.H., F.A.C.P.
Professor of Clinical Rehabilitation
School of Medicine;
Clinical Professor of Behavioral Sciences
and Community Health
Clinical Professor of Oral and Maxillofa-
cial Surgery
College of Dentistry
New York University;
Director of Rehabilitation Medicine
Goldwater Memorial Hospital
New York University Medical Center
Franklin D. Roosevelt Island
New York, New York 10044

J. Pierre Loebel, M.D., M.A.
Department of Psychiatry and Behavioral
Sciences
School of Medicine
University of Washington
Seattle, Washington 98195
at Harborview Medical Center
Seattle, Washington 98104

Marjorie W. Myers-Robfogel, Ph.D.
Assistant Professor of Pharmacology and
Oncology
University of Rochester Medical Center
School of Medicine and Dentistry
601 Elmwood Avenue
Rochester, New York 14642

Martha Taylor Sarno, M.D.hc
Associate Professor
Clinical Rehabilitation Medicine
Institute of Rehabilitation Medicine
School of Medicine
New York University Medical Center
400 East 34th Street
New York, New York 10016

Joyce Shapiro-Sabari, M.A., O.T.R.
Department of Occupational Therapy
New York University
34 Stuyevesant Street
New York, New York 10003

Sidney I. Silverman, D.D.S
Research Professor and Director of Geriatrics
New York University College of Dentistry;
80 Park Avenue
New York, New York 10016

Barbara Silverstone, D.S.W.
Executive Director
The Benjamin Rose Institute

636 Rose Building
Cleveland, Ohio 44115

John A. Spittel, Jr., M.D.
Mary Lowell Leary Professor of Medicine
Mayo Medical School
Consultant in Internal Medicine and Cardiovascular Diseases
Mayo Clinic
Rochester, Minnesota 14603

Nanette Kass Wenger, M.D.
Professor of Medicine (Cardiology)
Emory University School of Medicine;
Director, Cardiac Clinics
Grady Memorial Hospital
Atlanta, Georgia 30303

Introduction

Rehabilitation in the Aging: Philosophy and Approaches

Rehabilitation is an approach, a philosophy, and a point of view as much as it is a set of techniques. The aim of rehabilitation, "to restore an individual to his/her former functional and environmental status, or, alternatively, to maintain or maximize remaining function," should be at the heart of all care of aging persons in order to help them continue to live as full a life as possible.

As persons age there is a gradual, progressive loss of function that limits the maximum effort a person can achieve and limits the reserves with which to deal with stresses. But an aging person who is fortunate enough to be spared chronic disabling diseases should continue to have ample functional capabilities to carry out all ordinary living activities to very advanced ages. Continued regular performance of usual activities is essential to maintaining functional capabilities and is thus an important aspect of rehabilitation in the aging.

Unfortunately, most older persons acquire chronic diseases and disabilities and have complex problems of a physical, psychological, and social nature that call for specific efforts at treatment and restoration or maintenance of function. The rehabilitative approach must include simultaneous attention to varied problems by professionals from a number of fields. The team philosophy so well established in the field of rehabilitation in general is particularly important in the care of elderly persons.

Another major consideration in the rehabilitative approach to elderly persons is the importance of what may seem to be small gains in function. Such "small gains" can make all the difference in the degree of independence that a person can achieve, including the difference between being able to live in one's own home and requiring care in a long-term care institution. A simple example is acquiring the ability to transfer without assistance from bed to chair, commode, or wheelchair in a person recovering from a stroke. Such an ability could well permit independence in carrying out most activities of daily living even if the person were unable to walk and depended on a wheelchair for locomotion. Another example is the elderly person in whom a flare-up of osteoarthritis of the knees has made ambulation so slow and painful that he/she cannot even get to the bathroom without great difficulties. Here the proper treatment of the osteoarthritis with anti-inflammatory drugs and physical therapy may accomplish no more than restoring the osteoarthritis to its former moderately disabling status, but this may be sufficient to permit the person to manage his/her daily needs. Without such an accomplishment, modest in itself, the person would very likely come under increasing pressure to accept a different living setting, e.g., a nursing home.

What age ranges should be considered in discussing aspects of rehabilitation in the aging? It is necessary to interpret "aging" broadly, inasmuch as there is great variability in characteristics that can be associated with age among persons of a wide range of chronological age; in addition, the chronic disabilities so common in elderly persons, such as arthritis and stroke, often appear in the middle to late-middle ages.

This book is intended to deal in substantial ways with the application of the rehabilitation philosophy and approaches to the needs of aging persons. It should assist physicians and other health personnel who provide primary care for older persons to achieve more effective prevention of loss of function and maintenance of remaining function, as well as assisting professionals in the field of physical medicine and rehabilitation to accomplish restorative goals in older patients.

The first section lays the foundation in presenting aspects of health and disease in the aging that influence rehabilitation. Two chapters address areas of change associated with aging in the vital organ systems of the heart and lungs. Perhaps the most important observations are that the declines in stroke volume and maximum ventilatory capacity can be minimized by proper training and exercises. Specific cardiac and pulmonary diseases that affect rehabilitation potential and require their own rehabilitative approaches are also discussed in those chapters, as well as a later chapter on cardiac disorders.

Basic information on pharmacological changes associated with aging are next addressed, including the alterations in the delivery of drugs with aging to the target organs (changes in absorption, metabolism, excretion, and distribution), and altered cellular responsiveness to various drugs. The variation between aging individuals in responsiveness to drugs is emphasized.

Psychological factors that influence rehabilitation are next discussed, including both those of recent onset such as the influence of medications, alcohol, depression, stress, and "learned helplessness," and those more long-standing influences of personality type and motivation. Sociological factors underlying rehabilitation therapy are discussed, including the roles of informal support from family, friends, and neighbors (with emphasis on the importance of realistic assessment of their capabilities), as well as formal supports, the need for a continuum of care, and the problem of transfer trauma.

The first section of the book closes with a chapter on sexuality in aging as an until recently neglected aspect of quality of life that should be considered in any plan of rehabilitation.

The second major section presents approaches to rehabilitation in the aging. Here we deal first with the principles of physical, neuromuscular activity, which determine the limits of retraining and which must be a part of retraining plans. Approaches to achieving maximum isometric strength, aerobic or dynamic capabilities, and coordination are presented in quantitative terms. There is emphasis on the rapid losses that occur with disuse, and on the importance of the proper work/rest cycle.

The next two chapters deal with functional assessment as the first step in the rehabilitation process, and the development of a rehabilitation plan. The careful functional assessment should include attention to mobility, self-care, homemaking abilities, and environmental characteristics of the home that may have impact on function. The other necessary characteristics of the rehabilitation process, described in detail, include the role of the rehabilitation team, the use of case conferences and family conferences, the importance of setting specific goals, the place of home assessment, and the use of follow-up evaluations and of such support systems as day hospitals. Psychological and social considerations in planning rehabilitation strategies are also addressed in the earlier chapters on psychological and social aspects.

The third major section of this book deals with rehabilitation in specific disease entities commonly presenting in older persons, beginning with strokes. Special characteristics of patients with strokes that must be assessed and dealt with in rehabilitation are identified and discussed: truncal integrity (the ability to maintain sitting balance); problems of the upper extremity such as edema, glenohumeral dislocation, and need for assistive devices; ability to transfer; function of the lower extremity including a standing balance, ability to advance the paretic limb, and use of canes and braces; loss of perception of the paretic side; and emotional changes including depression and loss of affective expression. Disorders in communication, as seen in persons with strokes and in other diseases are the subject of a full chapter.

Arthritis in the elderly is discussed, with emphasis on adequate differential diagnosis and the importance of physical measures of rehabilitative treatment as well as precise use of medications. Other soft tissue disorders common in elderly persons are also considered. The very important topic of joint replacement in the elderly is addressed in a separate chapter, with attention to indications, principles of replacement, and coordination with other rehabilitative therapies.

The importance of restoring and maintaining vision, dentition, and the integrity of the feet in the overall rehabilitation and quality of life of elderly persons is recognized through separate chapters on these subjects. Perspectives not often noted are presented, including the importance of the teeth (one's own or prosthetic) in maintaining facial appearance and self-confidence, and the importance of comfort in walking on motivation to be active.

A chapter on specific cardiac disorders is followed by one addressing rehabilitative aspects of peripheral vascular disorders in the elderly.

The final chapter in the section on specific disorders addresses the significant urologic problems faced by many elderly persons, including the very common problem of urinary incontinence, which can in many instances be eliminated or controlled with adequate diagnosis and treatment.

This book closes with two chapters on specific rehabilitation therapies of importance to elderly persons: the use of assistive devices and the use of self-help devices. Assistive devices include measures for the relief of pain, for improvement of locomotion through splinting, orthoses, prostheses and mobility aids, and devices to aid in communication. Self-help devices are distinguished from assistive devices as being aids in making life safer, easier, and more enjoyable for older persons who are not overtly disabled. They include a variety of imaginative and often simple approaches to conserving energy expenditure, preventing accidents, and compensating for modest losses in coordination, dexterity or vision.

Almost everyone, in growing older, is beset with fears and concerns about losing previous capabilities, becoming chronically disabled, and facing a diminishing quality of life. To a large extent, much greater than is generally appreciated or attempted, such fears can be relieved and such outcomes prevented or realistically minimized through a comprehensive rehabilitation philosophy and the types of rehabilitative efforts presented in this volume.

T. Franklin Williams, M.D.

REHABILITATION IN THE AGING

Rehabilitation in the Aging edited by
T. F. Williams. Raven Press, New York © 1984.

Cardiovascular Status: Changes with Aging

Nanette Kass Wenger

Department of Medicine (Cardiology), Emory University School of Medicine; and Cardiac Clinics, Grady Memorial Hospital, Atlanta, Georgia 30303

Cardiovascular status is an important determinant of total performance ability. Cardiac changes in the elderly include both the physiologic alterations of aging and those due to associated cardiovascular disease.

The major alterations of cardiorespiratory function encountered with aging that influence activity performance include a decrease in maximal oxygen consumption, a decrease in maximal exercise heart rate, a decrease in exercise stroke volume, and a decrease in cardiac output (10,18) (Fig. 1). These result in a diminished capacity for work and a decreased ability to tolerate a variety of stresses (16).

However, even in the elderly, significant increases in endurance and work capacity can be achieved with physical training.

PATHOLOGY

Anatomic alterations in the cardiovascular system constitute an important component of the changes observed in cardiac status (5,13). Aging is characterized by a decrease in vascular distensibility, with aortoarterial elasticity at age

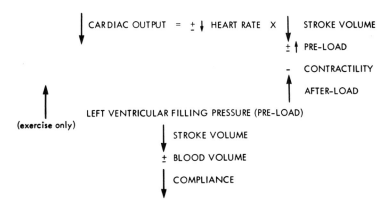

FIG. 1. Change in hemodynamics with aging. (From Noble and Rothbaum, ref. 18, with permission.)

70 reduced to half of its value at age 20. A widened tortuous aorta is common (7). The increase in aortic volume may partially compensate for aortic wall stiffness, which decreases the ability of the aorta to function as a compression chamber (9). The increased rigidity of the walls of the larger arteries and veins appears to render less effective the regulatory stretch receptors.

Heart valves typically become thicker and more rigid, have an increased collagen content, and may undergo degenerative calcification (20). Alternatively, valvular myxomatous degeneration may occur. Left atrial size tends to increase as does left ventricular mass (7), the latter possibly related to increased aortic impedance. The left ventricular wall at age 80 may be 25% thicker than at age 30. The increased myocardial wall stiffness of aging has been attributed to more rigid intercellular collagenous connective tissue.

The cardiac skeleton also becomes increasingly dense, with sclerosis of collagen. An increase in fibrous and elastic tissue in the conduction system, often with associated calcification, may result in conduction disturbances and atrioventricular block.

All these features place the aging heart at a mechanical disadvantage. There is only tenuous evidence for a cardiopathy of aging. It is therefore inappropriate to consider this as the etiology of heart failure in an elderly individual; rather, a specific and possibly remediable etiologic factor should be sought.

BLOOD PRESSURE

The blood pressure of the elderly individual is dependent on the balance between the loss of elasticity in the larger arteries that occurs with aging and the increased lability of vasopressor control. In general, there occurs an increase in the rate of rise of pressure, an increase in the peak systolic pressure, and a widening of the pulse pressure. The major change is in systolic blood pressure, which progressively increases to age 75 or 80, with subsequent stabilization of level. A marked widening of the range of systolic blood pressure occurs with increasing age. There is likewise a greater rise in exercise systolic blood pressure in the elderly (10), but this decreases with training (21). The problem of isolated systolic hypertension in the elderly is currently under intensive study. Diastolic blood pressure changes less, tending to increase slightly into the sixties, with a subsequent gradual but minimal decline. Most reviews of hypertension in the elderly use a blood pressure of 160/95 to 100 mm Hg as the indicator of hypertension.

Baroreceptor activity diminishes with aging, with a resultant decrease in the reflex tachycardia on assuming the upright position. This in part accounts for the increase in symptomatic orthostatic hypotension in the elderly (13). Again, decreased efficiency of the compensatory mechanism is a considerable component of the carotid sinus syncope, cough syncope, and micturition syncope more frequently encountered in elderly individuals.

CARDIAC OUTPUT

The causes of the decrease in cardiac output with aging have received considerable attention. Lean body mass, body surface area, and muscle mass all decrease with age. The decreased basal metabolic rate lessens the need for circulatory oxygen transport. Heart rate, thus, decreases with age. However, these features do not account for more than half of the observed decrease in cardiac output in the elderly (3). The decrease in stroke volume with aging accounts for the other half of the change. Stroke volume determinants are discussed subsequently.

It is necessary to examine the changes in cardiac output both at rest and with exercise, identifying differences in the supine and upright positions. In this way, the variations in the components of the change in cardiac output, the alterations in heart rate and stroke volume, can be defined.

The resting supine cardiac output varies considerably with age but tends to decrease about 1% per year after puberty (3,12,22) (Fig. 2). Only half of the decline corresponds to the decreased oxygen uptake with increasing age. Also, resting cardiac output is significantly lower in the sitting than recumbent position, despite the higher oxygen uptake (9). Interestingly, there is no difference between the resting stroke volume and cardiac output of older and younger individuals in the upright position because of the less marked decrease of stroke volume and cardiac output in the elderly when changing from the supine to the upright

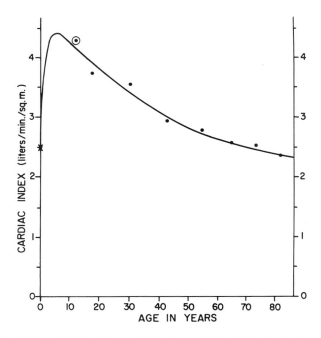

FIG. 2. Cardiac index at different ages. Data from K. Prec (×), L. Brotmacher (⊙), and M. Brandfonbrener (●). (From Guyton, et al., ref. 12, with permission of W. B. Saunders.)

position. Cardiac output in elderly men is less than in younger individuals with both sitting and supine exercise.

The increase in cardiac output and in oxygen uptake with an increased work demand is comparable in younger and older individuals. That is to say, a comparable increase in cardiac output and in oxygen uptake occurs between rest and activity in younger and older individuals. Thus, the difference is in work capacity, not in the efficiency of oxygen extraction. Nevertheless, for any given level of oxygen uptake, the cardiac output (as well as the stroke volume) is lower with increasing age, both at rest and with exercise. However, both the maximal cardiac output and the maximal oxygen uptake decrease less with increasing age in the physically active than in the sedentary (4).

Circulation time prolongs slightly with age. This decrease in blood flow velocity is consistent with the reduction in the volume of blood flow (3).

HEART RATE

No change occurs with aging in the resting heart rate or in the heart rate response to submaximal work loads (21); however, the maximal exercise heart rate decreases progressively with age (22) (Fig. 3). This inability of the elderly to reach a higher heart rate is not well understood. Fibrosis of the conduction system and pacemaker sites has been suggested, as has a decrease in myofiber catecholamine receptors. It may be related to the same mechanism that is responsible for the lesser increase in heart rate on assuming the upright position in the older individual (19). Additionally, there is prolongation of the time needed for the heart rate to return to normal after exercise (17). Because the mean heart rate at a given oxygen uptake is comparable in older and younger men, the lower mean cardiac output of the elderly results from a lower mean stroke volume, corresponding to the increased arteriovenous oxygen difference (10).

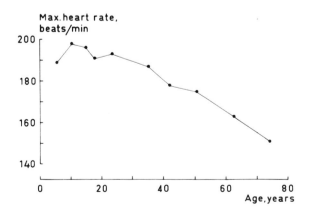

FIG. 3. Maximal heart rate during upright exercise in relation to age in 81 normal nonathletic men. (From Strandell, ref. 22, with permission of Plenum Press.)

Conway et al. (6) postulated that the exercise-induced sympathetic drive to the heart declines with age, accounting for the decreased cardiac output at all exercise levels. The basis for this concept was the lesser propranolol effect on exercise heart rate and cardiac output in older (age 50 to 65) than in younger (age 20 to 35) men. Systolic blood pressure also decreased after propranolol administration in both younger and older individuals with maximal exercise, but the decrease was greater in older than in younger individuals. Thus, propranolol administration to the young obliterates their improved response to stress as compared with the elderly. The decreased rate of systolic ejection as blood enters the stiffer vascular tree in older people may explain the lesser rise in pressure.

Nevertheless, the decrease in heart rate was partly compensated for by an increase in stroke volume; the older individuals achieved the same maximal stroke volume as the younger individuals (6). The aging hearts responded adequately to the demands of exercise, so that a decrease in cardiac performance did not appear responsible for the decreased physical capacity encountered with aging. Without beta blockade, younger individuals increased their cardiac output with increasing loads of exercise. With beta blockade, the cardiac output was comparable in older and younger individuals, with the propranolol effect becoming progressively more obvious as the exercise intensity increased.

STROKE VOLUME

The decrease in cardiac output with age, both at rest and with submaximal exercise, is influenced significantly by a decrease in the stroke volume (3,11). This is enhanced by the decrease in the maximal exercise heart rate response with aging. Stroke volume is lower in the aged at upright rest and with both recumbent and upright exercise (10) (Fig. 4). Only at sitting rest is stroke volume comparable in the old and young. With change from recumbent to sitting rest, stroke volume decreases 45% in the young and 21% in the aged (9). Stroke volume is inversely related to the arteriovenous oxygen difference. Arteriovenous oxygen difference is greater in the sitting than in the recumbent position, both at rest and with exercise, and stroke volume is significantly lower. A smaller increase in exercise stroke volume occurs in the older individual with change from the sitting to the supine position.

Contractile state, preload, and afterload influence stroke volume. Little change in contractility has been documented with aging in the absence of heart disease (7), although this aspect of myocardial function remains controversial.

The filling pressures at rest are comparable in older and younger individuals, but exercise produces an accentuated rise in the elderly. The increased exercise filling pressure in the aged increases myocardial fiber length and stroke volume in these individuals who have decreased wall compliance because of increased rigidity of the collagenous connective tissue. The increased exercise filling pressures of aging thus manifest an adjustment to the decreased cardiac wall distensi-

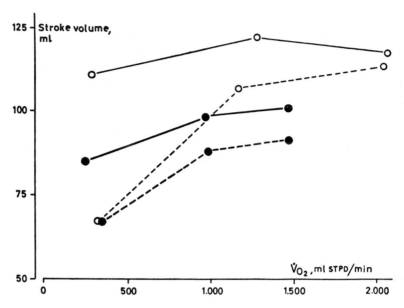

FIG. 4. Mean stroke volumes in relation to oxygen uptake (V_{O_2} at rest and during exercise in old (*filled circles*) and young (*open circles*) men in recumbent (*solid lines*, N = 16 and 23, respectively) and sitting (*broken lines*, N = 6 and 9, respectively) positions. (From Granath et al., ref. 10, with permission of S. Karger, AG, Basel.)

bility and should not be considered evidence of heart failure (9,11). With an increase in filling pressure, the ventricles increase their stroke volume and function in accordance with Starling's law of the heart. The increased exercise cardiac output in relation to oxygen uptake is produced by an increase in heart volume and an increase in pulmonary capillary wedge pressure.

Thus, the major determinant of the decreased stroke volume in the elderly is the afterload, the increased impedance to systolic ejection of both the right and left ventricles. This increased resistance decreases the stroke volume and increases the filling pressures by the increase in end-systolic volume, which results from the decrease in stroke volume. The increased rigidity of the aorta and other large vessels with aging compromises their function as a compression chamber and produces the increases in systolic arterial pressure, in pulse pressure, and in systemic resistance. Thus, systolic blood pressure and mean arterial pressure increase to a greater extent with exercise in older individuals, increasing the systolic pressure load on the left ventricle. Pulmonary and systemic vascular resistance indices are increased in the elderly both at rest and with exercise. Pulmonary artery distensibility also decreases with age, with a resultant increase in pulmonary artery systolic and mean pressures with exercise. Although pulmonary capillary wedge pressure is slightly lower in the aged individual at rest, pulmonary capillary wedge pressure, right ventricular end diastolic pressure, and pulmonary artery pressure are related to the degree of physical activity and are higher with exercise in the elderly (8). Trained elderly individuals have an increased exercise pulmonary capillary wedge pressure and right ventricular end diastolic pressure. Pulmonary ventilation correlates with exercise filling pressures, mediated through variations in central blood volume (9).

Measurement of left ventricular ejection time shows an increase of about 2 msec for each decade. Postulated causes include a decrease in sympathetic tone, a decrease in myocardial contractility, and/or an increase in aortic impedance. There is no significant effect of the heart rate or blood pressure on ejection time. These findings are compatible with prior reports of prolonged isometric contraction and relaxation with age (14). Decreased rate of calcium removal has been the suggested mechanism responsible for the increased relaxation time.

MAXIMUM OXYGEN UPTAKE WITH TRAINING

The maximal capacity of the cardiovascular system to deliver oxygen to exercising muscles as reflected by the maximal oxygen uptake decreases with age (21), about 0.45 ml/kg/year, regardless of habitual activity level (15) (Fig. 5). With the same initial aerobic capacity, less improvement occurs with training in older individuals. In general, training produces little or no increase in the maximal oxygen uptake in the elderly, but rather a decrease in the heart rate

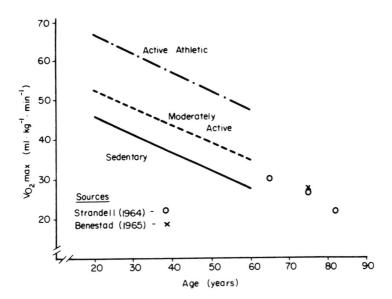

FIG. 5. The decrease of maximum oxygen consumption with age in men aged 20 to 60 years. Sedentary men: V_{O_2} max = 54.1 − 0.41 (age). Moderately active men: V_{O_2} max = 61.6 − 0.44 (age). Active athletic men: V_{O_2} max = 76.1 − 0.48 (age). (From Hodgson and Buskirk, ref. 15, with permission of the American Geriatrics Society.)

at any submaximal work load. However, with more intensive training, maximal oxygen uptake as well as stroke volume and cardiac output may increase modestly (21).

Benestad (2) trained 70- to 81-year-old men for a 5- to 6-week period, but did not alter the oxygen cost of exercise by the training (Fig. 6). Despite the lack of training effect on maximal oxygen uptake (aerobic capacity), an improved work efficiency was evident as a decrease in heart rate of about 14 beats/min. Because the oxygen cost was not altered, this heart rate change reflected an increase in the oxygen pulse (the amount of oxygen removed from the blood per heartbeat, calculated by dividing the oxygen intake by the heart rate over a given period of time). There was no effect of training on pulmonary ventilatory efficiency. There was, however, a tendency (nonsignificant) to increase the heart size and an increase in blood volume and hemoglobin concentration of borderline significance with training, suggesting an enhancement of the stroke volume. Stated another way, the effect of training in increasing the stroke volume with supine exercise appears due not to an increase in cardiac dimension related to the training, but rather to blood volume redistribution with exercise, with an ability to increase the central blood volume on exercising (9). In contrast to the training of young individuals, no change in maximal heart rate or aerobic capacity is achieved by training older individuals. However, training was associated with a general increase in well-being and an improvement in mental relaxation.

Endurance training of women aged 52 to 79 (1) showed a trainability similar to that of older men, with a decrease in resting heart rate, an increase in maximal oxygen consumption, and improved physical work capacity.

Because the energy expenditure of walking represents a larger percentage of the aerobic capacity with increasing age, walking becomes an effective physical conditioning stimulus (15) (Fig. 7).

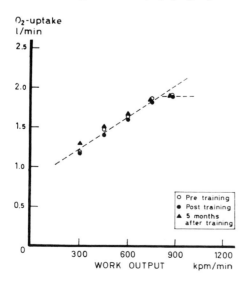

FIG. 6. Average oxygen uptake in 13 old men during bicycling at different loads. (From Benestad, ref. 2, with permission of Acta Medica Scandinavica.)

Premature ventricular contractions increase with age, but the effect of training on premature ventricular contractions in elderly persons has not yet been determined. Changes in static muscle strength and endurance (as measured by handgrip) occur in the aged individual. These decrease more from age 60 to 80 than from age 30 to 60. The heart rate response to static endurance work decreases with age, whereas the systolic blood pressure response increases. There is no change in diastolic blood pressure response.

CARDIAC OUTPUT DISTRIBUTION IN OLD AGE

The resistance to regional blood flow tends to increase with age but varies in the different vascular beds. The decrease in renal blood flow is related, at least in part, to the decrease in the number of nephrons. Renal blood flow may decrease 55% from the fourth to the ninth decades. This decrease in renal blood flow may explain the increased arteriovenous oxygen difference with aging. With a normal renal blood flow, a low arteriovenous oxygen difference is present. Calf blood flow in concomitant comparison studies remains essentially unchanged (9).

Also encountered is a decrease in cerebral blood flow. No major change in coronary blood flow, in the absence of coronary atherosclerotic heart disease, is encountered at rest and with moderate exercise. Information regarding coronary blood flow, however, is limited. Increased cardiac output with exercise, as in younger individuals, is distributed primarily to working muscles. The low skin temperature of the elderly is probably related to decreased skin blood flow. The inability to sweat efficiently with increased age, and limited temperature regulation with heat stress, may have a comparable basis. There is, however,

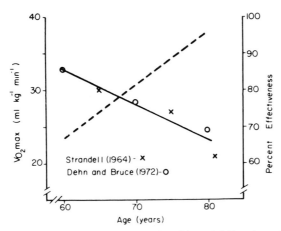

FIG. 7. The possible percentage effectiveness of walking at 3.5 mph on level ground as a conditioning stimulus for the elderly (*broken line*) related to the decrease in maximum oxygen consumption (*solid line*). (From Hodgson and Buskirk, ref. 15, with permission of the American Geriatrics Society.)

a lack of information on the distribution of the exercise cardiac output in elderly individuals.

EFFECTS OF PHYSICAL TRAINING

Maximal cardiac output and maximal oxygen uptake decrease less with increasing age in physically active individuals (15), documenting that regular physical activity helps maintain physical work capacity into old age.

Physical training of the elderly increases the stroke volume. Physically active elderly individuals have an increased stroke volume and increased pulmonary capillary wedge pressure with exercise. Very intensive training also increases the maximal oxygen uptake by about 10%, as well as decreasing the heart rate response (11).

The increase in stroke volume and maximal cardiac output with exercise appears largely due to the regulation of blood volume distribution, with the ability to increase the central blood volume with exercise. These changes are similar to those in younger individuals. In the elderly, however, the increase in maximal oxygen uptake seems due solely to this increase in stroke volume, and not as in younger persons to a simultaneous increase in the arteriovenous oxygen difference.

The limitation of physical work capacity with aging relates to the decrease in the maximal exercise heart rate and stroke volume, resulting in a decreased exercise cardiac output. The decrease in maximal oxygen uptake is more marked in sedentary individuals. Ventilatory factors do not appear to limit physical work capacity. However, no data are available in the aged regarding peripheral factors—muscle mass, muscle blood flow, cellular metabolic features such as mitochondrial changes—influencing physical work capacity.

SUMMARY

Cardiac changes that occur with aging, both physiologic changes and those associated with disease, must be appreciated in assessing the functional capacity of the elderly individual and in making recommendations for activity levels and energy expenditure.

REFERENCES

1. Adams, G. M., and de Vries, H. A. (1973): Physiological effects of an exercise training regimen upon women aged 52 to 79. *J. Gerontol.*, 28:50–55.
2. Benestad, A. M. (1965): Trainability of old men. *Acta Med. Scand.*, 178:321–327.
3. Brandfonbrener, M., Landowne, M., and Shock, N. W. (1955): Changes in cardiac output with age. *Circulation*, 12:557–566.
4. Brunner, D., and Meshulam, N. (1970): Physical fitness of trained elderly people. In: *Physical Activity and Aging*, edited by D. Brunner and E. Jokl, pp. 80–84. University Park Press, Baltimore.
5. Caird, F. I., and Kennedy, R. D. (1976): Epidemiology of heart disease in old age. In: *Cardiology*

in Old Age, edited by F. I. Caird, J. L. C. Dall, and R. D. Kennedy, pp. 1–10. Plenum Press, New York.

6. Conway, J., Wheeler, R., and Sannerstedt, R. (1971): Sympathetic nervous activity during exercise in relation to age. *Cardiovasc. Res.,* 5:577–581.
7. Gerstenblith, G., Frederiksen, J., Yin, F. C. P., Fortuin, N. J., Lakatta, E. G., and Weisfeldt, M. L. (1977): Echocardiographic assessment of a normal adult aging population. *Circulation,* 56:273–278.
8. Gerstenblith, G., Lakatta, E. G., and Weisfeldt, M. L. (1976): Age changes in myocardial function and exercise response. *Prog. Cardiovasc. Dis.,* 19:1–21.
9. Granath, A., Jonsson, B., and Strandell, T. (1964): Circulation in healthy old men, studied by right heart catheterization at rest and during exercise in supine and sitting position. *Acta Med. Scand.,* 176:425–446.
10. Granath, A., Jonsson, B., and Strandell, T. (1970): Circulation in healthy old men, studied by right heart catheterization at rest and during exercise in supine and sitting position. In: *Physical Activity and Aging,* edited by D. Brunner and E. Jokl, pp. 48–79. University Park Press, Baltimore.
11. Granath, A., and Strandell, T. (1964): Relationships between cardiac output, stroke volume, and intracardiac pressures at rest and during exercise in supine position and some anthropometric data in healthy old men. *Acta Med. Scand.,* 176:447–466.
12. Guyton, A. C., Jones, C. E., and Coleman, T. G. (1973): *Circulatory Physiology: Cardiac Output and Its Regulation,* pp. 8–20. Saunders, Philadelphia.
13. Harris, R. (1970): *The Management of Geriatric Cardiovascular Disease,* pp. 1–16. J. B. Lippincott, Philadelphia.
14. Harrison, T. R., Dixon, K., Russell, R. O., Jr., Bidwai, P. S., and Coleman, H. N. (1964): The relation of age to the duration of contraction, ejection, and relaxation of the normal human heart. *Am. Heart J.,* 67:189–199.
15. Hodgson, J. L., and Buskirk, E. R. (1977): Physical fitness and age, with emphasis on cardiovascular function in the elderly. *J. Am. Geriatr. Soc.,* 25:385–392.
16. Kolata, G. B. (1977): The aging heart: Changes in function and response to drugs. *Science,* 195:166–167.
17. Montoye, H. J., Willis, P. W., and Cunningham, D. A. (1968): Heart rate response to submaximal exercise: Relation to age and sex. *J. Gerontol.,* 23:127–133.
18. Noble, R. J., and Rothbaum, D. A. (1979): Heart disease in the elderly (geriatric cardiology). In: *The Heart, Update I,* edited by J. W. Hurst, pp. 211–234. McGraw-Hill, New York.
19. Norris, A. H., Shock, N. W., and Yiengst, M. J. (1953): Age changes in heart rate and blood pressure responses to tilting and standardized exercise. *Circulation,* 8:521–526.
20. Sell, S., and Scully, R. E. (1965): Aging changes in the aortic and mitral valves. *Am. J. Pathol.,* 46:345–365.
21. Skinner, J. S. (1970): The cardiovascular system with aging and exercise. In: *Physical Activity and Aging,* edited by D. Brunner and E. Jokl, pp. 100–108. University Park Press, Baltimore.
22. Strandell, T. (1976): Cardiac output in old age. In: *Cardiology in Old Age,* edited by F. I. Caird, J. L. C. Dall, and R. D. Kennedy, pp. 81–100. Plenum Press, New York.

Rehabilitation in the Aging edited by
T. F. Williams. Raven Press, New York © 1984.

Pulmonary Function and Disease in the Aging

Harold Keltz

*Montefiore Hospital; Respiration Laboratory, Veterans Administration Medical Center;
and Department of Medicine, Albert Einstein School of Medicine, Yeshiva University,
Bronx, New York 10461*

Respiratory function decreases with increasing age. The decrease is in part related to the long history of exposure to inhaled noxious agents such as tobacco smoke, air pollutants, and infecting agents. It is also, in part, related to the effect of aging in the various organs, which include not only the lungs but the muscles, brain, and heart. The relative contribution of the two factors is very difficult to measure since both are related to the passage of time.

Most data available on the effects of aging have been collected by studies of an aged population (cross-sectional) rather than studying individuals as they have gotten older (longitudinal studies). As a result, many of the conclusions are probably biased in favor of fit subjects who survive to an older age than the general population. There are also discrepancies in various studies but a consensus will be presented.

Normal lungs are usually sterile below the level of the carina. They assume the gross shape of the chest wall, which changes with increasing age because of changes in the spine, ribs, and cartilage. There is dilatation of the airways and the alveoli with occasional breakdown of alveolar walls suggestive of emphysema. The total content, by dry weight, of collagen and elastin, within the lung, appears to be unchanged with aging but there is an increase in the cross-linkage of the elastin. The pulmonary vessels also change with an increase in internal fibrosis and thickening of the vessel wall. All of these anatomic changes result in functional changes as well.

In addition to the changes in the lungs there are changes in the neuromuscular and cardiovascular systems that occur with aging. A properly functioning respiratory system requires proper function of the neuromuscular and cardiovascular system in order to maintain normal gas exchange between the tissues and the environment. Under normal circumstances, the central nervous system and peripheral receptors respond to changes in oxygen and carbon dioxide tensions, pH, and metabolic states with appropriate changes in ventilation. Abnormalities of either the nervous or muscular systems that occur with aging may result in abnormal respiration even if the lungs are normal.

Furthermore, gas exchange requires not only ventilation to maintain alveolar gases at normal levels, but an intact cardiovascular system to perfuse the pulmonary capillary bed so that normal gas exchange can take place at the alveolar capillary interface. Changes in cardiac output or distribution of blood flow in the lungs that result from abnormalities of the heart or blood vessels, frequently seen in the elderly, will also result in abnormal respiration even if the lungs are otherwise normal.

In the absence of disease, the decrease in respiratory function resulting from aging does not limit the elderly if the cardiovascular and neuromuscular apparatus is intact. Although the pulmonary function decreases with age, the loss is one of the reserve necessary during stress. The loss is not sufficient to interfere with ordinary activity. Even this decrease in reserve can be kept to a minimum if active efforts are made to maintain fitness.

CONTROL OF RESPIRATION

Unlike the heart, the muscles of respiration have no intrinsic rhythmicity and require stimuli from the central nervous system. With increasing age there is a decrease in response of the respiratory center to a lowered oxygen tension or an increase in carbon dioxide tension in the arterial blood, as well as a decrease in heart rate in response to hypoxemia (9). It is not clear whether this is due to changes in the peripheral receptors or central regulation. It has also been shown that sleeping men, but not sleeping women, have a decrease in ventilation and oxygenation with increasing age (3).

Cheyne-Stokes respiration is frequently seen in elderly subjects either because of brain damage or because of congestive heart failure with decrease in cerebral blood flow. This, however, does not result in alveolar hypoventilation. Both arterial oxygen and carbon dioxide tensions may be normal. Although the respiratory rhythm is abnormal, ventilation and gas exchange is adequate.

LUNG VOLUMES

As first shown by Hutchinson in 1846 vital capacity decreases in the elderly (8). Normal standards use an age correction factor. The measurement of vital capacity requires a maximal expiration after a maximal inspiration. Decrease in muscle strength, as part of aging, will result in a decrease in vital capacity independently of changes in the lungs. Residual volume (RV) increases with age (16). Since the total lung capacity (TLC), which is the sum of the vital capacity and RV, is relatively unchanged with age, the RV to TLC ratio is increased. The increase in RV/TLC is not necessarily indicative of emphysema but reflects the loss of elastic recoil noted with aging (12,16).

LUNG MECHANICS

During quiet inspiration the diaphragm and other inspiratory muscles contract, with the diaphragm providing the greatest force. The increase in thoracic volume with resultant decrease in pleural pressure results in a decrease in alveolar pressure. Air then flows from the environment at atmospheric pressure to the alveoli until alveolar pressure equals atmospheric pressure at the end of inspiration. Quiet expiration is passive with relaxation of the inspiratory muscles. Air is exhaled as a result of the elastic recoil of the lungs to a resting level at the end of expiration. At this point alveolar pressure is again atmospheric and the volume of air remaining in the lung is functional residual capacity.

Compliance is the measurement of the pressure change necessary for a given volume change in the lung and chest wall. Lung compliance tends to increase with increasing age. However, chest wall compliance decreases with increasing age (11). The decrease in chest wall compliance is greater than the increase in lung compliance so that total respiratory compliance decreases with age. This means that with increasing age a greater pressure must be exerted to get a given volume change. These measurements are made when there is no flow of air so that the pressure necessary to overcome airway resistance is not included.

During forced expiratory maneuvers the intercostal muscles and abdominal muscles provide the additional expiratory force. With increasing age all of the forced expiratory measurements decrease. Regardless of whether maximum voluntary ventilation, forced vital capacity, or flow volume curves are used as the measure of expiratory flow, there is a decrease with increasing age (14). Flow results from the driving pressure in the airways divided by the resistance of the airways. If the airway resistance is unchanged, the decrease in flow must result from the decrease in driving pressure. This decrease may be largely a result of muscle weakening with increasing age.

Measurements used to indicate small airway abnormalities such as closing volume and frequency dependent lung compliance show increasing abnormalities with age (2,4). This is probably related to small airway closure during forced expiratory maneuvers because of decreased elastic function in the lung.

VENTILATION

Ventilation is the process of moving air from the environment to the alveoli during inspiration and from the alveoli to the environment during expiration. Water vapor is added to the inhaled gases so that it is 100% saturated by the time it reaches the lung. Carbon dioxide is added and oxygen is removed from the alveolar gas, which is then expired. Ventilation consists of the sum of dead space ventilation plus alveolar ventilation with gas exchange occurring only in alveolar ventilation. Therefore, alveolar ventilation is the essential component for maintaining normal oxygen and carbon dioxide levels. Resting ventilation remains normal with increasing age as does the frequency of respiration and tidal volume. The distribution of ventilation in the elderly, however, is less uniform so that nitrogen washout curves indicate increasing abnormalities with increasing age (10). It also requires a greater degree of ventilation to wash out nitrogen with oxygen in the elderly (6). It is possible to obtain a greater uniformity in distribution in older men by increasing the tidal volume so that differences in uniformity of ventilation between younger and older men can be obliterated by deep breathing (6). Maximal ventilation decreases with increasing age.

GAS EXCHANGE

Normal gas exchange requires not only uniform ventilation of the alveoli but also blood flow distribution through the pulmonary capillary bed such that well-ventilated areas are also well perfused. Obviously, if a well-perfused area is poorly ventilated the blood will retain carbon dioxide and not gain oxygen. On the other hand, in areas that are well ventilated but poorly perfused, the ventilation is essentially wasted dead space ventilation. With increasing age a slight increase in dead space has been noted along with a decrease in the uniformity of ventilation. In addition to changes in ventilation there are changes in the pulmonary vascular bed with aging. As a result there is an increase in ventilation-perfusion imbalance with increasing age. There may also be mild abnormalities of diffusion that occur with aging so that gas exchange is impaired in the elderly. As a result of this the normal arterial oxygen tension tends to decrease with age (5). The carbon dioxide tension remains unchanged because it is possible to increase ventilation sufficiently to compensate for the impaired gas exchange of carbon dioxide resulting from mild ventilation-perfusion imbalances. A normal level of pH is maintained with aging.

ARTERIAL BLOOD GAS

The arterial oxygen tension tends to decrease with aging but saturation is normal or only slightly reduced. The relationship between oxygen saturation and oxygen tension is defined by the oxygen hemoglobin dissociation curve. A decrease in partial pressure of oxygen of 30 mmHg, from 100 to 70 mmHg, is associated with a decrease of saturation of only 4.7%, from 97.4 to 92.7%. The slope of the curve becomes more steep at this point so that further decrease in oxygen tension results in a more marked decrease in oxygen content of the blood. Therefore, the decrease of arterial oxygen tension seen in normal older subjects does not result in much decrease in oxygen content but results in the loss of reserve should there be a further decrease in oxygen tension for any reason.

The changes described with increasing age show a decrease in lung function as measured in the laboratory. These changes occur from the onset of adulthood and continue throughout life. However, they do not significantly interfere with ordinary activity if disease, obesity, and disuse are not added as burdens to the respiratory system. The nonsmoking, lean, physically active elderly person will not be limited by the effects that aging has on his pulmonary function.

EXERCISE

During exercise, ventilation increases and arterial oxygen tension, pH, and carbon dioxide tension remain within normal limits until extreme levels of exercise are achieved. The degree of exercise is usually measured by the oxygen consumption achieved. The greater the oxygen consumption, the greater the degree of exercise until a maximal level is achieved. The more fit and well trained the subject, the greater is the maximal oxygen consumption.

It has been shown that with increasing age there is a decrease of the maximal oxygen consumption (1,5). This is found even in subjects who have remained active physically and has been shown to be present both in longitudinal and cross-sectional studies. However, it has also been shown that trained subjects who are elderly have a greater maximal oxygen consumption than sedentary subjects who are younger (5). Thus, the ability to exercise decreases with aging both as a result of lack of training and the effect of aging itself.

In our present state of knowledge we are unable to modify the aging process. We can, however, readily modify fitness at any age by training. This has the advantage of both increasing the maximal oxygen consumption and also decreasing the oxygen cost of effort as efficiency also increases with training. As a result, more activity becomes possible with much less discomfort.

The fit person can engage in increasing activity levels with smaller increases in heart rate, cardiac output, oxygen consumption, and lactic acid production than the untrained person at the same level of activity. A greater reserve thus becomes available for a given stress situation, which then is easier to endure. In young healthy people, there is usually sufficient reserve in cardiopulmonary function to compensate for stress. In the elderly, the pulmonary and cardiac reserves are limited by age so it becomes increasingly important not to limit them also by inactivity. Training in the elderly, perhaps more than in young people, will help provide the cardiopulmonary reserve necessary to withstand future insults to the cardiopulmonary system. The tendency of physicians and society to emphasize decrease in activity among the elderly probably contributes more to poor pulmonary function than aging alone. This should be reversed and training for fitness at every age should be encouraged.

IMPACT OF DISEASE: PREVENTATIVE AND RESTORATIVE ASPECTS

Several common pulmonary diseases seen in the elderly will be discussed. It is frequently easier to prevent than to treat lung disease. Vaccines that offer some protection against influenza and pneumococcal pneumonia are available. Since both of these are fairly common infections and are potentially lethal, particularly in the elderly, both vaccines should be administered to older people. Not only should vaccines be used to help prevent disease but every effort should be made to keep the airways from being damaged in any way.

Elderly patients have had more time for inhalation of noxious agents so that effects of cigarette smoking, infections, air pollutants, and industrial exposure as well as aging become more significant. Unquestionably, cigarette smoking is the major contributor to pulmonary dysfunction.

Chronic Bronchitis and Emphysema

Chronic bronchitis and emphysema occur most frequently after the fifth decade of life. Chronic bronchitis is defined clinically by excessive mucus secretions resulting in a chronic cough. The chronic cough must be present for at least two years and occur three months of the year to meet the clinical criteria for bronchitis. Other causes of cough must be excluded. Emphysema is defined anatomically as abnormal enlargement of the air spaces distal to the terminal, nonrespiratory bronchiole, accompanied by destructive changes of the alveolar walls.

Bronchitis and emphysema usually occur together. Attempts to separate the two entities are difficult but in principle the bronchitic subject has obstruction to flow in the airways but is able to develop normal transpulmonary pressure. The emphysema patient has normal airway resistance but a reduction in transpulmonary pressure. Both diseases, therefore, result in decrease in airflow but in bronchitis it is due to an increase in resistance to flow whereas in emphysema it is due to a decrease in the driving pressure developed.

Pulmonary function tests will show a decrease in the various flow tests and an increase in RV in both diseases. However, in general, the TLC will tend to be normal in chronic bronchitis but increased in emphysema. The single breath carbon monoxide diffusing capacity ($DLCO_{SB}$) is usually normal in bronchitis but decreased in emphysema. It has also been shown that patients with chronic bronchitis have more severe ventilation perfusion imbalance at rest than emphysema patients with a resultant lower arterial oxygen tension at rest. During exercise, however, the arterial oxygen tension will remain the same or increase in bronchitis whereas the oxygen tension of emphysema patients tend to decrease with exercise.

Patients with chronic bronchitis and emphysema require vigorous attention to bronchial hygiene (7). Cigarette smoking must be stopped. Attempts are made to minimize the production of secretions and to maximize the clearance of the excess secretions, which are the hallmark of chronic bronchitis. The air should be well humidified and as free as possible from pollutants. Bronchodilators, by inhalation, will help reduce airway obstruction and help clear secretions. Isoproterenol has been the most widely studied sympathomimetic agent and is very effective. However, it has both beta-1 and beta-2 effects. Its major limiting factor is an increase in cardiac irritability. Isoetharine and metaproterenol sulfate are said to have more selective beta-2 effects and may, therefore, be less likely to produce toxic cardiac effects. Mucolytic agents have not been found to be helpful in clearing secretions and probably play no role in treating bronchitis.

Intermittent positive pressure breathing is not of particular benefit except as a pressure source to deliver bronchodilators. It has been shown that this is no more effective than simpler aerosols. Other measures, such as chest percussion and postural drainage, with the patient lying in the position he usually avoids and thus stimulating coughing, may also help to clear secretions.

Steroid therapy is of little value in bronchitis and emphysema. However, steroids do decrease edema and the inflammatory response of the bronchial tree and probably decrease mucus secretion. In patients with a large asthmatic component, steroids are useful during the wheezing episodes and will help clear the airways. The toxic effects of steroids, however, are a real threat to the elderly in whom they should be used only after other measures have failed.

Oxygen therapy may be necessary if significant hypoxemia is present. It must be emphasized that oxygen is a drug with toxic and dehydrating effects on the lungs. It should be used when necessary like other drugs, recognizing its potential toxicity. Since the normal elderly have a reduced oxygen tension associated with the aging process per se, older patients are more likely to require oxygen therapy during an acute illness.

Arterial oxygen tensions of 60 mmHg or above will usually provide saturation of 89% or better if the patient is not acidotic. This is sufficient to meet the needs of the various organs and supplemental oxygen is probably not necessary. It has been shown that pulmonary artery pressure will rise at saturations under 85%. Therefore, with oxygen tension between 50 and 60 mmHg, supplemental oxygen may be helpful. If the oxygen tension falls below 50 mmHg, oxygen should probably be used so as to bring the oxygen tension above 60 mmHg. Oxygen therapy may also be used during training programs to increase fitness in subjects with a low resting oxygen tension. Oxygen will not affect dyspnea except in those subjects in whom the dyspnea results from hypoxemia. When using oxygen therapy with patients with bronchitis and emphysema, the pH and carbon dioxide tension must be monitored to evaluate the possibility of respiratory acidosis developing as a result of the inhibition of ventilation associated with an increase in oxygen tension. The role of long-term oxygen therapy is not clear at this time and is under further evaluation. For patients who need oxygen therapy frequently or constantly, light-weight portable systems are available.

Since our efforts are directed toward encouraging cough and clearing bronchial secretions, cough depressants and sedating drugs should be avoided as they interfere with bronchial hygiene. The same principles that apply to the treatment of bronchitis and emphysema also apply to the other lung diseases that will be discussed. Appropriate antibiotics are necessary depending on the cause of the infection.

PNEUMONIA

Pneumonia is a common problem in the elderly. In a study of an elderly population it was shown to be the most common cause of death in a large autopsy series (13). Most pneumonias result from aspiration of the infecting organism, rather than from a blood-borne source. Although we ordinarily think of aspiration pneumonia as a specific entity with gastric or esophageal contents or a foreign body being aspirated, it must be kept in mind that "nonaspiration" pneumonia results from inhaling an infected particle into a normally sterile area of the lung. In the elderly this is more of a problem because the usual defense mechanisms such as cough and gag reflexes may be impaired. Difficulties with swallowing and decreased levels of consciousness also add to the risk of aspiration in the elderly. The ability to cough decreases with age since the maximal inspiratory effort decreases. In addition, the ability to obtain glottal closure and the forced expiratory maneuvers necessary to build up the high flow rates associated with coughing are also diminished.

Other difficulties of concern are poor dentition with resultant foci of infection, which can be a source of infecting particles. The edentate elderly individual is less likely to have this problem. Care of the remaining teeth, therefore, is necessary to help prevent pulmonary infection. The night time use of nose drops and mineral oil add to the incidence of aspiration with lipoid pneumonia noted at times in patients who have been using these products for years.

Some degree of aspiration probably accounts for many of the clinical pneumonias seen in the elderly. This is most often a problem among the bed- and chair-ridden patient and is less of a problem in the ambulatory patient. This again emphasizes the need for keeping the elderly as active as possible within the limit of their disability. Feeding patients who are not alert, either orally or with a nasogastric tube, increases the risk of aspiration.

In addition to the problems of increased aspiration, the symptoms and signs of pneumonia are more difficult to recognize. The elderly may not complain or the febrile and leukocyte response may not be very great. These patients must be observed carefully for early changes of function such as cough, increase in respiratory rate, and changes in respiratory pattern. They must be examined frequently.

In the treatment of pneumonia in elderly patients, vigorous, frequent respiratory therapy is important to aid in the clearing of bronchopulmonary secretions. Older persons, particularly those with other chronic disabling conditions and those living in homes for the aged or nursing homes, are more likely to have infections due to organisms other than the usual pneumococcus (in particular, gram-negative organisms) (17); it is important to identify the infecting organism(s) through obtaining, examining, and culturing a sample of the infected sputum and to treat with the appropriate antibiotic(s).

TUBERCULOSIS

Tuberculosis has become an increasing problem in the elderly. As infection rates have fallen markedly, the reservoir of infected people tends to be the elderly who were infected in the early part of the twentieth century. Exacerbation of this infection with clinically manifest disease occurring decades after the primary infection accounts for much of the tuberculosis seen today. The diagnosis should be considered in elderly patients in whom a chest X-ray suggests the possibility. Pleural effusions as a result of tuberculosis may occur in the elderly.

Therapy requires care since isonicotinic acid hydrazide (INH), the standard drug used in the treatment of tuberculosis, is associated with an increasing frequency of liver toxicity with increasing age. Therefore, I would not use INH prophylaxis in anyone over 35 years, but would rather reserve its use for those with active tuberculosis. Liver function tests should be monitored carefully in patients given INH. Two drugs should always be used in the treatment of tuberculosis.

CARCINOMA

Lung carcinoma is a disease frequently seen in elderly patients among those with a history of smoking. Tolerance for lung resection decreases over age 70 and a pneumonectomy after this age carries a high risk. Although age itself is not an absolute contraindication, it must weigh heavily in the surgical judgment.

PULMONARY EMBOLI

As elderly patients are not active and frequently have heart disease or require surgery, pulmonary emboli are a constant threat. The risks of anticoagulants in the elderly are also greater. There is some evidence that heparin in smaller than usual dosages, such as 5,000 units twice a day, may be effective in preventing significant pulmonary emboli during the postoperative period and during prolonged periods of bed rest after surgery or myocardial infarctions. Early ambulation remains important whenever feasible.

SUMMARY

In the evaluation of the aging respiratory system it is hard to separate out environmental factors and conditioning from the effects of aging alone. There tends to be a decreasing lung function with age such that there is little difficulty with ordinary demands, but some of the reserve has dissipated. This results not only from changes in the lung but from changes in the entire neuromuscular apparatus associated with ventilation.

Every effort should be made to maintain maximal respiratory function. This can best be provided by a pollutant-free environment, cessation of smoking, and a regular exercise program to maintain physical fitness. The sooner this is started the better with people of all ages included in any such program.

REFERENCES

1. Astrand, S., Astrand, O., Hallback, I., and Kilbom, A. (1973): Reduction in maximal oxygen uptake with age. *J. Appl. Physiol.*, 35:649–654.
2. Begin, R., Renezetti, A. D. Jr., Bigler, A. H., and Watanabe, S. (1975): Flow and age dependence of airway closure and dynamic compliance. *J. Appl. Physiol.*, 38:199–207.
3. Block, A. J., Boyden, R. G., Wynne, J. W., and Hunt, L. A. (1979): Sleep apnea, hypopnea and oxygen desaturation in normal subjects. *N. Engl. J. Med.*, 300:513–517.

4. Bode, F. R., Dosman, J., Martin, R. R., Ghezzo, H., and Macklem, P. J. (1976): Age and sex differences in lung elasticity and in closing capacity in non-smokers. *J. Appl. Physiol.,* 41:129–135.
5. Dehn, M. M., and Bruce, R. A. (1972): Longitudinal variations in maximal oxygen intake with age and activity. *J. Appl. Physiol.,* 33:805–807.
6. Edelman, N. H., Mittman, C., Morris, A. H., and Schok, N. W. (1968): Effects of respiratory pattern in age differences in ventilation uniformity. *J. Appl. Physiol.,* 24:49–53.
7. Fox, M. S., and Snider, G. L. (1979): Respiratory therapy. *JAMA,* 241:937–940.
8. Hutchinson, J. (1846): On the capacity of the lungs and on the respiratory functions. *Med. Clin. Soc. (Lond.) Trans.,* 29:137–252.
9. Kronenberg, R. S., and Drage, C. W. (1973): Attenuation of the ventilatory and heart rate responses to hypoxia and hypercapnea with aging in normal man. *J. Clin. Invest.,* 52:1812–1819.
10. Lewis, S. M. (1978): Emptying patterns of the lung studied by multiple-breath N2 washout. *J. Appl. Physiol.,* 44:424–430.
11. Mittman, C., Edelman, N. H., Norris, A. H., and Shock, N. W. (1965): Relationship between chest wall and pulmonary compliance and age. *J. Appl. Physiol.,* 20:1211–1216.
12. Niewoehner, D. E., Kleinerman, J., and Liotta, L. (1975): Elastic behavior of post-mortem human lungs; effects of aging and mild emphysema. *J. Appl. Physiol.,* 39:943–949.
13. Rossman, I., Rodstein, M., and Bornstein, A. (1974): Undiagnosed diseases in an aging population. *Arch. Intern. Med.,* 133:366–369.
14. Schoenberg, J. B., Beck, G. J., and Bouhuys, A. (1978): Growth and decay of pulmonary function in healthy blacks and whites. *Respir. Physiol.,* 33:367–393.
15. Sorbini, C. A., Grassi, V., Solinas, E., Muiesan, G. (1968): Arterial oxygen tension in relation to age in healthy subjects. *Respiration,* 25:3–13.
16. Turner, J. M., Mead, J., and Wohl, M. S. (1965): Elasticity of human lungs in relation to age. *J. Appl. Physiol.,* 25:664–671.
17. Valenti, W. M., et al. (1978): Factor predisposing to oropharyngeal colonization with gram negative bacilli in the aged. *N. Engl. J. Med.,* 298:1108–1111.

Rehabilitation in the Aging edited by
T. F. Williams. Raven Press, New York © 1984.

Clinical Pharmacology in the Aged: Aspects of Pharmacokinetics and Drug Sensitivity

Marjorie W. Myers-Robfogel and H. Bruce Bosmann

Department of Pharmacology and Toxicology and Cancer Center, University of Rochester, School of Medicine and Dentistry, Rochester, New York 14642

An increased risk of adverse drug reactions in the elderly has been recognized for centuries. Withering's treatise on the medical uses of foxglove (91) quotes an increased incidence of adverse reactions in older people. In 1956, Lasagna (47) reviewed the known effects of age on drug action and pointed out the need for increased research to solve the many questions unanswered at the time. Indeed in the past 25 years, a good deal of work has been done to clarify the effects of aging on the pharmacology of many drugs and appreciation for the necessity of such information has grown widespread. The principal contributions have been the study of both physiological changes associated with aging and the changes in pharmacokinetics of a variety of drugs when used by the elderly. Unfortunately these studies demonstrate that there are few simple rules to be applied in understanding drug effects in the aged. Although many specific questions regarding excretion, metabolism, or distribution have been answered for certain compounds, much more study will be required to comprehend the complex interactions between the aged individual and each particular drug or drug combination.

The magnitude of the problem of drugs and the elderly grows as the percentage of the "old" in our population increases. Although in 1976 only 11% of the population was over 65, 33% of expenditures for prescription drugs was accounted for by the elderly. Among patients discharged from the hospital, 25% of those over age 65 had prescriptions for six or more drugs as compared to only 3% for a younger group (17,76).

There are many studies which indicate that the elderly suffer an increased (perhaps twofold) risk of adverse drug reactions (39,55,70). For a variety of drugs, plasma concentrations are higher in elderly patients than in younger patients following comparable drug doses; serum half-life values are lengthened; and clearance is reduced (81). Thus both therapeutic and untoward effects may be higher in the elderly for a given dose of medicine. It is probable that many factors contribute to this problem. Foremost may be the normal physiological changes that accompany the aging process. Changes in organ perfusion, lean body mass, and body water contribute to a different set of determinants for the pharmacokinetic disposition of a compound in the elderly (63). It is also possible that during aging, tissues may develop altered sensitivity to a given amount of drug. The complexity of interrelationships between various disease processes manifested with aging may help create the need for multiple drug therapy and increased likelihood of drug interactions. Compliance with a prescribed regimen among the elderly may be poorer than in a younger group (76). However, even if the degree of compliance is similar, it may also be more important because of a smaller margin for error in dosage (87).

This chapter summarizes the aspects of clinical pharmacology of importance in aging and relevant to any comprehensive rehabilitation approach. The intention is to provide an understanding of the extent of what is and is not known about pharmocological changes with aging. As will be seen, because of limited research to date in a number of important areas, it is essential that the physician prescribing drugs for elderly persons (and other professionals observing for their effects) be aware of the principles of clinical pharmacology, and the effects that may be expected with aging, rather than trying to use a "cookbook" approach. Each older person must be considered individually and the individual variation is even greater in older than younger persons.

The principles of clinical pharmacology apply to all ages; these include pharmacokinetics, compliance, adverse reactions, and abuse. However, certain points need emphasizing: (a) the elderly are often much more frail than their younger counterparts, in part because chronic illness tends to be cumulative; (b) dementia adds to many of the problems associated with the elderly and drug use; and (c) the social context in which the elderly are taking their respective drugs, e.g., alone, in a family setting, or in a professionally supervised chronic facility such as a nursing home, contributes to the "clinical pharmacology" of the drug experience and the outcome.

Topics such as use of elderly in clinical trials for drug development, "drug-lag" of new drugs most suitable for the problems of the elderly, generic versus brand name drugs, third party reimbursements for drugs, and the various socioeconomic aspects of drug procurement for the elderly, will not be discussed here, although they are topics worthy of attention.

We will consider two machanisms for adverse drug function in the elderly. First is the *altered delivery* of drug to a target cell because of changes in absorption, metabolism, excretion, and distribution of the compound; however, in many of the clinical studies discussed, complete analysis of the pharmacokinetics of a drug has not been determined. Thus even though it may be reported that a particular drug concentration is elevated in the plasma of elderly persons, the factors contributing to that elevation may not be known. A summary of some demonstrated changes for drugs commonly used in the rehabilitation of the elderly is presented in Table 1. Second, there is the possibility that the elderly have *altered tissue sensitivity* to equivalent amounts of drugs. Changes in receptors and responses to equivalent amounts of drugs will also be discussed.

One of the problems of the studies discussed here is the selection of subjects. When human data exist, these have been discussed rather than data from animal

TABLE 1. *Pharmacokinetic changes associated with aging*[a]

Drug	Plasma concentration	Drug half-life	Volume of distribution	Probable critical parameter	Reference
Antibiotics					
Gentamicin		↑		Renal function	(51)
Kanamycin		↑		Renal function	(51)
Propicillin K	↑		↓	Renal function	(57)
Tetracycline	↑	↑		Renal function	(85)
Sedatives, tranquilizers, antidepressants					
Chlordiazepoxide		↑	↑	Hepatic metabolism; Lean body mass	(65)
Diazepam	—	↑	↑	Hepatic metabolism; Lean body mass	(46,52)
Nitrazepam		—			(10)
Imipramine	↑			Hepatic metabolism	(92)
Cardiovascular					
Digoxin	↑	↑	↓	Renal function	(14,21)
Lidocaine		↑	↑	Hepatic metabolism; Lean body mass	(53,83)
Metoprolol	↑	↑		Hepatic metabolism	(45)
Propranolol	↑	—	—	Hepatic metabolism	(9)
Others					
Phenylbutazone		↑		Hepatic metabolism	(60)
Cimetidine	↑	↑	↓	Renal function; Lean body mass	(61)

[a] ↑, parameter increased in elderly; ↓, parameter decreased in elderly; —, parameter unchanged in elderly.

models. In several studies the authors have been careful to examine drug response in healthy, elderly individuals in comparison to healthy, young people. In many studies, however, either/or both of the groups included patients undergoing therapy for a disease process. Equally difficult to assess and compare between studies is the definition of "aged." In some studies narrow age ranges are given, whereas in others, the "elderly" group encompasses any individuals beyond age 50. Comparisons between studies are often made difficult by these problems.

PHARMACOKINETICS

Absorption

Absorption of a drug often refers to absorption of the drug from the stomach or the intestine after oral administration. For convenience and economy oral administration of drugs is widely used; however, certain properties of drugs or specific diseases predicate other routes of administration. Thus absorption from intrathecal, topical, intramuscular, pulmonary, or other forms of administration could also be addressed. Limited data are available regarding parenteral absorption in the elderly. Although this review primarily discusses gastrointestinal absorption, two points should be made with regard to route of administration. First, the route of choice is usually that which is most convenient and also achieves desired blood levels for the appropriate time period; second, desired blood levels are those which achieve adequate levels of active drug moiety at the target tissue or cellular site with minimal risk of adverse reactions.

Relatively few studies have examined the rate or completeness of absorption of drugs in the elderly. Physiological changes of the gastrointestinal tract associated with aging might be expected to alter drug absorption from the gut. In fact, increases in gastric pH, reduction in splanchnic blood flow, altered absorptive surface, and decreased motility have been reported to occur with aging (3,4,13,76,78). A study of absorption following a single dose of digoxin demonstrated that rate of absorption was decreased in the elderly subjects, but the extent of total drug absorbed was not altered (14). Similarly, Shader et al. (73) reported a delay in reaching peak levels of plasma chlordiazepoxide after oral administration. However, many drugs that are absorbed by passive diffusion have been found to be taken up equally well by the young and elderly (78). Unchanged rates of absorption in old age have been reported for indomethacin (82), paracetamol, sulfamethizole (84), and lorazepam (34). In studies comparing the absorption of aspirin, an acid, and quinine, a base, absorption rate constants were comparable between healthy, young volunteers and geriatric patients. However, peak plasma levels were higher and were reached later in the elderly. These data indicate that gastric pH changes may not alter total absorption of the types of compounds most expected to be affected by pH changes. However, plasma half-time of the drug was longer and clearance rate slower in the aged, suggesting comparable rates of absorption but altered clearance of these compounds in the aged (78).

An interesting example of the effect of gut motility and gastric emptying time is seen with levodopa which undergoes degradative metabolism by decarboxylation in the stomach. In one elderly patient who was unsuccessfully treated with levodopa, it was found that he had very low gut motility. By therapy designed to hasten gastric emptying in this patient, increased serum levels of the unmetabolized drug were achieved. This converted that patient's response to the drug from unsuccessful to successful (7).

These studies indicate that absorption changes due to normal aging do not appear to be major determinants of drug response even though there are documented changes in the physiological function of the gastrointestinal system. However, these changes may lead to slower absorption and in certain persons, a physiologic failure to absorb the desired drug.

Metabolism

Metabolism of a given drug can range from essentially no metabolism, such as in the case of penicillin G which is excreted largely unchanged, through drugs that are conjugated and excreted as glucuronides, esters, or sulfates, to drugs such as chlorpromazine which has more than 130 metabolites already determined. Metabolism is important not only from the standpoint of excretion but also because it may activate or inactivate the drug. Study of the role of drug metabolism in the elderly is compounded by two problems: (a) most research on metabolism has been done on healthy normal animals or young human volunteers and these results may not necessarily be extended to the frail elderly; and (b) drug interactions involving metabolism changes may be more complex in the elderly with changes in metabolism of one or both drugs, and more frequent due to the increased use of drugs.

The ability of the liver to metabolize or excrete drugs may be decreased with aging. Early studies showed that liver mass declines with age, as does body weight. Uptake of bromsulfopthalein, a measure of liver function, is also lower in the elderly (8,80). Hepatic blood flow is reduced in aging (2) which may lead to a reduction in the rate of elimination of drugs that are avidly taken up by the liver, such as propranolol (25). In fact, in a clinical study of metoprolol, a β-adrenoceptor blocking agent which is eliminated largely after metabolism, it was shown that a group of elderly subjects had slower excretion and higher peak plasma levels of the drug (45).

Studies in rats and mice have shown species variations in the degree to which the drug-metabolizing enzymes in the liver decline with aging (42,44). Comparable data in elderly people are not available and so we cannot predict how a particular drug will be affected by possible changes in metabolic enzyme activity.

From clinical observation, it is known that a number of drugs metabolized by the liver have increased plasma half-lives in the aged. These include antipyrine (60), lidocaine (58), diazepam (13,52), chlordiazepoxide (65), aspirin (79), and phenylbutazone (6). However, studies of these drugs have measured overall clearance times; the rate of drug metabolism in a controlled system has not been determined. Other studies (79,83) suggest that drug metabolism by the liver may not change qualitatively with aging, but may be reduced quantitatively as a consequence of physiological changes resulting in reduced liver mass and hepatic blood flow. Furthermore, small changes in liver function would be magnified by a concomitant reduction in renal excretion of the drug and its metabolites resulting in presentation to the liver of an even larger amount of drug to be metabolized (27).

Table 1 shows commonly used drugs in which hepatic metabolism plays a prominent role in their disposition.

Renal Excretion

Renal excretion is generally the most important way in which many drugs are cleared from the body. Excretion in the feces often represents unabsorbed drug, although in certain instances biliary secretion is an important route of excretion. Aging is accompanied by several well-known changes in renal function which have direct consequences in the excretion of drugs and metabolites by the kidney (31). In 1950, Davies and Shock (15) demonstrated in men of various ages that both renal cortical mass and cortical blood or plasma flow decrease with age. Glomerular filtration rate was studied in a longitudinal prospective study and it was demonstrated that there is a progressive decline in filtration from the earliest age studied, 34 years. Sodium conservation, urine concentrating ability, and renal tubular secreting capacity have also been reported to decline with age (19).

Serum creatinine, however, does not rise in healthy older persons. This finding is attributed to the decrease in lean body mass which occurs upon aging and consequently there is decreased production of endogenous creatinine (41). This fact precludes a simple relationship between serum creatinine and the drug excreting capacity of elderly patients. Thus, unless there are also renal changes due to disease, the reduced capacity to excrete drugs as a result of normal aging processes is not obvious from serum creatinine levels. From their studies of both males and females between the ages of 20 and 99 years, Kampmann and Hansen (41) constructed a nomogram relating serum creatinine to creatinine clearance taking age, weight, and sex into account, which can be used in predicting clearance rates in the elderly. A conservative assumption in considering therapy with drugs that are largely excreted by the kidney, in persons aged 70 or older, in whom the serum creatinine is in the "normal" range, i.e., 1.1 mg/dl or less, is that the rate of excretion will be only one-half to one-third that of a younger adult.

Reduction of glomerular filtration decreases clearance of a large number of drugs which are either excreted unchanged or which are excreted as metabolites in the urine. Digoxin is a prime example of a drug where plasma concentration is primarily dependent upon glomerular filtration rate and for which severe clinical consequences of toxic levels may result if renal function is not considered with dosage. Ewy et al. (21) first studied digoxin elimination in the elderly and correlated increased half-life with decreased creatinine clearance. These studies have been confirmed and amplified by a large number of investigators and elaborate aids for dosage planning have been formulated that depend on creatinine clearance rates (14,64,77,79,89). Other drugs for which decreased glomerular filtration rate has been correlated with increased half-life include cephalothin, kanamycin, gentamicin, and phenobarbital (36,41,51,63). Decreased clearance of the metabolite of lidocaine, 4-hydroxyxylidine, has been related to decreased glomerular filtration (58,83). In this study, the relationship of volume of distribution to hepatic metabolism was also carefully evaluated to ascertain the origin of the observed increase in plasma half-life.

Clearance of drugs which are actively secreted by the kidney tubular cells such as benzylpenicillin also decreases with age (49). In 1979, Kampmann et al. (41) examined benzylpenicillin excretion in young subjects and elderly patients. Plasma half-life was twice as long in the elderly as in the young; however, probenecid tripled the penicillin half-life in the young subjects and doubled the half-life in the elderly such that after probenecid, the differences between clearance in the young and old were reduced in magnitude. These data indicate that not only is there reduced filtration of penicillin in the elderly but also reduced tubular secretion.

Table 1, again, indicates commonly used drugs in which the changing renal function with age (and any primary renal disease) would play a prominent role in disposition.

Distribution

The distribution of a given amount of drug into various body compartments determines the drug concentration at the target site. Distribution is affected by the perfusion ratio of a particular organ, the preferential sequestration of a drug in or from one compartment because of binding or solubility, and the total volume of a compartment such as total body water or lean cell mass. The physicochemical properties of a compound are the important determinants of drug distribution. Such properties as lipid solubility and ionic charge at physiological pH determine how readily a drug will cross membranes between compartments or into cells and how the drug will distribute between body water and body fat. The specific structure of a drug also determines how tightly the compound will associate with tissue or serum proteins restricting distribution into other compartments.Physiological changes associated with aging have been found to alter distribution of many drugs in the elderly. Generally, the percentage of body fat increases with age; there is a concomitant decrease in lean body or lean cell mass (22,35,59). Total body water also decreases in the aged; however, intracellular water, as a proportion of fat-free body mass does not change (50,59). Thus volume of distribution for a lipophilic compound may be increased in the aged or decreased for a polar, hydrophilic drug. This suggests that drugs which distribute in body water might reach elevated serum levels in the elderly as compared to younger persons, whereas drugs which are soluble in body fat might show decreased serum levels but increased tissue amounts. Thus serum levels of a drug in an elderly patient may not be comparable to those of a younger person when assessing body drug burden or possible toxicity.

Distribution of digoxin has been carefully studied in several groups of old and young patients. Ewy et al. (21) showed that the volume of distribution of digoxin during the first 24 hr following intravenous administration was smaller in the elderly subjects, which could explain the observed increased plasma drug levels. Digoxin is highly polar and, therefore, distributes in the lean body mass (20); there is also a fraction bound to tissue receptors. These data have been augmented and confirmed by others. Aronson and Grahame-Smith (1) demonstrated a reduced volume of distribution in a group of elderly patients at steady-state drug concentrations. Cusack et al. (14) also found a reduction in apparent volume of distribution following a single oral dose of digoxin to groups of young and older patients; this reduction correlated inversely with age. As discussed previously, plasma levels and clearance times of digoxin are increased partially because of reduced renal capacity in the elderly; however, increased plasma levels may also result from the smaller volume of distribution for digoxin in older patients. This suggests that age, independent of renal function, should be a consideration in the use of digoxin.

A similar study of the volume of distribution of propicillin K is described by Mitchard (57). Distribution is limited to the extracellular water which is decreased in the elderly. A corresponding increase in plasma concentration was observed. A significant but smaller decrease in volume of distribution has also been described for lorazepam, a benzodiazepine of intermediate solubility, following intravenous administration to elderly subjects (34).

Increases in volume of distribution have been reported for several lipophilic compounds. Triggs (83) has described the distribution of lidocaine in elderly subjects. The initial dilution space or volume did not differ between the young and elderly based on body weight; however, apparent volume of distribution and volume of distribution at steady state were significantly greater in the older group. Plasma drug half-life was prolonged but plasma clearance was not, suggesting that the increase in half-life was due to an increased body burden of lidocaine because of increased volume of distribution. Volumes of distribution are also increased in the elderly for diazepam and chlordiazepoxide (46,65,90). For diazepam, the most lipophilic of the benzodiazepines, both initial distribution space and volume of distribution at steady state is increased; however, for chlordiazepoxide which is more water soluble, initial distribution space is not significantly changed. For many other drugs, however, volume of distribution does not change in the elderly. Drugs for which data indicate no change include propranolol (9) and nitrazepam (10).

The concentration of albumin in plasma or serum is often decreased in the elderly (18,37,38,56); the magnitude of the changes in some studies has been as great as a decline from 4.7 g/dl at age 25 to 3.8 g/dl at 75. However, the possibility that these changes might be due to factors other than aging per se, such as malnutrition, has not been excluded. One study of apparently healthy elderly persons living at home reports no difference in albumin concentration between middle-aged persons, those aged 65 to 74 and those 75 and over; the mean values fall between 4.1 and 4.2 percent (48).

Nevertheless, to the extent that decreased serum albumin does occur in elderly patients on medications (37,38), the decrease in protein binding would be expected to increase free plasma or tissue levels of highly bound compounds. Increased free drug levels can lead to both increased rate of clearance or increased volume of distribution which would decrease drug effect; in another case, increased free plasma drug concentration might increase drug effect. Changes in plasma albumin drug binding can also affect drug interactions where one drug is highly bound and competes for binding sites with a more poorly bound drug. Reduction in albumin binding can affect the ratio of the bound forms of one or both drugs and thus alter the effects of both drugs.

Decreased protein binding leads to an increase in plasma-free drug concentration for a variety of compounds. Warfarin is highly bound to plasma albumin. In a study by Husted and Andreasen (40) the daily maintenance dose of phenprocoumon for patients over 60 years of age was significantly lower than for patients less than 60 years old; the plasma concentration of albumin was also significantly lower in the older group. A correlation with $p<.01$ was found between the daily maintenance dose of phenprocoumon and the albumin content of plasma. Similar studies suggest that protein binding of phenytoin (38) and of phenylbutazone (86) are decreased in the elderly. Wallace et al. (86) also showed that in patients on multiple drugs, the unbound proportion of salicylate and sulfadiazine was increased over that in younger subjects following phenylbutazone.

Triggs (83) has described the distribution of chlormethiazole following both oral and intravenous administration to young healthy males and to elderly male residents of long-stay health care facilities who were free of signs of heart disease and who had normal blood chemistries. The fraction of chlormethiazole free in plasma was 31% greater in the elderly subjects but the total chlormethiazole blood concentration was no different. The amount bound to plasma protein did not change but that bound to blood cells was decreased in the older subjects.

Chan et al. (12), however, have found that in the case of pethidine, which is highly bound by erythrocytes, older subjects have reduced binding of the drug. Hematocrits for the two groups were not different. A preliminary study of red blood cell proteins from young and older patients did not show any differences in the proteins, which might account for the decreased binding in the elderly (57).

Changes in tissue perfusion also affect drug distribution. Cardiac output declines with age; splanchnic and renal blood flow decreases about 40% in old age (2,5). Reduced perfusion of the kidneys and liver have the obvious consequence of reducing distribution of a drug in the excreting organs and thus prolonging its plasma half-life. However, there are few data which suggest that changes in perfusion of other organs alter drug distribution.

CELLULAR RESPONSIVENESS

Changes in sensitivity to drugs have been reported in the elderly. Sensitivity is used here to describe alterations in response when comparable amounts of drug are delivered to the target site. There are descriptions of such phenomenological changes for a variety of drugs including the diazepines, adrenergic agonists and antagonists, cardiac glycosides, antibiotics, anticoagulants, and antiarrhythmics. Study of the mechanisms behind such changes in responsiveness has lagged behind pharmacokinetic studies of drug delivery. Because this research involves the study of cellular responses rather than whole organism responses, far fewer data are available for humans than for animals. Until recently, many studies with laboratory animals have used widely different definitions of senescent or aged for the animals. Thus the data between various animal studies may not be directly comparable and, of course, may not necessarily predict the human situation. However, these studies and some work with human tissue have elucidated several mechanisms of altered sensitivity. For drugs that interact with receptors, receptor number or affinity may be responsible for the altered effect. In other cases, drug interaction with naturally occurring substances such as neurotransmitters or cellular enzymes may be changed because of alternations in the enzyme activity or amount of transmitter at the site. In many cases, however, it is not yet understood why the elderly exhibit a different response to drugs that reach cellular targets in the same concentration as in younger people.

Studies in isolated heart and blood vessels from older animals (rats) have shown decreased responsiveness, compared to tissue from younger animals, to drugs that produce vascular relaxation (isoproterenol) (28), inotropic response (ouabain) (26), and effects on cardiac rhythm (lidocaine, verapamil, quinidine) (29,30). Similar studies have not been reported with human tissues. In elderly humans, increased sensitivity has been reported to nitrazepam (11), in a study in which there was no explanation for increased loss of performance in a psychomotor test other than an increased sensitivity of the older subjects to equal amounts of the drug. Human lymphocytes have been found to have increasing sensitivity with age to the antiproliferative effects of bleomycin (71). And finally, the sensitivity of elderly patients to warfarin is increased over the younger, volunteer population. At equal plasma concentrations of warfarin, there is greater inhibition of vitamin K-dependent clotting factor synthesis among the elderly. However, in this study, there were no significant differences in the pharmacokinetics of the drug with respect to plasma half-life, apparent volume of distribution, plasma clearance, plasma protein binding, or plasma warfarin metabolites (74). The authors attribute these data to an unexplainable intrinsic sensitivity of the elderly to equal amounts of the drug. Although the discrepancy between these data and the data discussed previously of Husted and Andreasen (40) cannot be completely reconciled, the clinical message is the same. In the elderly, lower doses of warfarin or phenprocoumon result in greater anticoagulant response.

For drugs which act through interaction with receptors, change in receptor number or affinity during aging would be an important determinant of responsiveness to drugs. This is currently an area of active research both in animal models and in humans. In studies on animal and human brain tissue or lymphocytes there appears to be decreased binding with age for β-adrenergic antagonists (33,53,69,88) and dopamine antagonists (54,72). In all these studies the affinity constant for the receptors was unchanged, indicating an actual decline in the number of receptor sites rather than an alteration in the receptor. In a study of serotonin binding in cerebral cortex of young and old humans, total number of binding sites, classes of sites, and affinity of receptors for serotonin all showed changes with aging (75). Changes in affinity of binding were most striking. Affinity decreased with age and also shifted from two types of binding sites of high and intermediate affinity to a single class of sites of low affinity. However, the total number of binding sites increased with age. Whether this is compensatory in nature or relevant to other brain changes with aging remains to be elucidated. Changes in hormone receptors have also been reported. In both rat and human tissues there appears to be reduced binding sites with age for corticosteroids, androgens, and estrogens (67,68).

Activity of enzymes or amounts of interacting endogenous compounds near the active site for a drug may affect the responsiveness of the tissue to that drug. Monoamine oxidase (MAO) activity has been found to increase with age in a number of human and rat tissues (brain, platelets, plasma, heart) but not in other tissues, e.g., blood vessels (23,24,32,66). Changes in MAO activity might directly alter responsiveness to drugs metabolized by that enzyme, might alter response to MAO inhibitors, or might indirectly affect activity of compounds which interact with endogenous monoamines near the active site of the drug. The activity of acetylcholinesterase in human brain (putamen) has been reported to be decreased in aging (62). Activity of enzymes contributing to the synthesis of neurotransmitters may also change with age. Enzymes involved in the synthesis of catecholamines, dopamine, acetylcholine, and gamma-aminobutyric (GABA) acid all decrease in human brain with aging (16). Thus, it is possible that the physiological changes of the nervous system during aging contribute to drug complications by complex changes in drug-receptor or drug-endogenous ligand interactions which account, in part, for age-related alterations in drug sensitivity.

TWO IMPORTANT EXAMPLES

Digoxin

Digoxin represents a drug widely used by the elderly. The principles and data outlined above have led to improved and rational therapeutic usage of this drug. The association of increased incidence of digoxin toxicity with age is old and clinically accepted dogma. The fact that the therapeutic ratio for digoxin is low has meant that toxic events have been well chronicled and are widely recognized. The basis for increased toxicity in the elderly is the increased levels of digoxin which result from doses appropriate for younger patients. As detailed above, little change is seen in absorption, metabolism, or protein binding for digoxin. The volume of distribution is reduced in the elderly (1,14), which may contribute to increased plasma levels of drug. However, it is widely recognized that a major determinant of digoxin levels, and thus toxicity, is renal clearance. Because clearance of both digoxin and creatinine is largely a function of glomerular filtration rate, creatinine clearance is used as a tool to predict rates of digoxin elimination. Therapeutic regimens based solely on patient sex, age, weight, and creatinine clearance have been devised by computerized systems to adjust digoxin dosage to the individual patient in a rapid and accurate manner.

In cases where creatinine clearance is not measured directly, age, sex, and weight variables are used to predict clearance from serum creatinine values as discussed above (89). This type of analysis has provided a basis for rational therapy which used the best of the pharmacological data obtained from studies in the elderly.

Benzodiazepines

The benzodiazepines are an important class of drugs, often prescribed during rehabilitative phases of illness in the elderly. These drugs have similar mechanisms of action and are widely accepted to have high therapeutic margins. However, data are accumulating which suggest that use of the benzodiazepines in the elderly is associated with increased frequency of untoward effects. Increased response with a host of central nervous system depressive effects has now been recognized as a common result of benzodiazepine therapy in the aged. As a class of drugs, the correct dosing is quite complex and illustrates many of the principles discussed above.

Two factors contribute to the difficulty of adjusting dosage to reduce the incidence of side effects. First, the nature of CNS effects—psychomotor impairment, ataxia, confusion, lassitude—may not easily be perceived by the patient or by health-care professionals in certain settings but is particularly important to the overall health of the aged. Secondly, the pharmacokinetic properties of the drugs may differ subtly but widely in spite of their similar chemical and pharmacologic properties. This makes prediction of drug toxicity for a particular elderly patient of unknown physiologic status very difficult. For example, absorption studies have indicated that absorption of lorazepam is unchanged from either the gastrointestinal tract or from an intramuscular site (34). However, absorption of chlordiazepoxide from the gut is delayed (73). Plasma half-lives of chlordiazepoxide and diazepam are increased with age but half-lives of oxazepam or lorazepam, a more polar metabolite of both chlordiazepoxide and diazepam are not (90). Volume of distribution at steady state is increased for chlordiazepoxide and diazepam but initial distribution space of chlordiazepoxide is not decreased. Volume of distribution is unchanged for nitrazepam or lorazepam (10). Hopefully, these types of data will in the near future be useful in determining optional regimens for benzodiazepine therapy. However, the complexity of a particular drug's pharmacokinetic disposition and the concept that sensitivity of receptors toward benzodiazepines in the elderly (11) may be altered do not allow simple formulas to be used in the prescription of these drugs for use by the aged.

A final comment is needed about the role of measurement of concentrations of drugs in the serum, as a guide to appropriate drug therapy. The capabilities of clinical laboratories to provide such information is continually increasing and is often helpful in assessing the net effects of the pharmacokinetic factors (discussed in this chapter) in the individual elderly patient. However, drug levels cannot be used as the only, or even primary, measure of appropriateness of a given drug dosage regimen. Other variables including degree of protein binding and end-organ responsiveness will also have major influences on the therapeutic effects (and side effects) obtained. Thus the clinical determination of therapeutic effectiveness in the individual patient remains the ultimate guide for decision about drug therapy in older persons.

SUMMARY

Although it is recognized that the elderly are at especially high risk for drug complications, the complete elucidation of the pharmacodynamics of many drugs is yet to come. Aging is accompanied by a vast number of physiological changes which alter drug activity. Important among those changes are a decline in renal function, a decline in lean body mass, and the accumulation of multiple pathologies. However, it has been impossible to predict the pharmacologic behavior of many drugs based on a few simple rules of aging. Often, qualitative changes in organ or receptor physiology are not found; more likely it is a number of interacting quantitative alterations which result in the unexpected pharmacokinetics of, or sensitivity to, a particular compound in the elderly individual. Thus although the study of the physiology of aging is necessary for the understanding of alterations in drug behavior, the actual accumulation of data for each problem drug in elderly people will be required for accurate and safe use of those drugs and for the determination of drug levels associated with untoward effects in the aged. Until the time arrives when we have all of the required data to prescribe with knowledge, that is, complete pharmacokinetic data, defined physiologic patient status and known toxic and therapeutic drug levels, the awareness of the likelihood and nature of problems which might be encountered in the elderly, and the watchful monitoring of patient responses and physiological status are still the physician's major concerns.

ACKNOWLEDGMENTS

This work was supported in part by Research Development funds of the University of Rochester Cancer Center Core Grant 5-P30-CA 11198–12. M.W.M. is a Scholar of the Alexandrine and Alexander L. Sinsheimer Foundation. H.B.B. is a Geriatric Academic Medicine Awardee of N.I.A.

REFERENCES

1. Aronson, J. K., and Grahame-Smith, D. G. (1977): Monitoring digoxin therapy: II. Determinants of the apparent volume of distribution. *Br. J. Clin. Pharmacol.,* 4:223–227.
2. Bender, A. D. (1965): The effect of increasing age on the distribution of peripheral blood flow in man. *J. Am. Geriatr. Soc.,* 13:192–198.
3. Bender, A. D. (1968): Effect of age on intestinal absorption in the elderly. *J. Am. Geriatr. Soc.,* 16:1331–1337.
4. Bender, A. D. (1974): Pharmacodynamic principles of drug therapy in the aged. *J. Am. Geriatr. Soc.,* 22:296–303.
5. Brandfonbrener, M., Landowne, M., and Shock, N. W. (1955): Changes in cardiac output with age. *Circulation,* 12:557–566.

6. Brodie, B. B., Gillette, J. R., and La Du, B. N. (1958): Enzymatic metabolism of drugs and other foreign compounds. *Annu. Rev. Biochem.,* 27:427–454.
7. Calimlim, L., Dujovne, C. A., Morgan, J. P., Lasagna, L., and Bianchine, J. R. (1970): L-Dopa treatment failure: Explanation and correction. *Br. Med. J.,* 4:93–94.
8. Calloway, N. O., and Merrill, R. S. (1965): The aging adult liver: I. Bromsulphothalein and bilirubin clearances. *J. Am. Geriatr. Soc.,* 13:594.
9. Castleden, C. M., and George, C. F. (1979): The effect of aging in the hepatic clearance of propranolol. *Br. J. Clin. Pharmacol.,* 7:49–54.
10. Castleden, C. M., and George, C. F. (1979): Increased sensitivity to benzodiazepines in the elderly. In: *Drugs and the Elderly,* edited by J. Crooks and I. H. Stevenson, pp. 169–178. University Park Press, Baltimore.
11. Castleden, C. M., George, C. F., Marcer, D., and Hallett, C. (1977): Increased sensitivity to nitrazepam in old age. *Br. Med. J.,* 1:10–12.
12. Chan, K., Kendall, M. J., Mitchard, M., Wells, W. D. E., and Vickers, M. D. (1975): The effect of age on plasma pethidine concentrations. *Br. J. Clin. Pharmacol.,* 2:297–302.
13. Crooks, J., O'Malley, K., and Stevenson, I. H. (1976): Pharmacokinetics in the elderly. *Clin. Pharmacokinet.,* 1:280–296.
14. Cusack, B., Kelley, K., O'Malley, K., Noel, J., Lavan, J., and Horgan, J. (1979): Digoxin in the elderly: Pharmacokinetic consequences of old age. *Clin. Pharmacol. Ther.,* 25:772–776.
15. Davies, D. F., and Shock, N. W. (1950): Age changes in glomerular filtration rate, effective renal plasma flow, and tubular excretory capacity in adult males. *J. Clin. Invest.,* 29:496–507.
16. Davison, A. N. (1978): Biochemical aspects of the ageing brain. *Age Ageing,* 7 (Suppl.):4–11.
17. Davison, W. (1978): The hazards of drug treatment in old age. In: *Textbook of Geriatric Medicine and Gerontology,* edited by J. C. Brocklehurst, pp. 651–669. Churchill Livingstone, London.
18. Ehrnebo, M., Agurell, S., Kalling, B., and Boréus, C. O. (1971): Age differences in drug binding by plasma proteins: Studies in human foetuses, neonates, and adults. *Eur. J. Clin. Pharmacol.,* 3:189–193.
19. Epstein, M. (1979): Effects of aging on the kidney. *Fed. Proc.,* 38:168–172.
20. Ewy, G. A., Bertron, M. G., Ball, M. F., Nimmo, L., Jackson, B., and Marcus, F. (1971): Digoxin metabolism in obesity. *Circulation,* 44:810–814.
21. Ewy, G. A., Kapadia, G. G., Yao, L., Lullin, M., and Marcus, F. I. (1969): Digoxin metabolism in the elderly. *Circulation,* 39:449–453.
22. Forbes, G. B., and Reina, J. C. (1970): Adult lean body mass declines with age: Some longitudinal observations. *Metabolism,* 19:653–663.
23. Fowler, C. J., and Callingham, B. A. (1978): The effect of age on the number of monoamine oxidase active centres in the rat heart. *Biochem. Soc. Trans.,* 6:955–956.
24. Fuentes, J. A., Trepel, J. B., and Neff, N. H. (1977): Monoamine oxidase activity in the cardiovascular system of young and aged rats. *Exp. Gerontol.,* 12:113–115.
25. George, C. F., Orme, M. L. E., Burnanapong, P., Macerlean, D., Breckenridge, A. M., and Dollery, C. T. (1976): Contribution of the liver to overall elimination of propranolol. *J. Pharmacokinet. Biopharm.,* 4:17–27.
26. Gerstenblith, G., Spurgeon, H. A., Froehlich, J. P., Weisfeldt, M. L., and Lakatta, E. G. (1979): Diminished inotropic responsiveness to ouabain in aged rat myocardium. *Circ. Res.,* 44:517–523.
27. Gillette, J. R. (1979): Biotransformation of drugs during aging. *Fed. Proc.,* 38:1900–1909.
28. Godfraind, T., and Dieu, D. (1978): Influence of ageing on the isoprenaline relaxation of aortae from normal and hypertensive rats. *Arch. Int. Pharmacodyn.,* 236:300–302.
29. Goldberg, P. B., and Roberts, J. (1978): Physiological and pharmacological changes of rat cardiac pacemakers with increasing age. *Adv. Exp. Med. Biol.,* 97:315–318.
30. Goldberg, P. B., Stoner, S.-A., and Roberts, J. (1978): Influence of age on activity of antiarrhythmic drugs in rat heart. *Adv. Exp. Med. Biol.,* 97:309–313.
31. Goldman, R., Rockstein, M., and Sussman, M. L. (1975): *The Physiology and Pathology of Human Aging.* Academic Press, New York.
32. Gottfries, C. G., Adolfsson, R., Oreland, L., Ross, B. E., and Winblad, B. (1979): Monoamines and their metabolites and monoamine oxidase activity related to age and to some dementia disorders. In: *Drugs and the Elderly,* edited by J. Crooks and I. H. Stevenson, pp. 189–198. University Park Press, Baltimore.
33. Greenberg, L. H., Dix, R. K., and Weiss, B. (1978): Age-related changes in the binding of ^{3}H-dihydroprenolol in rat brain. *Adv. Exp. Med. Biol.,* 97:245–249.

34. Greenblatt, D. J., Allen, M. D., Locniskar, A., Harmatz, J. S., and Shader, R. I. (1979): Lorazepam kinetics in the elderly. *Clin. Pharmacol. Ther.,* 26:103–113.
35. Gregerman, R. I., Gaffney, G. W., and Shock, N. W. (1962): Thyroxine turnover in euthyroid man with special reference to changes with age. *J. Clin. Invest.,* 41:2065–2074.
36. Hansen, J. M., Kampmann, J., and Laursen, H. (1970): Renal excretion of drugs in the elderly. *Lancet,* 1:1170.
37. Hayes, M. J., Langman, M. J. S., and Short, A. H. (1975): Changes in drug metabolism with increasing age. I. Warfarin binding and plasma proteins. *Br. J. Clin. Pharmacol.,* 2:69–79.
38. Hayes, M. J., Langman, M. J. S., and Short, A. H. (1975): Changes in drug metabolism with increasing age. II. Phenytoin clearance and protein binding. *Br. J. Clin. Pharmacol.,* 2:73–79.
39. Hurwitz, N. (1969): Predisposing factors in adverse reactions to drugs. *Br. Med. J.,* 1:536–539.
40. Husted, S., and Andreasen, F. (1977): The influence of age on the response to anticoagulants. *Br. J. Clin. Pharmacol.,* 4:559–565.
41. Kampmann, J. P., and Hansen, J. E. M. (1979): Renal excretion of drugs. In: *Drugs and the Elderly,* edited by J. Crooks and I. H. Stevenson, pp. 77–87. University Park Press, Baltimore.
42. Kato, R., and Takanaka, A. (1968): Effect of phenobarbital on electron transport system, oxidation, and reduction of drugs in liver microsomes of rats of different age. *J. Biochem.,* 63:406–408.
43. Kato, R., Takanaka, A., and Onoda, K.-I. (1970): Studies on age difference in mice for the activity of drug-metabolizing enzymes of liver microsomes. *Jpn. J. Pharmacol.,* 20:572–576.
44. Kato, R., Vassanelli, P., Frontino, G., and Chiesara, E. (1964): Variation in the activity of liver microsomal drug metabolizing enzymes in rats in relation to age. *Biochem. Pharmacol.,* 13:1037–1051.
45. Kendall, M. J., Brown, D., and Yates, R. A. (1977): Plasma metoprolol concentrations in young, old, and hypertensive subjects. *Br. J. Clin. Pharmacol.,* 4:497–499.
46. Klotz, U., Avant, G. R., Hoyumpa, R., Schenker, S., and Wilkinson, G. R. (1975): The effects of age and liver disease on the disposition and elimination of diazepam in adult man. *J. Clin. Invest.,* 55:347–359.
47. Lasagna, L. (1956): Drug effects as modified by aging. *Proc. Assoc. Res. Nerv. Ment. Dis.,* 35:83–94.
48. Leask, R. G. S., Andrew, G. R., and Caird, F. I. (1973): Normal values for sixteen blood constituents in the elderly. *Age Ageing,* 2:14–23.
49. Leikola, E., and Vartia, K. O. (1957): On penicillin levels in young and geriatric subjects. *J. Gerontol.,* 12:48–52.
50. Lesser, G. T., and Markofsky, J. (1979): Body water compartments with human aging using fat-free mass as the reference standard. *Am. J. Physiol.,* 235:R215–R220.
51. Lumhultz, R., Kampmann, J., Siersbaek-Nielsen, K., and Hansen, M. (1974): Dose-regimen of kanamycin and gentamicin. *Acta Med. Scand.,* 190:521–524.
52. Macleod, S. M., Giles, H. G., Bengert, B., Liu, F. F., and Sellers, E. M. (1979): Age and gender-related differences in diazepam pharmacokinetics. *J. Clin. Pharmacol.,* 19:15–19.
53. Maggi, A., Schmidt, M. J., Ghetti, B., and Enna, S. J. (1979): Effect of aging on neurotransmitter receptor binding in rat and human brain. *Life Sci.,* 24:367–374.
54. Makman, M. H., Ahn, H. S., Thal, L. J., Sharpless, N. S., Dvorkin, B., Horowitz, S. G., and Rosenfeld, M. (1979): Aging and monoamine receptors in brain. *Fed. Proc.,* 38:1922–1926.
55. Melmon, K. L. (1971): Preventable drug reactions; causes and cures. *N. Engl. J. Med.,* 284:1361–1368.
56. Misra, D. P., Loudon, J. M., and Staddon, G. E. (1975): Albumin metabolism in elderly patients. *J. Gerontol.,* 30:304–306.
57. Mitchard, M. (1979): Drug distribution in the elderly. In: *Drugs and the Elderly,* edited by J. Crooks and I. H. Stevenson, pp. 65–75. University Park Press, Baltimore.
58. Nation, R. L., Triggs, E. J., and Selig, M. (1977): Lignocaine kinetics in cardiac patients and aged subjects. *Br. J. Clin. Pharmacol.,* 4:439–448.
59. Novak, L. P. (1972): Ageing, total body potassium, fat free mass and cell mass in males and females between the ages of 18 and 85 years. *J. Gerontol.,* 27:438–443.
60. O'Malley, K., Crooks, J., Duke, E., and Stevenson, I. H. (1971): Effect of age and sex on human drug metabolism. *Br. Med. J.,* 3:607–609.
61. Redolfi, A., Borgogelli, E., and Lodola, E. (1979): Blood level of cimetidine in relation to age. *Eur. J. Pharmacol.,* 15:257–261.
62. Reichlmeier, K., Eng, A., Iwangoff, P., and Meier-Ruge, W. (1978): Age-related changes in

human brain enzyme activities: A basis for pharmacological intervention. *Adv. Exp. Med. Biol.*, 97:251–252.

63. Richey, D. P., and Bender, A. D. (1977): Pharmacokinetic consequences of aging. *Annu. Rev. Pharmacol. Toxicol.*, 17:49–65.

64. Roberts, M. A., and Caird, F. I. (1976): Steady-state kinetics of digoxin in the elderly. *Age Ageing*, 5:48–67.

65. Roberts, R. K., Wilkinson, G. R., Branch, R. A., and Schenker, S. (1978): Effect of age and cirrhosis on the disposition and elimination of chlordiazepoxide. *Gastroenterology*, 75:479–485.

66. Robinson, D. S. (1975): Changes in monoamine oxidase and monoamines with human development and aging. *Fed. Proc.*, 34:103–107.

67. Roth, G. S. (1975): Reduced glucocorticoid responsiveness and receptor concentrations in splenic leukocytes of senescent rats. *Biochem. Biophys. Acta*, 399:145–156.

68. Roth, G. S. (1979): Hormone receptor changes during adulthood and senescence: Significance for aging research. *Fed. Proc.*, 38:1910–1914.

69. Schocken, D. D., and Roth, G. S. (1978): Age-associated loss of beta adrenergic receptors from lymphocytes *in vivo*. *Adv. Exp. Med. Biol.*, 97:273–276.

70. Seidl, L. G., Thornton, G. F., Smith, J. W., and Cluff, L. E. (1966): Studies on the epidemiology of adverse drug reactions. III. Reactions in patients on a general medical service. *Bull. Johns Hopkins Hosp.*, 119:299–315.

71. Seshadri, R. S., Morley, A. A., Trainor, K. J., and Sorrell, J. (1979): Sensitivity of human lymphocytes to bleomycin increases with age. *Experientia*, 35:233–236.

72. Severson, J. A., and Finch, C. E. (1980): Age changes in human basal ganglion dopamine receptors. *Fed. Proc.*, 39:508a.

73. Shader, R. I., Greenblatt, D. J., Harmatz, J. S., Franke, K., and Koch-Weser, J. (1977): Absorption and disposition of chlordiazepoxide in young and elderly male volunteers. *J. Clin. Pharmacol.*, 17:709–718.

74. Shepherd, A. M. M., Hewick, D. S., Moreland, T. A., and Stevenson, I. H. (1977): Age as a determinant of sensitivity to warfarin. *Br. J. Clin. Pharmacol.*, 4:315–320.

75. Shih, J. C., and Young, H. (1978): The alteration of serotonin binding sites in aged human brain. *Life Sci.*, 23:1441–1448.

76. Smith, C. R. (1979): Use of drugs in the aged. *Johns Hopkins Med. J.*, 145:61–65.

77. Smith, T. W., and Haber, E. (1970): Digoxin intoxication: The relationship of clinical presentation to serum digoxin concentration. *J. Clin. Invest.*, 49:2377–2386.

78. Stevenson, I. H., Salem, S. A. M., and Shepherd, A. M. M. (1979): Studies on drug absorption and metabolism in the elderly. In: *Drugs and the Elderly*, edited by J. Crooks and I. H. Stevenson, pp. 51–64. University Park Press, Baltimore.

79. Taylor, B. B., Kennedy, R. D., and Caird, F. I. (1974): Digoxin studies in the elderly. *Age Ageing*, 3:79–84.

80. Thompson, E. N., and Williams, R. (1965): Effect of age on liver function with particular reference to BSP excretion. *Gut*, 6:266–269.

81. Thompson, J. F., and Floyd, R. A. (1978): Effect of aging on pharmacokinetics. In: *Drugs and the Elderly*, edited by R. C. Kayne, pp. 143–155. Monograph of the Ethel Percy Andrus Gerontology Center. University of Southern California Press, Los Angeles.

82. Traeger, A., Kunze, M., Stein, G., and Anckerman, H. (1973): Zur Pharmacokinetik von Indomethacin bei alten Menschen. *Z. Alternsforsch.*, 27:151–155.

83. Triggs, E. J. (1979): Pharmacokinetics of lignocaine and chlormethiazole in the elderly; with some preliminary observations on other drugs. In: *Drugs and the Elderly*, edited by J. Crooks and I. H. Stevenson, pp. 117–132. University Park Press, Baltimore.

84. Triggs, E. J., Nation, R. L., Long, A., and Ashley, J. J. (1975): Pharmacokinetics in the elderly. *Eur. J. Clin. Pharmacol.*, 8:55–62.

85. Vartia, K. O., and Leikola, E. (1960): Serum levels of antibiotics in young and old subjects following administration of dihydrostreptomycin and tetracycline. *J. Gerontol.*, 15:392–394.

86. Wallace, S., Whiting, B., and Runcie, J. (1976): Factors affecting drug binding in plasma of elderly patients. *Br. J. Clin. Pharmacol.*, 3:327–330.

87. Weintraub, M., Au, W. Y. W., and Lasagna, L. (1973): Patient compliance as a determinant of the serum digoxin. *JAMA*, 224:481–485.

88. Weiss, B., Greenberg, L., and Cantor, E. (1979): Age-related alterations in the development of adrenergic denervation supersensitivity. *Fed. Proc.*, 38:1915–1921.

89. Whiting, B., Lawrence, J. R., and Sumner, D. J. (1979): Digoxin pharmacokinetics in the elderly. In: *Drugs and the Elderly,* edited by J. Crooks and I. H. Stevenson, pp. 85–101. University Park Press, Baltimore.
90. Wilkinson, G. R. (1979): The effects of ageing on the disposition of benzodiazepines in man. In: *Drugs and the Elderly,* edited by J. Crooks and I. H. Stevenson, pp. 103–116. University Park Press, Baltimore.
91. Withering, W. (1785): *An Account of the Foxglove, and Some of Its Medical Uses: With Practical Remarks on Dropsy, and Other Diseases.* G. G. J. and J. Robinson, London.
92. Nies, A., Robinson, D. S., Friedman, M. S., Green, P., Cooper, T. B., Ravaris, C. L., and Ives, J. O. (1977): Relationship between age and tricyclic antidepressant plasma levels. *Am. J. Psychiatr.,* 135:790–793.

Rehabilitation in the Aging edited by
T. F. Williams. Raven Press, New York © 1984.

Psychological and Psychiatric Factors in the Rehabilitation of the Elderly

*J. Pierre Loebel and **Carl Eisdorfer

*Department of Psychiatry and Behavioral Sciences, School of Medicine, University of Washington, Seattle, Washington 98195, at Harborview Medical Center, Seattle, Washington 98104; and **Montefiore Medical Center, Bronx, New York 10467

Much has been made of the biomedical advances of the past century that have enabled us to diagnose disease in many cases, to treat it to a point of cure in some cases, and to prevent disease occurrence in a number of other cases. Perhaps insufficient attention has been paid, however, to an equally important set of developments—that of functional improvement or maintenance in the increasingly large group of the population whose diseases are chronic rather than curable and where the sequelae of a disease leave persistent if not permanent disability.

The rhythm pattern from cure to care is particularly important in our approach to elderly patients who are likely to suffer from chronic illnesses and a significant proportion of whom have functional disability. The clinical care of these patients requires a different set of strategies designed to maximize function at minimal risk to the patient and the caring system. This strategy of rehabilitation requires a high degree of patient collaboration and motivation, which as a rule exceeds that of compliance with medication regimes or the other relatively short-lived procedures usually associated with acute diseases.

An understanding of personality and psychosocial factors in patient care then becomes of particular importance in the context of rehabilitation. The particular problem of aging complicated by societal attitudes and personal beliefs (as well as those of health care professionals) enlarges the need for more information about such factors in patient management.

Rehabilitation is described in the 15th edition of the *Encyclopaedia Britannica* as the use of (medical and vocational) techniques to enable a sick or handicapped person to live as full a life as remaining abilities and degree of health will allow (17). In subscribing to this general point of view we will assume in what follows that primary illnesses and handicaps have received their appropriate initial diagnosis and treatment. Our focus will be on the psychiatric concomitants that then require attention in the longer-term process of rehabilitation.

It might be argued that a certain degree of "wear and tear" is a concomitant of the (normal) aging process and that since we cannot rejuvenate the patient it is pointless to speak of rehabilitation for older persons. We do not agree. In

41

many cases it has been shown that decrements that had been accepted as a result of inevitable aging had in fact emerged as an instance of a modifiable pathological process. Even where such a process cannot be adduced, an attempt to achieve the optimal pleasure and productivity of the person concerned, within the constraints acting on him or her, is the proper and legitimate aim of the clinician. As Braceland once stated, "I submit that we are striving to return to society a 'compleat person,' skilled and perhaps newly skilled in important techniques and especially in the art of living. . . . the rehabilitation of the aging individual is indeed one of the most meaningful fields of modern medicine" (6).

In the following review we shall examine, first, some of the factors affecting the rehabilitation process that reside in the individual, and, secondly, some that arise in the individual's setting. Finally, we shall comment on a number of programs and approaches to the issues that have emerged and show promise for improving patient care.

FACTORS RELATING TO THE INDIVIDUAL

Psychological factors influence the goals and pace of change and often the limits of rehabilitative efforts in the elderly. They may be categorized as falling into two broad groups, those of relatively recent onset and those of more long-standing duration.

Psychological Factors of Recent Onset

A cardinal factor relating to rehabilitation potential is the sense of loss. This often pervades the impression made by the individual needing help. Although there is a multitude of specific losses that may be applicable to any elderly person, what is lost, as a common factor, is a part of the self that has cared for ("been invested in") something believed to be gone and irretrievable. It should be understood that restoration of a particular loss may never be completely achieved, despite the fact that new friends, facilities, or faculties approximate the ones that are no more and may do much to restore the individual's sense of integration.

Although the specific objects of loss are, of course, manifold and the validity of the foregoing point stands, it may still be valuable to address each major loss to the maximum extent feasible. Suggestions for so doing will be made later, in the section on "Programs". Losses span the range from the loss of valued personal belongings (a particularly distressing issue within institutions where the loss of familiar surroundings compounds the problem); the loss of valued others and the roles played in relation to them; the loss of faculties, both physical (e.g., sight, hearing, agility, sexuality) and psychological (e.g., memory); to, finally, the expectation of the loss of life itself.

The loss then may be best understood as relating to an initial loss of a part of the sense of self and a secondary loss related to the missing object, person, or ability. The primary loss may initiate the psychological state of depression (discussed in detail below), which will compromise rehabilitation efforts. The secondary loss, i.e., loss of specific abilities and functions or relationships, may generate a chronic depressive state, which the clinician may recognize as feelings of sadness, futility, lack of futurity, and hopelessness.

Psychiatric Syndromes

The next group of factors includes the formal psychiatric syndromes of affective (e.g., depression, anxiety), cognitive (e.g., organic brain syndrome), and delusional (e.g., paranoid) disorders, and their combinations. The occurrence of these syndromes should be regarded as indicating a need for specific treatment. They are mentioned here also to draw attention to the fact that elements of these syndromes are often present albeit disguised either during the resolution phases of the disorders themselves, or as personality derivatives. Whatever the origin, cognizance should be taken of these affective, cognitive, and delusional symptoms whose occurrence can impose severe limitations on rehabilitative efforts. We have found no specific references in the literature to the incidence of these syndromes, at subclinical levels of severity, in a population of the elderly receiving rehabilitative help. But, by extrapolation from studies of what are sometimes referred to as minor mental illnesses in the general population, we can conclude that their incidence is high (4), and even higher when we allow extension to include, for example, existential sadness as well as depression, anger as well as anxiety, suspiciousness as well as paranoia, and reduction in mental acuity as well as disorientation or frank memory failure.

Of particular cogency are the depressive syndromes. Depressive disorders, the major disturbances of affect, are the most prevalent psychiatric conditions among all patients. Although the major depressive (endogenous) illnesses (i.e., bipolar, unipolar, and schizoaffective disorders) appear to be no more frequent among the aged than younger patients, depressive symptomatology increases in later life (5). There is also a tendency for depression in older persons to be less frequently diagnosed in the United States, as compared with Great Britain (30), in contrast to dementia.

Reactive or secondary depressive disorders are doubtless even more frequent, although not well documented. Such reactive disorders stem from a range of medical conditions, from several classes of medication (the most notorious of which are reserpine-containing antihypertensive drugs), and from any important loss. Several issues relevant to reactive depression warrant review. Recent trauma or loss as the precipitant for any of the endogenous depressions may well be the rule rather than the clinical exception. Although the response is almost invariably a far more exaggerated reaction than the precipitant warrants, the alert clinician should be cautious in evaluating the sequelae of loss and grief.

The persistence of a pattern of sadness and the failure of the individual to recover from the loss and reinstate work, self-care, and leisure activities after a reasonable period (i.e., several weeks after the loss), even in the absence of the familiar patterns of endogenous depression (15), may indicate a level of chronicity that bodes poorly for further adaptation in the absence of help.

Assistance for the grieving should emphasize supportive care, techniques for reentry, and counseling. The use of psychotropic medication, clinically indicated for major affective disorders, is not appropriate for the patient with reactive illness unless untoward clinical changes occur. Obviously, a careful medical examination, including a meticulous scrutiny of all drugs being taken by the patient, is a first requirement.

The recent emergence of the "learned-helplessness" (64) paradigm of depression has particular relevance for older persons with physical (or psychological) losses in ability. As mastery over one's environment is lost the cognitive style of the depressed individual emerges.

Eisdorfer (14) has recently elaborated a similar model of suspiciousness and paranoia in the aged. In such instances, the value of a contingency approach coupled with cognitive therapy and environmental changes that enhance personal control seem worthy of attempt. Clinical research is lacking to provide data on therapeutic efficacy but the empirical underpinning of the model makes it worthy of considerable interest and effort.

The role of alcohol or other substance misuse either as a continuation of a lifelong pattern or as a new condition in later life should be considered. Alcohol use to ward off the symptoms of depression is not uncommon and frank alcoholism may occur as a problem in later life. It is interesting that, if detected, rehabilitative efforts on behalf of the alcoholic aged patient are more successful than those among the young (3).

The misuse of medication for a variety of reasons including dependency should also concern the clinician caring for aged patients. Not only multiple prescriptions per patient but also borrowing, hoarding, and mixing of medications can be a problem causing psychological states resembling dementia and depression as well as untoward physical reactions. The latter may range from unanticipated side effects of medication and alterations in blood levels of medications to a range of physical disorders.

Dealing with the patients' belief systems concerning their medications can be helpful in understanding the basis for non- or poor compliance and can prevent distress to all concerned.

Other Distress Reactions

There are some emotional difficulties that are not typically regarded as formal psychiatric syndromes, but that are certainly prevalent among the elderly requiring rehabilitation. These include feelings of loneliness, isolation, rigidity, disengagement, and powerlessness. These are not necessarily normal constituents of aging and, although their expression may be a means of soliciting help, it is also evident that they bring about problems in their own train. The issue of dependency, or the adoption of a "sick" role, is an obvious example of this.

Physical Impairments

Finally, note must also be taken of the high incidence of physical impairment that occurs among the elderly (49). The particular issues and techniques of rehabilitation that relate, for instance, to patients who have suffered cardiac damage or strokes are beyond the scope of this chapter, but suffice it to draw attention to a closely related issue, the hazards of polypharmacy in the aged (66).

Factors of More Long-Standing Duration

Personality

The chief of these factors concerns personality traits, that constellation of propensities to feel and respond in ways that are generally believed to be relatively stable and enduring over time (and that are popularly believed to become exaggerated or more openly delineated with the passage of the years) (42,50,59,63).

A good recent review is that of Neugarten (52). She remarks that although much has been written in this area, little has been established, and cogently reviews some of the conceptual and methodological reasons for this. One study showed that personality, as assessed by means of the Cattel 16 Factor Personality Questionnaire (7), was a significant predictor of psychological well-being among 380 white men and women aged from 50 to 76 years (23). Another study was able to identify characterological profiles in older men who adapted well (the Mature, Rocking Chair, and Armored types), and badly (the Angry and the Self-Hating types) (57). Yet another study, from West Germany, investigating 220 men and women aged from 60 to 79 years, demonstrated that the personality feature identified as *rigidity* remained stable over a five-year period (67). Finally, Neugarten's own group reported eight patterns of aging: the Reorganizers, the Focused, the Disengaged, the Holding On, the Constructed, the Succorance Seeking, the Apathetic, and the Disorganized (53).

Although we are not aware of any studies that have attempted to relate these personality clusters to the outcome of rehabilitative efforts as such, there is an *a priori* case to be made that these factors would, indeed, have an important bearing on relearning and adaptation. Neugarten quotes Havighurst as claiming that "from a social psychological perspective aging is better viewed, not as a process of engagement or disengagement, but as a process of adaptation in which personality is the key element" (33). We suggest that what is probably true for aging also applies to the results of attempts to rehabilitate the aged. To adapt Henry Miller's dictum regarding head injuries, it is not so much the nature of the pathology in the aged as the nature of the aged person affected, which dictates the rehabilitative problem that must be addressed.

Motivation

Also central in determining the response to rehabilitation, but no easier to pin down than the contribution of personality, is the motivational factor (8, 43,70).

The clinical picture is well described by Clark:

> Motivation is a key factor in the management of old patients in home or hospital. It represents a quality and attitude of mind imparting a sense of direction and purpose, a keenness to participate, an interest in current affairs and events—a *joie de vivre*. The patient wants to be independent and to maintain mental and physical activity.
>
> Its antithesis is an air of physical weariness and lassitude. Physical and mental inertia lead to the vicious circle of apathy-inactivity-sloth-apathy. A daily routine becomes stereotyped, with increasing exhaustion and disinterest, the sufferers adopting a lifestyle more in keeping with their calendar than their biological age (8).

It could be defensible to regard this presentation as indicative of a depressive disorder and to manage that on its own merits. But there are two other aspects that may be at work and that could yield to other approaches.

The first is one to which Eisdorfer and co-workers have pointed in the past (13). Their series of investigations demonstrated that decrements in performance, especially the errors of omission that are so readily ascribed to low motivation, may, in fact, be due to the converse, i.e., to heightened arousal interfering with effective performance in the environment. Recent studies of autonomic nervous system functioning have supported this hypothesis particularly as it involves increased sympathetic nervous system activity (plasma catecholamines) among aged men (73).

The second has to do with the influence that stimulus-response contingencies and schedules of reinforcement have on behavior. From this perspective, performance does not only depend on inner springs to action but also represents the impact on the agent of the field. Then the "low motivation" may be said to reside in the effects of the environment on the individual rather than in the individual. This point will be taken up further in the section below dealing with "milieu" issues, but we feel that it should be a major issue in the evaluation of the patient's behavior. Reference is made to the work of Filer and O'Connell who showed the beneficial effect on self-care and general engagement in the program in a rehabilitation hospital, of a group of elderly patients, when a system of rewards clearly contingent on their behavior was instituted (19).

Belief

The patients' beliefs about their conditions, causes, appropriate treatments, and outcomes (with or without treatment) may be of paramount importance in compliance and in motivation. It is proper to investigate the patients' assumptions, because age, experience, social class, education, and ethnic factors all play important roles in beliefs about health, disease, and prognosis for certain disorders (40).

FACTORS OUTSIDE THE INDIVIDUAL

Institutionalization

Of all the extrinsic factors that have been regarded as having a psychological impact on rehabilitation in the elderly, perhaps the most important is the emotional climate of the setting within which the individual is treated. Early analysis of this factor stems from observation of what became termed *institutionalization* because this related to chronic mental patients living in institutions (24,74). As it is clear that many of the handicaps shown by institutionalized patients were a function of a less than enriching or enhancing environment, it may be supposed that the behaviors of elderly persons exposed to similar influences are similarly affected. One of many accurate descriptions is that of Townsend in a review of institutions for the aged.

> In the institution people live communally with a minimum of privacy and yet their relationships with each other are slender. Many subsist in a kind of defensive shell of isolation. Their mobility is restricted and they have little access to a general society. Their social experiences are limited and the staff leads a rather separate existence from them. They are subtly oriented toward a system in which they submit to orderly routine, non-creative occupation, and cannot exercise much self determination. They are deprived of intimate family relationships and can rarely find substitutes which seem to be more than a pale imitation of those enjoyed by most people in a general community. The result for the individual seems fairly often to be a gradual process of depersonalization. He has too little opportunity to develop the talents he possesses and they atrophy through disuse. He may become resigned and depressed and may display no interest in the future or in things not immediately personal. He sometimes becomes apathetic, talks little, and lacks initiative. His personal habits and toilet may deteriorate. Occasionally he seems to withdraw into a private world of fantasy (68).

Another review of elderly persons residing in institutions finds that they "tend to be docile, submissive, show a low range of interests and activities, and to live in the past rather than the future. They are withdrawn and unresponsive in relationship to others" (44).

Although much is made of the thrust to develop rehabilitative settings in which these deleterious effects are minimized, the nature of much institutional care remains "custodial" rather than therapeutic and even in therapeutically accented settings the age of the patient is likely to be a major factor in staff attitudes toward the patient's rehabilitation potential.

The efficacy of programs like reality therapy is a challenge to the milieu since it represents a replacement of interpersonal care and environmental stimuli that should never have been missing to begin with (11). Another question is raised by the issue of a variable impact of the environment on the patient. Do all people exposed to these influences respond similarly? If not, why so? Are some aspects more injurious than others (e.g., stimulus deprivation, degree of control over personal autonomy and mastery over the environment) or are factors relating to the patient of greater pathoplastic importance (e.g., degree of preparedness for the move into an institution, premorbid personality) (46,64)? Another way of conceptualizing these issues is to inquire into the effect of improving the "matching" between an individual's abilities and the demands made by the environment in a "demanding" rather than a "prosthetic" environment. When the match is poor a degree of functional incapacity may emerge that outweighs the limitations specifically related to, say, the impaired integrity of a person's central nervous system (45).

It is evident that methodological difficulties in investigating these and many other pertinent specifics abound, but whatever answers emerge, there can be no doubt that the setting has a significant bearing on presentation and outcome and that it will influence rehabilitation efforts.

Life Event Stresses

Holmes and Rahe (37), and other investigators, have reported on the damaging influence on mental as well as on physical health of the accumulation of relatively nonspecific stresses. With the passage of time the elderly are, of course, particularly prone to the quantitative accumulation of these stresses. Any list of major life changes would include an array of losses to which the elderly are prone and to which allusion has already been made. These include losses of relatives and friends, social roles, income and personal possessions, physical energy, sensory faculties, general health, and sexual functions. In addition, changes of abode, the impact of physical ill health, and iatrogenic difficulties all can bring about a heightened propensity to affective and cognitive pathology.

Social Support Systems

Those without families and other interpersonal attachments are overrepresented in mental hospital populations. This is no less true among the aged in institutions (28,39,60). The social impairments that antecede admission are numerous but it follows that rehabilitative efforts need to address these specifically. An elderly person whose self-care has deteriorated, owing, for example, to difficulties in dressing and bathing caused by arthritis or postural problems, will deteriorate much more rapidly if another person is not available to help with these tasks. In the absence of friends or family prepared to provide these services, these services must be purchased, or the elderly person may be neglected. Since financial support by governmental agencies is largely lacking for such needs in many countries, progression to institutionalization is predictable, and rehabilitative efforts may founder on the same financial obstacles. Even when family support is available, their efforts on behalf of the patient may be inappropriate to the extant level of ability because of a wish to deny impairment, or from a sense that greater pressure will overcome what appears to be growing apathy, or the family's own mounting frustration and fear of future burden. This situation is likely to bring about increasing anxiety in the elderly relative, whose performance will then show further deterioration. Rehabilitation must include education and support for the family with the aim of achieving a closer fit between expectation and performance (58).

Labeling and Prejudice

The effects of labeling of the patient are insidious and far reaching. They range from philosophical conclusions (that to label something is not only to describe what we have seen but also to understand the patient's condition and "know" the prognosis of the particular patient) to such specifics as the infliction of a cardiac neurosis (34).

The elderly are particularly prone to these damaging effects of labeling since the ascription of "dementia" or "senility" rings with such finality in popular awareness, despite the fact that cognitive impairments may be patchy, not global, progression not inevitable, and the very diagnosis itself often erroneous (47,61). Nor is it only the lay public who take this attitude about possible organic brain syndromes in the elderly. Prejudice and antitherapeutic nihilism among professionals is as well recognized as it is poorly countered, and rehabilitative efforts are further hampered by this (12,18).

Clearly, then, a host of proactive psychological traits and premorbid states interact with the vicissitudes of aging and the environment in which the individual finds him- or herself to affect therapeutic and rehabilitative outcome. A program of careful psychiatric evaluation of aged persons is warranted for all patients in rehabilitation.

APPROACHES TO CARE

This section will examine a number of therapeutic approaches, to some of which allusion has already been made. Programs that respond to the many needs that have been identified are increasingly being devised and only a limited review is therefore possible. The topic is in its infancy. Many questions are being asked and it is not surprising that answers are given that are more in the nature of proposals and descriptions than established research findings. The dearth of properly planned and controlled evaluations of the interventions and approaches to be described below may be among the most serious deficits we face in patient care.

The ensuing review will address four main areas: psychotherapy, the milieu, the multiple strategy approach, and some specific interventions.

Psychotherapy

The role of psychotherapy in rehabilitation is an essential but still poorly investigated one, with a growing number of process reports, but few outcome studies (16). Psychotherapy plays a part in the general issues of establishing an active and forward-looking attitude, of attempting to reawaken hope in the "demoralized" patient (21), as well as dealing with specific problem areas such as the expression of anger, reduction of guilt, and overcoming the sense of loss (35). Although it may be argued that these pose specific difficulties and are not in themselves particularly related to rehabilitation, there is also a growing literature on, for example, the encouragement of an acceptance of the process of aging (32) and an analysis of dependency (62).

One approach that often has a fundamental bearing on rehabilitative problems is that which has been developed by Seligman and his co-workers (64). It identifies "learned helplessness" as a core difficulty. Since one of the problems frequently associated with aging has been noted to be the loss of a role, it follows that there is likely to be a major decrement in approval received and a loss in the sense of mastery over the environment. These developments then become expressed in the helplessness that is often a prime target of rehabilitative efforts.

Techniques that have been found to be applicable with the elderly range widely and include insight-oriented, transference-related, and behavioral techniques. They are well reviewed by Knight (41).

Milieu Aspect

"Milieu treatment attempts to alter the total environment in ways that will change the behavior of persons who are not acting according to acceptable social standards" (26). This description by Gottesman, adapted for our present purpose by adding "or to their optimal levels," is an apposite introduction to an element in the rehabilitation of the elderly, which is of paramount importance.

The literature on environmental restructuring to bring about desired behavioral changes has a recent origin in the works of Maxwell Jones and others writing in the period soon after World War II and was given impetus by the observations of Goffman, as well as the deinstitutionalization movement in the United States and the United Kingdom (24,29,38). Much remains to be investigated in detail but the general movement away from institutional wards that Whitehead described as "annexes to the mortuary" (72) to environments in which the atmosphere is one of expectancy of improvement, and that judicious blend of support and challenge required in order to bring this about, has been a salutary one (27). It seems self-evident that if patients are to regain self-respect and a spark of *joie de vivre* is to be rekindled, the emotional tone around them as set by the staff must be that of respect, enjoyment, and a belief in their eventual recovery. The necessity for optimism, enthusiasm, and some dash are frequently referred to in the literature on rehabilitation. The total environment needs to be bent to this aim.

It is therefore vital that an atmosphere of activity and optimism exists in the geriatric wards of the hospital. The right climate, which has such powerful effects on the expectations and progress of the individual patient, depends on many different groups: other patients, relatives, nurses, doctors, voluntary helpers, ward orderlies, porters, ministers of religion, social workers, and paramedical therapists. This very large group of individuals forms a "therapeutic community" and it is this— and not just the "rehabilitation team" of physiotherapists, occupational therapists, speech therapists, and doctors—which determines the quality of rehabilitation in the hospital ward. Good communication is needed if rehabilitation is to thrive (36).

All members of the staff have a role to play and although the professional staff are important group leaders who need to create and maintain the right attitudes of enthusiasm and optimism around them, others are needed to form "the therapeutic community." A pattern of mutual support and a positive attitude are vital ingredients in this regard. Of course, an overly challenging approach, if it leads to an experience of failure, must also be guarded against and it is therefore equally important for staff to have the capacity for patience, perseverance in the face of slow progress, as well as compassion for periods of failure. These attributes of a therapeutic milieu are far easier to describe than prescribe and an energetic administrator, stable yet receptive and creative, is a central asset (25). (See also G. S. Clark and G. P. Bray, *this volume.*)

The physical conditions of the milieu are as important as the emotional tone. Proper lighting by day and night, comfortable and homelike furniture, facilities that have due regard to physical infirmities, appropriate noise and temperature levels, and readily visible and available informational sources and signs are necessities that are as essential as they have been often ignored in the past. For those with physical disabilities, the creation of appropriate environmental supports can not be emphasized enough. A considerable growth in function will follow personal physical supports, e.g., improved wheelchairs, automobiles, stores, and even eating and writing utensils.

Multiple Strategy Approach

A widely held conviction is that the multiple needs of the elderly person, and indeed of the chronically infirm in general, whether in body or mind, are best met by a multiple strategy or "team" approach. A representative listing of such team members is that given by Rao (56) who lists the following services and personnel in the team approach to care of the aged.

1. Administrative Services
2. Recuperative Services
   Medical (physicians, consultative, surgical and nonsurgical specialists), nursing, pharmaceutical, dietary, dental, podiatric, psychological.
3. Restorative Services
   Physical therapy, occupational therapy, speech therapy, audiology, respiratory therapy.

4. Investigatory Recording
   Results of laboratory tests, results of roentgenography, medical records.
5. Patient Activities
   Activity therapy, recreation, volunteer functions, religious.
6. Public Relations
   Patient representatives, educational services, family and friends.
7. Social Services
   Institutional, community, governmental.

There are important omissions, even to this compendious tabulation, for example, hairdressers and cosmetologists! A more fully detailed list is beyond the scope of this section, but a useful analysis of many of these roles is that given by Whanger and Busse, writing from a perspective of care within the hospital (71). Emphases may change after discharge from the hospital or institution but the basic requirement is that a broad spectrum of care be continued if hard won gains are not to be eroded. Once living again in the community, the elderly patient may require ongoing assistance by formal mental health services (psychiatric and social work consultation), volunteer visitors, transport, a telephone hotline, activity programs, home helpers including meals-on-wheels, and assistance with laundry and residential facilities covering the whole range of increasing support. It is noteworthy that many of these needs have been identified, and programs designed, by persons working from the standpoint of concerned citizens groups and not by the traditional professional organizations as such (48,65). Perhaps we in the professions must make ourselves more aware of the importance of the range of abilities required for self-care, and the importance of doing for one's self in having a sense of personal integrity and psychological health.

Although there can be little doubt that an array of services may be germane to the multiple needs of the incapacitated elderly, major questions relate to the efficient application, coordination, and funding of these services. With these questions, organizations both in the United States and the United Kingdom are currently struggling and clearly no one ideal set of solutions has emerged (22). Traditionally, for instance, it has been expected that a medically qualified person should act as the team leader, with the rationale that such a person is the one best prepared to assess the complex interplay between biomedical and psychosocial factors at work in the patient (9). This is, however, only one paradigm and, in part because doctors are not as a group invariably effective collaborators with members of other disciplines, or in part for economic efficiency, other models should continue to be explored.

SPECIFIC INTERVENTIONS

Motivation/Socialization

A prime target for rehabilitative efforts and one that has been alluded to frequently above, concerns the tendency toward social disengagement of the elderly person. In addition to the general comments that have already been made, attention must be drawn to the increasing number of reports of the beneficial effects of providing the elderly with a role. It is clearly insufficient to provide a stimulating environment and a sense of challenge if no emotional rewards are forthcoming when levels of activity do become raised. Such reinforcement of behavioral changes does, however, occur when, for example, elderly persons are provided with opportunities to be of assistance to others. There are a number of reports of the effective use of groups of elderly volunteers in assisting other more incapacitated persons, or assisting children (1,51,69).

Reality Orientation

Since the disorientation of the elderly, whether suffering from cognitive or perceptual impairment, is believed to be one of the antecedent conditions leading to disengagement and apathy, intensive efforts to reorient such persons to their environment have been devised and found to be beneficial (20). As described by Olsen (54) quoting the results of a study by Parker on the outcome of a program of reality orientation,

> At the beginning all the patients were unresponsive, apathetic, perseverating and vacant. None was an individual person viewed from the door; all were a ward group. Some needed much help. In 8 weeks mannerisms had minimized, folk looked to see who had come into the ward, they moved within the ward, incontinence did not exist. In 12 weeks all were said to be eating less (an improvement), all had lost weight and were judged to be in better physical shape. In 18 weeks occupations had been established about which some could converse. Greater recall was evident in all patients I talked with (55).

Other advantages were also reported. The persistence of these effects has been questioned but the clinical value of stimulating and of spending more time with these patients cannot be doubted. Changing the socialization pattern on a ward by using various reinforcers has been similarly demonstrated to be of positive value to the morale of patients.

Cognitive Training

Another approach intended to increase the elderly person's sense of independence, in this instance over the internal environment (and specifically over a sense of anxiety), is sometimes referred to as the psycho-educative one (2). It essentially attempts to bring about an improved understanding of the origin of common psychosocial stressors and to teach improved coping strategies in response to these. This emphasis on the rational and cognitive distinguishes the approach from the traditional psychotherapeutic one. One such program was described by Hall (31). A group of persons whose mean age was 76.3 years assessed the stresses impinging on themselves by means of the Holmes and Rahe Life Stress Schedule. Classes were held, teaching specific stress reduction techniques. At 6 months follow-up 80% reported improvement.

Involvement of the Family

An important element in successful psychological rehabilitation is the proper preparation of the family members amongst whom it is hoped that the elderly individual will again be able to take a place. This preparation is needed to advise the family of resources in the community that are available to assist them. This may permit them to greet the returning relative with some optimism rather than a fearful expectation, likely to become self-fulfilling, of failure. Perhaps even more important, it is also needed to inform the family of functional levels attained by the relative, so that appropriate demands may continue to be made, and effective rewards continue to be provided (36).

CONCLUSION

What fundamental features may be said to emerge from a review of some of the approaches that have been attempted in the field of ameliorating the psychological obstacles to rehabilitation in the elderly?

Attention is directed to two features. First, independent of the particular service being performed for the elderly individual, it is the attitude of the agent that plays a significant role in the outcome. "The most important aspects of rehabilitation of the elderly, however, are conveying hope, establishing confidence, and overcoming undue fear of death" (75). Closely related to this is that efforts be directed specifically at overcoming the demoralization that comes particularly with the sense of loss of autonomy. Simone de Beauvoir has written,

> The aged brood upon dangers that they have no means of averting. Even if no particular threat hangs over them, it is enough for them to know that they are defenseless to be filled with anxiety; the peace they enjoy seems to them precarious; and since they are no longer the master of it, the future is heavy with frightening possibilities (10).

The second, and probably closely related, feature is that rehabilitative efforts and conditions should be specifically directed toward providing the patient-client with the sense that he or she is still valued by others.

Mastering the environment, whether internal or external, and **mattering** to others are two of the basic foundations on which successful psychological rehabilitation rests. In these conclusions we are restating matters that have long been recognized as of fundamental importance in medicine. "During the war observers noted two influences which, when operating on the personalities of men, were of the greatest importance in preventing neuroses and chronic disability. These influences were high individual motivation and high group morale" (6). The diagnosis of specific psychiatric syndromes and their treatment should be part of an attitude that aging *per se* does not mean that careful and concerned clinical care is unnecessary or wasteful. The therapeutic strategies that work at younger ages are effective for the aged with the same *caveat*. They only work if they are employed.

REFERENCES

1. Abrahams, J. P., Wallach, H. F., and Divens, S. (1979): Behavioral improvement in long-term geriatric patients during an age-integrated psychosocial rehabilitation program. *J. Am. Geriatr. Soc.*, 27:218–221.
2. Armstrong, H. E., Jr. (1980): An educational approach to psychiatric day care. In: *Behavioral Group Therapy: An Annual Review*, edited by D. Upper and S. M. Ross, pp. 125–146. Research Press Co., Champaign, Ill.
3. Atkinson, J. H., Jr., and Schuckit, M. (1981): Alcoholism and over-the-counter and prescription drug misuse in the elderly. *Annu. Rev. Gerontol. Geriatr. (in press).*
4. Bebbington, P., Hurry, J., and Tennant, C. (1980): Recent advances in the epidemiological study of minor psychiatric disorders. *J. R. Soc. Med.*, 73:315–318.
5. Blazer, D., and Williams, C. D. (1980): Epidemiology of dysphoria and depression in an elderly population. *Am. J. Psychiatry*, 137:439–444.
6. Braceland, F. J. (1957): The role of the psychiatrist in rehabilitation. *JAMA*, 165:211–215.
7. Cattell, R. B., Eber, H. W., and Tatsuoka, M. M. (1970): *Handbook for the 16 Personality Factor Questionnaire (16PF)*. 4th ed. Institute for Personality and Ability Testing, Champaign, Ill.
8. Clark, A. N. G. (1978): Morale and motivation. *Practitioner*, 220:735–737.
9. Cohen, G. D. (1977): Approach to the geriatric patient. *Med. Clin. North Am.*, 61:855–866.
10. de Beauvoir, S. (1972): *The Coming of Age.* G. P. Putnam's Sons, New York.
11. Duffy, M., and Weinstein, C. E. (1978): Architectural design characteristics of public housing and well-being of the elderly. Gerontological Society: 31st Annual Scientific Meeting, *18*(5,2), 66.
12. Eichler, M. (1977): Report from Israel. *J. Geriatr. Psychiatry*, 10:243–248.
13. Eisdorfer, C. (1968): Arousal and performance: Experiments in verbal learning and a tentative theory. In: *Human Aging and Behavior*, edited by G. A. Tallard, pp. 189–216. Academic Press, New York.
14. Eisdorfer, C. (1980): Paranoia and schizophrenic disorders in later life. In: *Handbook of Geriatric Psychiatry*, edited by E. W. Busse and D. G. Blazer, pp. 329–337. Van Nostrand Reinhold Co., New York.
15. Eisdorfer, C., Cohen, D., and Veith, R. (1981): Overview of aging, the challenge to medicine and society. In: *Psychiatric Aspects of Aging: A Clinical Guide*, edited by C. Eisdorfer. Springer, New York *(in press).*
16. Eisdorfer, C., and Stotsky, B. A. (1977): Intervention, treatment and rehabilitation of psychiatric disorders. In: *Handbook of the Psychology of Aging*, edited by J. E. Birren and K. W. Schale, pp. 724–748. Van Nostrand Reinhold Co., New York.
17. Encyclopaedia Britannica (1978): *Micropedia*, Vol. 8, 15th edition, p. 484. Encyclopaedia Britannica, Inc., Chicago.
18. Exton-Smith, A. N., and Evans, J. G. (1977): *Care of the Elderly*. Grune & Stratton, New York.
19. Filer, R. N., and O'Connell, D. D. (1964): Motivation of aging persons in an institutional setting. *J. Gerontol.*, 19:15–22.
20. Folsom, J. D. (1968): Reality orientation for the elderly mental patient. *J. Geriatr. Psychiatry*, 1:291–307.
21. Frank, J. D. (1973): *Persuasion and Healing.* Johns Hopkins University Press, Baltimore.
22. Gaitz, C. M., and Hacker, S. (1970): Obstacles in coordinating services for the care of the psychiatrically ill aged. *J. Am. Geriatr. Soc.*, 18:172–182.
23. George, L. K. (1978): The impact of personality and social status factors upon levels of activity and psychological well-being. *J. Gerontol.*, 33:840–847.
24. Goffman, E. (1961). On the characteristics of total institutions. In: *Asylums: Essays on the Social Situations of Mental Patients and Other Inmates.* Doubleday, Garden City, N.Y.
25. Gottesman, L. E. (1970): Organizing rehabilitation services for the elderly. *Gerontologist*, Winter (1), 287–293.
26. Gottesman, L. E. (1973): Milieu treatment of the aged in institutions. *Gerontologist*, 13:23–26.
27. Gottesman, L. E., Quarterman, C. E., and Cohn, G. M. (1972): Psychosocial treatment of the aged. In: *APA Task Force on Aging Report*, edited by C. Eisdorfer and M. P. Lawton. American Psychological Association, Washington, D.C.

28. Grad de Alarcon, J. (1971): Social causes and social consequences of mental illness in old age. In: *Recent Developments in Psychogeriatrics,* edited by D. W. Kay and A. Walk. Headley Brothers, Ashford, Kent.
29. Greenblatt, M., York, R. R., and Brown, E. L. (1955): *From Custodial to Therapeutic Care in a Mental Hospital.* Russell Sage Foundation, New York.
30. Gurland, B. J. (1976): The comparative frequency of depression in various adult age groups. *J. Gerontol.,* 31:289–292.
31. Hall, R. C. W. (1979): *Life Stress Approach to Rehabilitation in the Elderly.* American Psychiatric Association Annual Meeting, Chicago.
32. Hammer, M. (1972): Psychotherapy with the aged. In: *The Theory and Practice of Psychotherapy with Specific Disorders.* Charles C Thomas, Springfield, Ill.
33. Havighurst, R. J. (1968): A social-psychological perspective on aging. *Gerontologist,* 8:67–71.
34. Haynes, R. B., Sackett, D. L., Taylor, D. W., Gibson, E. S., and Johnson, A. L. (1978): Increased absenteeism from work after detection and labeling of hypertensive patients. *N. Engl. J. Med.,* 292:741–743.
35. Hiatt, H. (1971): Dynamic psychotherapy with the aging patient. *Am. J. Psychother.,* 25:591–600.
36. Hodkinson, H. M. (1973): Rehabilitation of the elderly. *Br. Med. J.,* 4:777–778.
37. Holmes, T. H., and Rahe, R. H. (1967): The Social Readjustment Rating Scale. *J. Psychosom. Res.,* 11:213–218.
38. Jones, M. (1953): *The Therapeutic Community: A New Treatment Method in Psychiatry.* Basic Books, New York.
39. Kay, D. W. K., Beamish, P., and Roth, M. (1964): Old age mental disorders in Newcastle-upon-Tyne. Part II. *Br. J. Psychiatry,* 110:668–681.
40. Kleinman, A. (1980): *Patients and Healers in the Context of Culture.* University of California Press, Berkeley.
41. Knight, B. (1978): Psychotherapy and behavior change with the non-institutionalized aged. *Int. J. Aging Hum. Dev.,* 9:221–236.
42. Kuhlen, R. G. (1964): Personality change with age. In: *Personality Change,* edited by P. Worchel and D. Byrne, pp. 524–555. Wiley, New York.
43. Kumpel, Q. (1979): Rehabilitation in geriatric psychiatry. *Rehabil. gerontopsy.,* 13:53–55.
44. Lieberman, M. A. (1969): Institutionalization of the aged: Effects on behavior. *J. Gerontol.* 24:330–340.
45. Lindsley, O. R. (1964): Geriatric behavioral prosthetics. In: *New Thoughts on Old Age,* edited by R. Kastenbaum, pp. 41–60. Springer, New York.
46. Luria, A. R. (1973): The Working Brain. Basic Books, New York.
47. Marsden, C. D., and Harrison, M. J. G. (1972): Outcome of investigation of patients with presenile dementia. *Br. Med. J.,* 2:249–252.
48. Meyer, J. (1977): Cardinal Ritter Institute provides care with flair to St. Louis elderly. *Aging,* 272–273:8–10.
49. Mezey, A. G., Hodkinson, H. M., and Evans, G. J. (1968): The elderly in the wrong unit. *Br. Med. J.,* 3:16–18.
50. Mischel, W. (1969): Continuity and change in personality. *Am. Psychol.* 24:1012–1018.
51. Mulligan, M. A. (1978): A friendly visitor program: Its impact on the social and mental functioning of the elderly. *Issues Ment. Health Nurs.,* 1:1–11.
52. Neugarten, B. L. (1977): Personality and aging. In: *Handbook of the Psychology of Aging,* edited by J. E. Birren and K. W. Schaie, pp. 626–649. Van Nostrand Reinhold Co., New York.
53. Neugarten, B. L., Havighurst, R. J., and Tobin, S. S. (1968): Personality and patterns of aging. In: *Middle Age and Aging,* edited by B. L. Neugarten, pp. 173–177. University of Chicago Press, Chicago.
54. Olsen, R. (1979): Services for the elderly mentally infirm. In: *Community Care for the Mentally Disabled,* edited by J. K. Wing and R. Olsen, pp. 152–170. Oxford University Press, Oxford.
55. Parker, F. (1974): *Second Childhood.* Times Educational Supplement, August, 3089:12–13.
56. Rao, D. B. (1977): The team approach to integrated care of the elderly. *Geriatrics,* February, 88–96.
57. Reichard, S., Livson, F., and Petersen, P. G. (1962): *Aging and Personality.* Wiley, New York.
58. Reifler, B. V., and Eisdorfer, C. (1980): A clinic for the impaired elderly and their families.

Am. J. Psychiatry, 137:1399–1403.
59. Riegel, K. F. (1959): Personality theory and aging. In: *Handbook of Aging and the Individual,* edited by J. E. Birren, pp. 797–851. University of Chicago Press, Chicago.
60. Ross, H. E., and Kedward, H. B. (1976): Demographic and social correlates of psychogeriatric hospitalization. *Soc. Psychiatry,* 11:121–128.
61. Ron, M. A., Toone, B. K., Garralda, M. E., and Lishman, W. A. (1979): Diagnostic accuracy in presenile dementia. *Br. J. Psychiatry,* 134:161–168.
62. Rouch, J. L., and Maizler, J. S. (1977): Individual psychotherapy with the institutionalized aged. *Am. J. Orthopsychiatry,* 47:275–283.
63. Schaie, K. W., and Marquette, B. (1972): Personality in maturity and old age. In: *Multivariate Personality Research: Contributions to the Understanding of Personality in Honor of Raymond B. Cattell,* edited by R. Dreger, pp. 612–632. Claitor's Publishing, Baton Rouge.
64. Seligman, M. E. P. (1975): *Helplessness.* W. H. Freeman & Co., San Francisco.
65. Sluyter, E. H. (1977): Planning and implementation of a comprehensive community services program for the elderly. *Aging,* 272–273:13–17.
66. Stotsky, B. A. (1970): Use of psychopharmacologic agents for geriatric patients. In: *Clinical Handbook of Psychopharmacology,* edited by A. DiMascio and R. Shader, pp. 265–278. Science House, New York.
67. Thomae, H. (ed.) (1975): *Patterns of Aging: Findings from the Bonn Longitudinal Study of Aging.* Karger, Basel.
68. Townsend, P. (1962): *The Last Refuge—A Survey of Residential Institutions and Homes for the Aged in England and Wales.* Routledge & Kegan Paul, London.
69. Wallach, E., Kelley, F., and Abrahams, J. (1978): Psychosocial rehabilitation for chronic geriatric patients. Gerontological Society: 31st Annual Scientific Meeting, *18(5:2),* 136.
70. Wallen, V. (1970): Motivation therapy with the aging geriatric veteran patient. *Milit. Med.,* 135:1007–1010.
71. Whanger, A. D., and Busse, E. W. (1975): Care in hospital. In: *Modern Perspectives in the Psychiatry of Old Age,* edited by J. G. Howells, pp. 450–485. Brunner/Mazel, New York.
72. Whitehead, A. (1970): *In the Service of Old Age.* Penguin, Harmondsworth.
73. Wilkie, F., Halter, J., Eisdorfer, C., Benedetti, N. and Prinz, P. (1980): Effects of age on metabolism and metabolic effects of epinephrine in man. Paper presented at the Gerontological Society of America Meeting, San Diego.
74. Wing, J. K., and Brown, G. W. (1970): *Institutionalism and Schizophrenia: A Comparative Study of Three Mental Hospitals.* Cambridge University Press, Cambridge.
75. Wolff, K. (1971): Rehabilitating geriatric patients. *Hosp. Community Psychiatry,* January, 24–27.

Rehabilitation in the Aging edited by
T. F. Williams. Raven Press, New York © 1984.

Social Aspects of Rehabilitation

Barbara Silverstone

The Benjamin Rose Institute, Cleveland, Ohio 44115

Even under the best of circumstances, rehabilitation efforts seldom return a disabled old person to fully independent functioning. The risks and vulnerabilities associated with old age, and the complexity and multiplicity of ailments, militate against the more dramatic successes commonly associated with short-term amelioration. Furthermore, unlike the younger patient who has made functional gains, the elderly, because of more limited social roles, are given fewer opportunities to engage in rewarding activities that enable them to maintain self-care skills (17).

This is not to dismiss the need to take a hard look at those concepts of rehabilitation that can be successfully utilized in the care of the elderly. Lawton (6) notes that realistic goal setting and acceptance of small successes are viewed as necessary components of the rehabilitation process: "The probability of improvement is highest when the goal for the old person is set successively at only the next step higher than the current level of functioning."

The advantage of this approach lies in its broad inclusiveness of the wide range of severe and chronic disabilities common to a significant number of older persons. If modest efforts are valued as much as dramatic improvements, then even the most disabled person can make significant improvements. A realistic rehabilitation framework of this type holds much promise for a population viewed as hopeless and candidates only for custodial care. Small improvements in functioning may reduce dependence on others to the extent that less direct caregiving is needed. Even if the change is indiscernible to the caregiver, the psychological benefits that accrue from feelings of greater self-reliance may be reward enough for the patient.

Particularly unfortunate are funding policies which exclude from rehabilitation those elderly with diagnoses of organic brain syndrome (even when the primary condition for which rehabilitation is being recommended is a physical condition such as a hip fracture). Although learning skills might be presumed lost, the failure to attempt modest improvements is both nihilistic and expensive, for the lack of intervention will most probably result in a further deterioration in functioning and the necessity for costly nursing care.

This chapter will examine the importance of the social environment in rehabilitation of the elderly, highlight the need for psychosocial assessment, review the components of the psychosocial plan, evaluate social and health care planning, and address financial considerations.

IMPORTANCE OF THE SOCIAL ENVIRONMENT

The social environment—those persons, groups, and organizations who interact with the elderly rehabilitation client—plays a crucial role in the rehabilitation process. There are older persons with internal resources that enable them to surmount all obstacles including the lack of support from others. But for many, the result of illness and impairment is increased dependence on others. The economic, social, and psychological depletions often accompanying old age exacerbate this increased dependence. Thus, cues from the social environment can have a profound effect on the attitudes and behavior of elderly rehabilitation clients.

For many, the psychological impact of disabling illness and the toll it takes on self-esteem can result in depression and a waning of motivation. The vicious cycle of lowered self-esteem, depression, and reduction in motivation often can only be broken by external interventions.

The long-term needs of the elderly underscore the importance of the social environment. Despite the strong emphasis placed on self-reliance and greater self-mastery, numerous social supports are required by the elderly rehabilitation client, first, simply, to learn new skills, and then maintain them. A social commitment that includes organizational provisions is essential. These provisions range from personal care and homemaker services to the enabling features of the physical environment, whether they are provided in an institutional setting or in the home to which the rehabilitation client returns.

The rehabilitation philosophy in and of itself makes explicit demands on the social environment. The very specific, step-by-step goals of rehabilitation, and the importance of objective assessment of functioning with feedback to caretakers, calls for clarity in communication from the onset of the disabling condition to postdischarge adaptation.

The implications of this philosophy for the social environment are profound. The entire therapeutic team of physicians, nurses, nurse assistants, physical therapists, occupational therapists, social workers, family, and friends—who interact with the older person in the home, the community, or the institution—must be attuned to the explicit rehabilitative goals. For example, the well-intentioned efforts of a rehabilitation team can be subverted by well-meaning but confused family members who simply do not understand the rehabilitative process.

On a more subtle level there are varying social interactions between the chronically disabled older person and others, which can enhance or disrupt the rehabilitative process. Role behavior is useful in understanding these interactions. The variety of roles assigned to most persons carry with them a set of expected behaviors. One of the serious depletions associated with aging is the decrease in the number of roles the elderly experience during their adult lives. If disabled, the role of patient may be one of the few left to them.

The term *patient role* is used here to denote an exclusive set of behaviors that are commonly expected of a person who is disabled and requires the care of others. It is closely akin to the *sick role* formulated by Parsons (9) to denote a set of behaviors on the part of the patient, presumably adaptive to the relationship with the physician during an illness. These behaviors include dependency, cooperation in the treatment process, and motivation to get well.

The term patient role in contrast to the sick role denotes a set of behaviors that can outlive an acute episode and thus more appropriately describe the chronically disabled. These behaviors, which are readily apparent in institutions but which also can occur within the family setting, include conformity, dependency, and receptivity to care, and exclude aggressiveness and attempts at self-reliance. Such behaviors are seen as adaptive for the long-term client in that they enhance care and/or organizational efficiency.

Just as the sick role is antithetical to rehabilitation philosophy because the chronically disabled cannot recover, so is the patient role. Older persons who see themselves as only being cared for are poor candidates for rehabilitation. Independent strivings and active participation are crucial components of rehabilitation. The adage "you can lead a horse to water but you can't make it drink" is only too applicable here. Redefinition, expansion, and revitalization of roles for the chronically disabled are needed.

The establishment or reinforcement of such roles for some elderly may not be an easy task in view of their constricted social world. The older person who returns to the community may pick up former roles such as housekeeper, spouse, grandparent, or church member, all of which have the potential for providing alternatives to the patient role. On the other hand, the discharge of an elderly person to a long-term care facility is an occasion fraught with danger because of the not uncommon tendency of these facilities to treat the older patient within the acute care model and, paradoxically, also as a permanent ward.

The importance of the social environment in rehabilitation cannot be overemphasized, particularly for those elderly individuals who are highly dependent on the environment for nurturance and cues, whose needs for care are long-term, and whose roles and potential roles are limited. Specific interventions by the rehabilitation team are called for in order to alter the social environment.

In most instances, the social worker is charged with these intervention tasks. All staff, however, must be attuned to the impact of the social environment and be prepared to respond accordingly. Social intervention can take place only within the context of the total rehabilitation effort. It is a social worker's task to make a psychosocial assessment, to acquaint the full team with the background and needs of the rehabilitation patient at all phases of the rehabilitative process, and to develop a plan for direct intervention with the older person, family, staff, and significant organizations.

The work of the rehabilitative team ideally begins at the time a physical or mental disability is identified—in the acute hospital, the doctor's office, the community agency, or nursing home—and is extended to these settings in the latter phases of the rehabilitation process. The rehabilitation team usually functions only within a recognized rehabilitation setting although, as noted, some skilled nursing and intermediate care facilities have adopted a rehabilitative philosophy. It behooves the social worker in the acute hospital or community agency to embark on a psychosocial assessment plan even when rehabilitation efforts are deferred because of organizational constraints. This early effort will enhance the rehabilitative process once it is formally initiated. Where no formal rehabilitative effort is in the offing, such as in a nursing home or community, the task of the social worker reaches beyond the needs of individual clients to community organization and planning efforts directed at revitalizing or creating new services.

PSYCHOSOCIAL ASSESSMENT

It is essential that the interaction between the rehabilitation client and his or her social environment be clearly understood and evaluated. The behavioral patterns of the client must be identified as well as those aspects of the social environment that impinge on that behavior: the family, staff, and significant organizations. The psychosocial assessment is an essential evaluative tool in planning the social aspects of rehabilitation. Components of this assessment may be contributed by other members of the team such as the psychologist or psychiatrist. A clinically trained social worker may also undertake a behavioral evaluation. In any event, the psychological and social elements of an individual's adaptation must be viewed conceptually as a whole and, of course, integrated with the physical and biological aspects of the older person's condition.

Individual Behavior

Important behavioral elements to identify in the elderly person are typical patterns of adaptation to stress, loss, illness, and disability over the life span. Aside from the impact of the social environment and the increased vulnerabilities of old age, these are the factors, not aging alone, that will help explain the client's current adaptation.

This chapter does not permit a full account of the vagaries and complexities of human behavior in relation to illness and disability. However, one important clue to the adaptive capacities of older persons is their demonstrated ability in the past and present to cope with their problems realistically, both cognitively and emotionally. Persons who have exercised a great deal of denial throughout their lives in relation to crises or losses beyond the initial impact, may attempt to deny over time the reality of the present illness or disability and thus refuse to take the necessary steps. Others may respond with so much anxiety and depression that they are immobilized. Yet another group, although understandably upset and concerned about their plight, are able to make "the best of the situation" and move ahead.

A closely related, yet distinctive, characteristic is the older person's capacity to use the help of others. Older persons, like younger ones, may perceive the social environment as hostile and not helpful and reject attempts at positive feedback and support. They may interact with the social environment in a purely utilitarian way avoiding warm, personal involvements, thereby diminishing staff gratification. Or they may feel so helpless and dependent on others that an inordinate amount of staff time is involved and progress impeded by the older person's unceasing desire for nurturance.

To be taken into account, of course, are changes in adaptive capacities over the life course. On the one hand, the elderly are seen by Steger (17) as exercising less denial in relation to disability and illness because they are at a time of life when these "insults" are bound to occur. On the other hand, they are often seen as more dependent because of depletions commonly associated with aging. In either case, adaptive patterns have been modified over the life course, but the clues they offer should be carefully weighed. Individual variations can be extensive even when the physical disability and age level are similar.

Two cases help to illustrate this point:

Afflicted with a stroke, this was the first serious illness in the life of a 75-year-old man, Mr. M., who typically throughout his life denied the emotional importance of crises such as the loss of jobs and the death of his wife and generally "bounced back" quickly with an optimistic view of the future. He suffered periodic depressions in his life, but these were viewed as separate and apart from these crises and losses both by him and his family whose support and help he seemed not to need. Rehabilitation seemed at first particularly hopeful for this man in view of his optimism, eagerness, and seemingly independent character. Although small goals were initially set by the rehabilitation team, more extensive goals seemed realistic as well. The man's cheerful outlook that had affected staff positively were put into a more realistic perspective by an examination of the psychosocial history. The severe depression he had suffered years ago after the death of his wife served as a warning to staff that rushing ahead too quickly might only exacerbate a serious depression.

An 80-year-old woman, Mrs. K., suffering from a hip fracture seemed at first to need a great deal of nurturing from staff although little progress took place. Her social history revealed a lifelong pattern of utilizing physical ailments to gain an undue amount of attention from others. Unconsciously, the secondary benefits gained from this behavior outweighed the benefits of good health. Thus, she continually complained of minor ailments. This historical pattern of behavior suggested to staff that functional recovery from her hip fracture might not be seen by her to be in her best interests. They embarked on a very matter-of-fact approach to her disability and gave positive support and feedback only to healthful gains.

An examination of the interaction of both these individuals with their social environments revealed one case of seeming independent behavior and the other dependent behavior; in one case the emotional impact of the disability was denied and in the other it was exaggerated. A close look at the history of these interactions added invaluable dimensions to the staff's understanding and development of a rehabilitation strategy.

A number of other factors enter into the formulation of a psychosocial strategy, which in turn extends beyond immediate rehabilitation efforts and interaction with the older person. These include family, friends, and the various organizations that impinge on the course of recovery and long-term care.

Informal Supports

The informal social structure surrounding a person in everyday life can profoundly influence behavior in relation both to handling of illness and disability and also in relation to the adjustment that person will make in the future. This informal social structure includes the older person's family, friends, and neighbors—those primary relationships that can provide affection, socialization, and highly individualized care and support.

The spouse remains a close family relation particularly for men in the later years. Fifty-five percent of the elderly over 65 are married and most couples live alone. However, 68.2% of women over 75 are widowed in contrast to only 22.1% of men over 75. The extended family structure is important for the elderly as well; 40% of those over 65 have great-grandchildren. Although older couples and widows tend to live apart from their families, 52% live within easy traveling distance from one or more children (11,12,18).

Friendships for widows and widowers are important components of their social lives. These informal groups may be found in apartment houses for the elderly, in old neighborhoods where the elderly are still living, or within organizational structures such as churches, synagogues, and senior centers.

Most older persons are actively involved with family, friends, and neighbors in a variety of social and traditional activities, contradicting the common myth that older persons are abandoned by family or isolated from social contacts. In fact, over 80% of the care given to older persons is provided by the family (11). There is also a sizeable group of older persons who have remained isolated from others all their lives or who have outlived family and friends and have been unable to develop new relationships (16).

An important task of the psychosocial assessment is to determine the actual presence and strengths of these informal supports for they will be a crucial factor in determining the rehabilitative plan for an elderly patient. Without some types of informal support, a return to the patient's home in the community may be impossible. When the presence and number of supports have been determined, then the type, quality, quantity, and reliability of the supports must be evaluated both from the client's and professional's perspectives. There are great variations among families, ranging from adult children or spouses who can and will provide total support to aging kin, to those whose contribution, although well-meaning, may be minimal.

The presence of family does not necessarily suggest there are persons ready or able to perform a variety of tasks for an older person. A daughter living in the same city as an elderly mother suffering a hip fracture may be the mother's confidant and very concerned about her welfare but unable to help with activities of daily living such as cooking, cleaning house, providing personal care, or arranging transportation to a day rehabilitation program. The daughter herself may be ill, working, or caring for others.

Family members may be ready to take on more tasks for an older person, but hastily drawn assumptions should not be made about this readiness. For instance, a loving daughter may be already burdened with the care of her own immediate family or perhaps another elderly family member. The spouse of an older person may also be disabled. The effects on the family over time must be assessed. Caregiving, supervision of care, the provision of minor tasks, and emotional support to the older person can produce stress for the family and affect several generations. An examination of the family's coping strategies in the past may be enlightening.

The assessment of the informal social structure must extend beyond measuring the practical supports that family and friends can or cannot provide and the toll this may take. In addition, emotional and social relationships exist that can significantly affect the patient's attitudes and alter the course of rehabilitation. As previously noted, most elderly interact with, and rely on, their relatives. As a result, the family is an important determinant in the development of attitudes and role expectations.

Attitudes about aging, disability, illness, and death and dying are shaped and reinforced within the extended family structure (1). Often such attitudes are positive ones similar to those found in the rehabilitation philosophy. However, it is equally possible that the family belief system is antithetical to rehabilitation goals. Family members can strongly reinforce the "patient role" for an older member. Such adages as "you can't teach an old dog new tricks" can be deeply ingrained in a family's belief system and can successfully inhibit rehabilitative measures. Thus, their impact bears consideration perhaps even before rehabilitative steps are initiated. These family beliefs usually focus on such notions as "mother is too old or weak" or "should be protected at this time of her life." Such attitudes, in addition to being rooted in a belief system, can sometimes emanate from hostility on part of the family toward the older person and other feelings that distort a realistic appraisal of the situation.

At the other extreme are those families whose belief structure dictates that no matter how old an individual is, he or she can accomplish meaningful tasks. Once again, these attitudes may be primarily rooted in a particular family's own denial of the seriousness of a disability. The family may demand or seek unrealistic goals that counteract a basic tenet of rehabilitation—to take one step at a time and be satisfied with small successes.

The close interplay between the individual behavior of the rehabilitation client and the social environment is vividly exemplified in family relationships. The older person's reliance on family help in the past may be perpetuated into the later years. The 75-year-old man, Mr. M., who alone bravely extricated himself from crises earlier in life may still refuse family aid despite their willingness. The 80-year-old woman, Mrs. K., who for years exploited her family's concern through hypochondriacal complaints may no longer find them responsive. On the other hand, the relationship between the generations may be mutually respectful and helping ones, enabling the family to adapt—relatively conflict-free—to the demands of the present situation.

The complexities, subtleties, and variations in the behavior of older rehabilitation clients and their families and friends extend far beyond the limitations of this chapter, which attempts only to identify certain broad directions. A thorough assessment of the situation from the viewpoint of patient and family within a historical, dynamic, and contemporary framework establishes the necessary foundation for evaluating the broader social environment and planning the social aspects of future rehabilitative care.

Formal Settings and Services

An assessment of the formal system of care that impinges on rehabilitation clients and their families is essential. On the most basic level, such an assessment can determine whether rehabilitative services, inpatient and outpatient, and other services are available and accessible. If so, the assessment can determine the quality of those services with regard to the psychosocial needs of the elderly patient and family. Finally, the assessment will gauge the transitions required in the older person's life and the effects of these changes on the individual's stability.

The presence or absence of rehabilitation services may determine the future course of an older person's life. By the same token, the absence of other services may render rehabilitative efforts useless. Mr. M., 75 years old, may wish to return to his own home, but find it impossible to receive on-going physical rehabilitation because of a lack of transportation. He may be unable to care for himself, refuse family help, and/or cannot find available agency services. The family of 80-year-old Mrs. K. may require special counseling to sustain their support of her. The availability of such professional help must be determined.

At the same time, consideration must be given to the accessibility and affordability of services. The willingness of client and family to pay for services is a paramount issue, as is their eligibility for government subsidized and third party reimbursed programs. (See section on financing.) The willingness to pay for services should not be assumed even when personal resources exist. The "rainy day" for an older person who lived through the Depression may still be around the corner and the present crisis not seen as meriting rehabilitative efforts.

If services are available, accessible, and affordable to older persons and their families within or outside of the rehabilitative setting, the psychosocial components of this care must be assessed. The rehabilitation effort, which must be sustained indefinitely for the elderly in greater or lesser degrees, needs to be an integral part of staff philosophy regardless of the setting in which the older person is being helped. The attitudes that accompany this philosophy are a vital component of staff interaction with older persons and their families.

Staff, as well as the client and family, must envision roles other than the patient role. Staff attitudes should convey a belief in the small successes that can be achieved and in the older person's capacity for growth and change regardless of the degree of debilitation.

A homemaker assigned regularly to assist an older person who is enrolled in an outpatient rehabilitation program for a mending hip may unwittingly undermine treatment efforts by performing tasks which the elder is actually able to do. The staff member admitting an older person to a nursing home may contradict the rehabilitative progress being made by omitting that person from the decision-making process accompanying admission.

This concern with staff attitudes and interactions in the variety of settings in which an older person receives help is reflected in the continuum of care concept. As noted, rehabilitative efforts are maximized if they are made at each step of the continuum of care: the acute hospital, extended care facility, nursing home, and accessible community facilities that serve patients who return to their homes.

Often, these various "levels of care" are not viewed as a continuum that should provide a consistent plan of intervention as the patient's condition improves. Unfortunately, in the American health care system, these institutions usually function as discrete entities. The transition from one to another is frequently abrupt in nature and the care defined more by the program of the institution than by the needs of the patient (14).

Particularly for the elderly, these levels of care must be viewed as crucial ingredients of a long-term care system of care that recognizes the chronic ailments of the elderly and their need for ongoing continuing help. These levels of care are not necessarily synonymous with particular institutions since old people may receive very intensive care in their own homes and minimal care, for example, in a boarding home. Usually, however, the course is viewed as a linear progression from community to nursing home with the acute hospital frequently an intermediate stop.

This state of affairs is particularly unfortunate in view of the fact that many elders can be rehabilitated to less restrictive and intense levels of care. Rehabilitation centers that admit and discharge old people from and to the community are few and far between. Following the acute phase of a chronic illness, discharge is made to the home with little or no consideration for rehabilitation and support to the family. If there is no available family, discharge is made to a nursing home, which seldom is equipped to expedite discharge at a later time when the older person is more ready. Given an institutional readiness for effective discharge, there are often insufficient community supports to sustain the older person at home at a higher level of functioning.

The disjointed fashion in which the elderly move from one level of care to another reflects our fragmented system of social and health care. It is not unusual for an older person to be hospitalized in an acute setting and then to be discharged to the community, the home, or a nursing facility by a discharge planner whose chief concern may be that of freeing a hospital bed. Some hospitals have their own home care programs that provide home services to an older person for a prescribed number of days following hospitalization. As will be noted later, reimbursement restrictions often limit this coverage.

When discharge is made from the acute hospital to a nursing facility, little more may pass between the discharge planner and the intake clerk of a nursing facility than an exchange of records and vital statistics. Some of the more advanced nursing facilities plan carefully for the admission of residents and have good working relationships with hospitals, which mitigate this fragmented effort. However, these are serendipitous events that occur as the result of the quality and resources of a particular institution and not because of a widespread commitment to a continuum of care. The needs of mentally impaired older persons, when measured against this confusing array of services, are particularly poignant.

In addition to the discontinuities of care between facilities and settings, which must be carefully assessed, there are the striking contrasts among institutions in their commitments to rehabilitative efforts on behalf of older persons. These institutional commitments can strongly affect staffs that interact with resident and family.

Some of the pessimistic attitudes and belief systems held by the family and older person are also held by some caregivers and professionals. An acute hospital may overlook the immediate rehabilitation steps for a stroke victim, thus making it much more difficult for a rehabilitation center to pick up after discharge. The acute hospital may also overlook the needs of the family whose attitude might be difficult to reverse at a later time. Patients discharged to a nursing home may receive only the most cursory rehabilitative care, undoing whatever successful efforts were initiated at an earlier time.

A complete psychosocial assessment, in summary, requires an examination of individual and family behavior, historically, currently, and its potential for the future; a determination of the supports available formally and informally; and an appraisal of the attitudes and commitment of the variety of actors who play a role in the rehabilitation scenario. The complex interplay among these various factors serves as an important determinant of realistic goal setting and rehabilitation planning for the elderly person.

SOCIAL REHABILITATION PLAN

A social plan of care should evolve from the assessment and, of course, be modified accordingly as reassessment takes place. As with the assessment, the plan of care may be developed and implemented primarily by the social worker. However, both consensus and implementation should be viewed as a task of the entire rehabilitation team.

A social rehabilitation plan should be closely interwoven with physical, psychological, and nursing rehabilitative efforts. It can be viewed as a process that may begin either with a catastrophic incident such as a stroke or hip fracture or at a point of deterioration for an older person when the need for rehabilitation is recognized. Unfortunately, such recognition is frequently delayed too long for optimal intervention. The process is usually time-limited for older persons who, though rehabilitated to higher levels of functioning, do require ongoing reinforcement and supportive feedback to counteract the unrelenting social, psychological, and physical assaults that accompany advanced age.

The role of the social worker in developing and implementing the social rehabilitation plan is multifaceted. He or she can serve as counselor, enabler, coordinator/liaison, and advocate (10). Under the best of circumstances, the worker's relationship with patient and family extends through the entire rehabilitation process. Continuity of care is achieved to the extent that at least one professional relationship is sustained for the patient and family.

Unfortunately, organizational constraints usually limit a social worker's role to one setting. The social rehabilitation plan, regardless of the setting from which it originates, should nevertheless encompass the entire rehabilitation process with some attempts made at continuity.

Social aspects of the rehabilitation process can be divided into three phases that closely parallel the physical aspects of rehabilitation. These phases can arbitrarily be divided into the acute or recognition phase, the recuperative phase, and the maintenance phase.

Acute Phase

Not all elderly rehabilitation clients necessarily experience an acute phase of illness or disability. Rather, their disability may be the result of slow ongoing deterioration as typified by chronic brain disorders, encroaching arthritis, or progressive sensory impairment.

The acute phase of an illness usually results in hospitalization and is a crisis period for the older person and family. It is a time that may signal a shift in an older person's life from independence to dependence, causing a drastic change in lifestyle, fears for the patient's future, and severe disruption for the family. It is often a crisis for the hospital staff whose task is regarded as a life-saving one.

Crisis resolution can set the stage for patterns of care that may complement or contradict the rehabilitative process. Crucial decisions are often made at a time of crisis that overlook the long-range picture and even omit elderly clients from the decision-making process because of their debilitated condition.

It is during the acute phase that the psychosocial assessment can be initiated. Generally, however, the emotional turmoil that accompanies this period obscures typical client and family behavior patterns. Thus hastily drawn conclusions about the lack of potential for rehabilitation should be avoided.

Given some receptivity on the part of client and family, however, the first stage of any social rehabilitation plan can be initiated: sensitizing the client and the client's social environment to the rehabilitation philosophy. Attitudes of hopelessness and fear about the future can be gently questioned. The client, family, and staff can be acquainted with the small but important successes other older persons have achieved through rehabilitation. They can be alerted to the social worker's plan for mobilizing external resources. This important second stage of planning must necessarily take place during the acute phase, particularly when a client is hospitalized, because of organizational requirements for discharge once the acute phase is over.

The involvement of the client and family in preparation for discharge, another important planning stage, can be a rehabilitation measure in and of itself if they participate actively in the decision-making process. The ambiguity and distress that may characterize client and family at this time can, through staff encouragement, be replaced by clarity of decision. The next highest level of functioning may be achieved in keeping with the rehabilitation point of view (6).

Precipitous discharge planning can lead to inappropriate nursing home placements, or return to an ill-prepared family and home in the community. Ideally, physical rehabilitation is initiated before discharge where the acute hospital has a rehabilitation unit or beds to which a patient can be transferred. Or, discharge is made expeditiously to another inpatient or outpatient facility that can provide intensive rehabilitation care: a rehabilitation center, a nursing home, or extended care facility equipped to provide this care. The sooner a rehabilitative strategy is introduced, the better the chances of averting the more typical downward course of events.

In summary, several important planning stages should first be implemented during the acute phase of a client's disabling illness: sensitization of the client and the client's social environment to the rehabilitative philosophy, mobilization of rehabilitative resources, and involvement of client and family in decision making relevant to discharge.

The recuperative phase should not be sharply demarcated from the acute phase in terms of a rehabilitation strategy although organizational constraints often make it impossible to avoid such a demarcation. The interventions suggested here may help to bridge this situation for client and family.

Recuperative Phase

The recuperative phase is the one in which the most intense rehabilitative efforts are made. This phase may represent the first step in the rehabilitation process for those older persons whose physical and/or mental deterioration has been gradual. They may be residents in a nursing home, clients of a social agency, or simply living alone or with families receiving no services at all. If a rehabilitation strategy is viewed as potentially helpful by clients, family, staff and/or physician and if resources are available, an important step has already been accomplished. The lack of recognition of a rehabilitation need—particularly in cases of progressive deterioration, which are so closely associated in the minds of many with the aging process—can interfere with further planning.

If the client has moved into the recuperative phase of rehabilitation care from an acute or deteriorating condition, the following stages of the social rehabilitation plan can next be implemented: intense sensitization of staff, client, and family to the rehabilitation philosophy and the specifics of the actual process; resocialization of the client; and making provisions for long-term care and living arrangements. A high degree of involvement of all staff as well as client and family, to the rehabilitation effort is crucial. Rehabilitation efforts cannot be consigned to one or two professionals such as the physical or occupational therapists. Floor staff, nurses, and aides must constantly reinforce and encourage newly learned skills and be sensitive to the value of small successes.

Lawton (6) emphasizes the importance of defining standards for measuring improvement in the client and utilizing tools to measure this improvement. He notes that the members of the therapeutic team must know the results of their treatment since this feedback provides very powerful motivation for future efforts. Staff is gratified by the knowledge that actual progress has been made or alerted to change their techniques if progress has not been made. He notes that the lack of systematic observation obscures knowledge of results. Furthermore, the use of a measuring instrument that can make fine discriminations is conducive to setting realistic goals, rather than goals so far removed from the client's level of functioning that attainment is impossible. Thus, clarity and specificity of communication to all in the social environment of the rehabilitation client is a necessity.

In addition to receiving accurate and specific information about the progress or lack of progress a client may be making in the rehabilitation process, staff must be sensitized to client and family idiosyncracies and behavioral patterns. It is here that the psychosocial assessment of client and family is an indispensable tool. The subjective reactions of staff, which can create tensions between client, family, and staff, can be avoided when historical and dynamic dimensions are treated as an integral part of understanding the client's recovery. The tempo of rehabilitation, regardless of the small incremental steps being taken, may be inhibited or hastened depending on the personality of the older person and his interactions with the family. By the same token, understanding of staff frustrations, difficulties, and attitudes about rehabilitation is necessary to build a positive feedback system between client, family, and staff.

The inclusion of family members in the rehabilitation effort not only involves them positively and meaningfully, but sets the stage for the therapeutic role they will play, particularly if the elderly return to the home environment. Family and client idiosyncratic reactions to the progress or lack thereof, regardless of their acceptance of the rehabilitation philosophy, must be handled. The disappointments, frustrations, and anxieties aroused when it is recognized that complete recovery may not be achieved must be aired and handled.

For the staff as a whole, meetings and informal consultation serve as the means by which a respect for small successes is encouraged. Deeply ingrained attitudes about acute medical care and the aging process must be confronted day in and day out. The rehabilitation philosophy must be painstakingly fostered.

Paralleling staff meetings are family meetings. In addition to individual counseling with the patient and family members, it is desirable at the earliest possible juncture (sometimes even in the acute settings) for the social worker to meet with significant family members, including the patient, to discuss the nature of the illness (which families often do not understand) and the facets of the rehabilitation process. Ideally, other team members should also participate, contributing their expertise.

The particular advantage of this approach is that all members of the family who interact regularly with the older person are hearing the same message from staff, and staff in turn are receiving feedback from the family as a whole. Individual differences communicated privately often result in divisiveness. Consensus of all significant persons is essential to establish immediate rehabilitative goals. In addition, the sooner all persons feel "a part of the action," the more ready they may feel to continue their involvement.

The organization of relatives' groups has been found to be a useful intervention in rehabilitation programs (7,15). Although counseling by a social worker or psychologist is considered necessary for relatives having major difficulties making an adjustment to the new situation, the group experience is appropriate for others in offering education and emotional support. Families typically may have difficulty in accepting the changes in an elderly relative, the necessary role changes (particularly for spouse) that they must make, and handling very practical problems such as finances and respite care.

The resocialization of an elderly rehabilitation client is a specific intervention that must be carefully planned for and, of course, is closely interrelated with the measures just discussed. Of significant importance is the need for the client to learn and relearn a variety of social skills to negotiate the new level of functional adjustment that has been achieved. These social skills may involve adapting to different types of dependences, developing new recreational and perhaps vocational activities, acquiring new methods of communication, adjusting to one's new self-image as a more disabled person, rethinking the impact this has on one's capacity for friendships and family relationships, and developing roles other than that of patient. Finally, an important step in resocialization is reorganizing one's view of the future in light of the changed physical or mental condition and ordering one's life accordingly.

Individual counseling is a useful intervention and appropriate for many clients. Once again, the psychosocial assessment can be a valuable tool in gauging the appropriateness of individual counseling. The very process of talking with a trusted person about the various feelings triggered by the situation and one's fears and plans for the future may be all that some individuals need in order to reorder their lives. Others may need more direction and suggestions, or may need to share this process with their peers.

There are pros and cons about the benefits of group meetings to clients in rehabilitation center. Intense periods of socialization can mitigate against early discharge of a person who may become too attached to the peer group. However, the dangers of this type of fostered dependency may be overshadowed by the benefits of having clients meet and share with each other their own struggles, difficulties, and attempts at resocialization in a world that is now different for them. Open-ended, time-limited membership groups might be the best solution to this dilemma.

The group meeting may also be an important format for clients in the recuperative phase to participate in their own treatment program. Any type of participatory activity on the part of clients, be it directly in their own rehabilitation care or in the environment around them, encourages feelings of competence so necessary to improvement.

If the older person is to return to the home or family following recuperation, the home visit is a very useful resocialization tool. Periodic visits increasing in frequency and duration give client and family the opportunity to test out gradually the new adaptations they must make. Problems can be brought back to staff and client and family groups and, hopefully, further resolved.

Rehabilitation day programs offer another excellent opportunity for the resocialization of the rehabilitation client. In the maintenance phase of rehabilitation, they may serve as a continuing reinforcement for rehabilitation gains achieved and as respite for families.

Finally, an important stage of planning in the recuperative phase includes practical arrangements for long-term care or living arrangements for the older person. The total psychosocial assessment should outline these particular needs, which may include protective housing, skilled nursing care, homemaker services, personal care, and prosthetic supports in a client's own home.

The complexity and difficulty of making these types of plans cannot be overemphasized. The sooner plans are initiated, the better the chance that some type of long-range plan can be made. The involvement of family and client in this decision-making process is crucial. For the client alone, it conveys the importance of continuing participation in the rehabilitation process.

Maintenance Phase

Ongoing care for the older person has been strongly emphasized. Whereas younger clients are more able to return to milieus and ways of life that reinforce their thrust toward increased independence, older persons will return to settings, even their own homes, where more regressive behavior may be subtly encouraged by others or readily accepted by those elderly who view themselves as too old for change. Thus, conscious and deliberate rehabilitative efforts can never cease. They will vary, of course, according to the assessment of the environment to which the person is returning. The abilities of the older client to overcome environmental obstacles are crucial factors and must be carefully monitored.

An important intervention in the maintenance phase of social rehabilitation is the persuasion of all significant others, as well as the client, that this phase is a necessary one. Setbacks such as an acute illness or loss of a loved one must be anticipated, and rehabilitative goals adjusted accordingly rather than abandoned.

Another crucially important provision of the maintenance phase are social and physical supports in the home. The level of functioning achieved by an elderly person may still require assistance from others in housekeeping and personal care as well as prosthetic appliances and/or furnishings. If the family or friends cannot provide these services, formal arrangements should be made with appropriate community agencies. Fully independent functioning is often an unrealistic goal. If it is actively pursued or implicitly taken for granted, undue stress and anxiety on the part of the elderly client can result and impede or undermine the rehabilitative process.

This assistance in the home, however, should be considerably less than that required if rehabilitative goals had not been pursued. The cost benefits are apparent to the older person, family, and hopefully third party payers. Less apparent are the benefits that accrue from the judicious use of services and even physical supports. A fine line divides that amount of necessary care essential to maintaining a decent quality of life free of inordinate anxiety and an excessive amount of care, which deprives the client of the challenge and stimulation necessary for optimal functioning.

This balance must be continually weighed in the case of the elderly because of the subtle changes in functioning that can occur in the later years for better or worse. Thus, reassessments are a crucial ingredient of the maintenance phase. Dramatic changes for the worse, of course, may require more intense care and a return to the restorative phase of rehabilitation.

If available, long-term day programs can serve an important function in the maintenance phase. Although these day programs need not necessarily provide rehabilitation services, per se, as required in the restorative phase, they can serve as a social milieu that encourages and reinforces functional gains as well as providing socialization and recreation for the older person and respite for the family.

With or without such formal programs, it is essential that maintenance be regarded as an integral part of rehabilitation for the elderly. Lack of sufficient input, particularly for the very old person, can result in regression. Elderly clients and their social networks should be monitored regularly and indefinitely and/or the client and family be strongly encouraged to seek help when frustrations or difficulties arise. While the old person living alone without family requires special attention, ongoing consideration of involved families is essential.

Long-Term Care Facility

Approximately fifteen percent of the elderly over the age of 75, and a much higher proportion of the mentally and physically disabled, live in long-term care facilities. In the opinion of some, this proportion could be significantly reduced if sufficient rehabilitation and community services were available to the elderly living in their own homes or congregate housing. Given such fortunate circumstances, however, the nursing home will still remain an important option for many very old people, particularly those who are widowed, poor, and without available family.

The long-term care facility is an important setting for the maintenance phase of rehabilitation, and in some cases the acute and recuperative phases as well. Expectations of optimal functioning on the part of even the most mentally and physically disabled resident can help to reduce abject dependency on staff on the one hand and enhance the older person's self-esteem on the other hand (19).

Long-term care facilities, however, vary greatly in the amount of rehabilitation services and programs provided to elderly residents, and different facilities emphasize different aspects of rehabilitation. Furthermore, the custodial and acute medical and nursing models of care that tend to characterize long-term institutional care may obscure rehabilitation goals if they do exist. "Excess disability," that amount of disability in a resident not accounted for by his or her actual physical or mental impairment, is viewed as a product of some nursing home environments (2).

On the other hand, the opportunity for successfully operationalizing rehabilitation goals is enhanced by the fact that all staff are located in one setting and under one administration. Consistent care in the community, with its greater variety of formal and informal services, may be more difficult to achieve.

Long-term care facilities to a large extent are severely constrained in their social rehabilitation efforts by organizational and financial considerations that often prohibit professional involvement. Within these constraints, however, some steps can be taken to enhance psychosocial functioning among residents with the encouragement of staff. Attitudes respecting the person's individuality, privacy, and functional gains as well as setbacks is one endeavor that does not require large expenditures of funds, but rather imaginative leadership on the part of the administrator and top staff.

Another endeavor is the expansion of roles and social and participatory activities for the long-term resident. Organizations such as a resident council can provide an excellent framework for meaningful participation and development of leadership roles (13).

The potential for long-term care facilities to serve not only as permanent homes for the disabled old, but as a resource for the elderly and their families living in the community is yet to be widely realized. If space is available, day programs can offer physical rehabilitation, occupational therapy, social services, recreation, and nursing and medical care to the end of maintaining the older person living in the community at an optimal level of functioning. Day programs and the temporary use of long-term beds can offer respite to families. The closer integration of long-term care facilities into a rational system of long-term care is consistent with the principles of social rehabilitation outlined in this chapter.

PROFESSIONAL, INSTITUTIONAL, AND FINANCIAL CONSTRAINTS

The barriers to comprehensive rehabilitation care for elderly persons are formidable. They are partially rooted in professional and institutional traditions alien to rehabilitation principles.

To a large extent, a client's future course will be set by the personal physician. The family, as well, may rely heavily on the physician's opinion. If the physician enthusiastically views rehabilitative goals as useful ones, the implementation of a rehabilitation plan is feasible, offering excellent leverage for mobilizing staff, patient, and family in maintaining care. If not, rehabilitative efforts and maintenance may be impossible. Cognizance must be given to the fact that medical and other practitioners in the United States have only begun in the past few years to view geriatric care as a distinct body of knowledge and to recognize the rehabilitative potential of the aged.

Cited repeatedly in this chapter as a chief source of the difficulties encountered in achieving a continuity of care for the elderly rehabilitation client is the acute health care model which institutions as well as professions tend to adhere to. Some settings may offer rehabilitation services without espousing a true rehabilitation philosophy. There may be a lack of coordination between organizations and facilities that a patient may have to traverse. Even the cluster of services that may or may not be available to persons living in their own home within the community may be fragmented and not consonant with one another.

Over and above these professional and institutional constraints are the lack of rehabilitative services per se, reflecting inadequate funding, and third-party reimbursement. Physical therapy, speech therapy, occupational therapy, rehabilitative nursing, and social services are in short supply in acute hospitals, in intermediate-care and skilled nursing facilities, and in outpatient and community settings. Although a minority of elderly are able to purchase rehabilitation services if available, the overwhelming number must rely on health insurance and/ or government assistance.

Medicare, a federal health insurance for persons over 65, was considered at its inception in 1965 to be a hallmark in the development of comprehensive services for the elderly. In reality, it provides partial coverage for acute care and reimburses rehabilitation services limited to acute and/or recent conditions. Maintenance care is excluded.

Medicare has two parts: Part A, hospital insurance, and Part B, medical insurance. Part A provides inpatient hospital care, medically necessary care in a skilled nursing facility after a hospital stay, and home health care. Within these settings, covered rehabilitation services include physical and occupational therapy and medical appliances. Medical social services and home health aid services may also be included.

Although these services at first glance seem comprehensive, their limitations lie in the fact that reimbursement is time-limited. For example, after 90 days of hospitalization, the program makes no further payment and the patient is forced to pick up all expenses if their lifetime reserve of 60 days has been exhausted. Extended care in a nursing home or patient's home is limited to several months after a hospitalization, thus seriously hampering the long-term maintenance needs of older persons either in a facility or their own homes. Furthermore, in terms of rehabilitation services only some conditions are covered.

Medicare Part B helps pay for doctor's services, outpatient hospital care, outpatient physical therapy and speech pathology services, home health care, and some other services and supplies not covered by Medicare hospital insurance. Physical therapy and speech pathology services are partially covered if provided in a doctor's office or by an independent physical therapist if prescribed by a doctor. These services may also be provided on an outpatient basis by hospitals, skilled nursing facilities, and home health agencies if prescribed and reviewed by a physician. The permitted frequency of these extended services is far less than that which can be provided in the acute hospital. Extended rehabilitation is also short-term in duration.

Although all older persons over 65 on Social Security are eligible for Medicare and those not receiving Social Security can make special application, it is important to note that deductible and co-insurance features create inequities in access to medical care and distribution of benefits. The cost of care increases for a person the longer they are hospitalized. Certain persons and/or conditions, such as chronic brain disease, may be exempt from coverage (3).

Private insurance for coverage of rehabilitation is extremely limited. Supplemental insurances that cover co-insurance and deductible payments are available to some older persons. These plans vary, however, and are usually as limited in scope as Medicare.

Medicaid is a government-sponsored program of direct financial assistance to the medically indigent. Supported by federal, state, and local funds, Medicaid is administered through the states. Thus, eligibility requirements and services vary widely from state to state with the exception of federally mandated programs. The most extensive of these is reimbursement for nursing home care. Much of the 20.6 billion dollars now being spent annually on nursing home care is supported by Medicaid.

In most states, Medicaid programs will pay for acute rehabilitation services but not on an ongoing basis. A few states provide extensively for related services such as home health care. Other states are very restrictive. It should also be recognized that clients may receive similar treatment in a variety of settings— in an acute rehabilitation center, a long-term care hospital, or a skilled nursing facility–but that Medicare or Medicaid may only reimburse certain types of facilities for these treatments.

These deficits in services and funding are of great concern to planners in the field of geriatric care because of the growing numbers of people expected to survive to advanced old age in the future and the increasing disabilities that will accompany this trend. If functional improvements are not encouraged through a system of rehabilitation care, it is likely that the custodial population will increase disproportionately in numbers, the economics of which will be staggering. Hirschberg (4) summarizes the problem for the elderly hemiplegic patient:

> The greatest obstacle to rehabilitating the elderly hemiplegic patient is access to an appropriate rehabilitation program. Private and government hospitalization insurance strictly limits the amount of physical therapy and rehabilitation that can be given in an acute hospital. The Department of Health, Education, and Welfare has stringent guidelines for rehabilitation programs that many hospitals cannot meet. In addition, most hospitals do not have staff skilled in the rehabilitation of the elderly hemiplegic. Few hospitals have rehabilitation centers, and neither the patient nor the physician favors referral to a distant center soon after a stroke. Many stroke patients are sent to nursing homes, the majority of which are not equipped for rehabilitating the elderly hemiplegic.

SUMMARY

This chapter has advocated an approach that supports an understanding of various levels of functioning among the disabled elderly and argues for a rehabilitation philosophy that values small gains and sustained support. Thus, rehabilitation of the elderly has been viewed within the framework of long-term care which "consists of those services designed to provide diagnostic, preventive, therapeutic, rehabilitative, supportive and maintenance services for individuals of all age groups who have chronic physical and/or mental impairments, in a variety of institutional and noninstitutional care settings, including the home, with the goal of promoting the optimal level of physical, social, and psychological functioning (20)."

Emphasis has been placed on the crucial role of the social environment in the rehabilitation process and the explicit demands of a rehabilitation philosophy—for the client, family, and staff. Since it is imperative that interaction between the rehabilitation client and the social environment be clearly understood and evaluated, the psychosocial assessment has been cited as an essential tool in planning the social aspects of rehabilitation. Such an assessment must include a consideration of individual behavior, informal supports, and formal settings and services. All of these elements impinge on and profoundly influence the rehabilitation process.

A social and health care plan for the rehabilitation client derives from the psychosocial assessment. This plan should deal specifically with the three rehabilitation phases: the acute phase, the recuperative phase, and the maintenance phase. These phases have been viewed from a psychosocial perspective ranging from a consideration of the individual client and family involvement to community and societal issues on an organizational policy level.

Professional, institutional, and financial constraints present a significant barrier to the implementation of an appropriate rehabilitation philosophy. Deficits in services and funding are of serious concern to planners and providers. Conceptual blinders that have obscured the chronic needs of the very old have significantly influenced the organization and funding of rehabilitation resources.

Successful rehabilitation efforts on behalf of the elderly in the future will rest on society's willingness to invest sufficient resources for this purpose. Unquestionably, greater self-esteem and dignity accrue to the older person who can maintain a reasonable level of functioning. In addition, cost-effective benefits of rehabilitative efforts must be considered. Custodial care is very expensive, as documented by present and projected nursing home budgets. To invest meaningfully in rehabilitative measures offers the promise of reducing long-term dependency of the old and encouraging a philosophy that will better serve the growing numbers of frail elders in our society.

REFERENCES

1. Bengston, V. L., and Treas, J. (1980): The changing family context of aging and mental health. In: *Handbook of Mental Health and Aging,* edited by J. E. Birren and R. B. Sloane, pp. 400–428. Prentice-Hall, Englewood Cliffs, N.J.
2. Brody, E. M., Kleban, M. H., Lawton, M. P., and Silverman, H. (1971): Excess disabilities of mentally impaired elderly: Impact of individualized treatment. *Gerontologist,* 2:124–133.
3. Davis, K. (1974): *Lessons of Medicare and Medicaid for National Health Insurance,* General Series Reprint #295, The Brookings Institution, Washington, D.C.
4. Hirschberg, G. G. (1976): Ambulation and self care are goals of rehabilitation after stroke. *Geriatrics,* 31:61–65.
5. Isaacs, B., Neville, Y., and Rushford, I. (1976): The stricken: The social consequences of stroke. *Age Ageing,* 5:188–192.
6. Lawton, M. P. (1968): Social rehabilitation of the aged: Some neglected aspects. *J. Am. Geriatr. Soc.,* 16:1346–1363.
7. Mykyta, L. J., Bowling, J. H., Nelson, D. A., and Lloyd, E. J. (1976): Caring for relatives of stroke patients. *Age Ageing,* 5:87–90.
8. NASW Committee on Aging (1979): *Long Term Care for the Elderly, Chronically Ill and Disabled.* National Association of Social Workers, Washington, D.C.
9. Parsons, T. (1951): *The Social System.* Free Press, New York.
10. Rusk, H. A. (1977): *Rehabilitation Medicine.* C. V. Mosby, St. Louis.
11. Shanas, E. (1979): Social myth or hypothesis: The case of the family relations of old people. *Gerontologist,* 19:3–9.
12. Shanas, E., Townsend, P., Wedderburn, D., Friis, H., Milhoj, P., and Stehouwer, J. (1968): *Old People in Three Industrial Societies.* Atherton Press, New York.
13. Silverstone, B. (1974): *Establishing Resident Councils.* Federation of Protestant Welfare Agencies, Division of Aging, New York.
14. Silverstone, B. (1978): Multilevels and options in chronic care: Myth or reality? *Bull. N.Y. Acad. Med.,* 54:271–275.
15. Silverstone, B. (1978): The family is here to stay. *J. Nurs. Adm.,* 7:47–51.
16. Silverstone, B., and Miller, S. (1980): The isolation of the community elderly from the informal social structure: Myth or reality? *J. Geriatr. Psychiatry,* 13.
17. Steger, H. G. (1976): Understanding the psychological factors in rehabilitation. *Geriatrics,* 31:68–73.
18. *Statistical Abstracts of the United States* (1982): Department of Commerce, Bureau of the Census, Washington, D.C.
19. Stone, L. B. (1969): Provision of rehabilitation in nursing homes. *J. Am. Geriatr. Soc.,* 17:576–594.
20. *The Future of Long Term Care* (1977): National Conference on Social Welfare, Division of Long Term Care, Health Resources Division, Public Health Service, U.S. Department of Health, Education, and Welfare, Washington, D.C.

Rehabilitation in the Aging edited by
T. F. Williams. Raven Press, New York © 1984.

Sexuality in the Aging

Grady P. Bray

Monroe Community Hospital and the Department of Preventive, Family, and Rehabilitation Medicine, University of Rochester School of Medicine, Rochester, New York 14642

During the last twenty years there has been considerable change in our sexual knowledge, attitudes, and behaviors. As a society we have demonstrated a willingness to discuss sexual practices, lifestyles, and relationships in part because of our increasing understanding of sexuality and its role in our lives and culture. As a result of this sexual evolution it is easier to accept the sexuality of people with disabilities, to understand the sexual pressures of young people, and to secure the sex counseling, education, or therapy needed by couples experiencing sexual dysfunction.

Unfortunately these changes in sexual awareness have not altered the prevailing views or treatment of geriatric sexuality. Aging patients continue to be described as "acting out" when they attempt physical closeness and are often viewed as humorous, a nuisance, or a danger to themselves or others when they express their sexuality.

To alleviate such misconceptions and erroneous views it is important to understand aging and sexuality from three perspectives: physiological, psychological, and sociological. This chapter will describe the implications of these three areas for geriatric sexuality, discuss the role of sexuality in geriatric rehabilitation, and identify who should be responsible for addressing sexual issues with the aging patient.

HISTORICAL PERSPECTIVE

Given the repressive nature of society in dealing with sexual issues before the 1940s it is not surprising that the majority of our aging population function with limited sexual information, experience, or expectation. Most of today's geriatric population grew up in an era replete with myths and misinformation concerning sexuality and aging. The majority of the aged reached maturity and established sexual relationships before the advent of the sexual revolution with the work of Kinsey in the 1940s. Before Kinsey, a few researchers, such as Van de Velde (24), had attempted to address the issue of sexuality but most were rebuffed by a Victorian society.

The population of the early twentieth century viewed sexuality as primarily male oriented. Sex existed for procreation and the enjoyment of the male. Women were conditioned to submit to the desires of their husbands and were taught to endure their "beastial natures." Sexual options were quite limited and sexual practices deviating from the norm were considered "abominable." Those who dared to experiment sexually often did so at the risk of legal harassment, extreme anxiety, and guilt (21).

Despite their early orientation, today's geriatric population should not be viewed exclusively in terms of their minimal sexual insight for they too have been exposed to society's changing view of sexuality. Frequently elderly patients have acknowledged long-standing questions concerning sexuality that originated with exposure to mass media and its treatment of sexual issues. Although their awareness of sexual issues had been increased, they remained silent because they were not sure who would respond appropriately to their questions. Perhaps in not so subtle ways, health care providers have communicated discomfort, a lack of knowledge, and a rejection of sexuality for the elderly.

This limited experience and knowledge of an aging population offers tremendous opportunities for sexual growth and development. During the process of helping older people gain additional insight into their sexual function, health professionals can assist them in redefining sexuality in much broader terms. Sexuality can be conceptualized and discussed with these patients in terms of communications, sharing, and intimacy.

It is also important for aging people to understand that sexuality is a normal and natural part of their life development process. Each person is born a sexual being. Within hours of birth the male child will experience his first erection and the female infant will experience the biological counterpart to erection, vaginal lubrication. However, it would be erroneous to consider the etiology of sexual identity as only biological. Sexual identity is a complex interplay of biology, psychology, and sociology. Symbolically, the color of the infant's blanket communicates a subtle message of identity and the statements of the parents concerning their son or daughter serves to confirm the sexual identity of the infant.

These messages are so effectively transmitted to the child that by the age of 18 months most children have a well-defined gender identity (7). It is usually difficult for most people to separate the issues of gender and sexuality but this distinction is important to make because the issue of gender emerges again in later life. Just as the young child is reinforced in a gender role by social interactions and expectations, the adult is affirmed by social contacts and role models. Through our culture, education, and family orientation the meanings of masculine and feminine are crystalized into rigid definitions. These definitions ultimately contribute to stereotypes, and the propagation of myths concerning roles, functions, and aging.

Our culture emphasizes that the sexually desirable person should be young, beautiful, and healthy. Millions of dollars are spent annually on cosmetics whose sole purpose is to deny the reality of aging. As a person ages they are confronted with the beliefs of society, and often begin to view themselves as less than a complete man or woman. When one no longer meets the gender identity requirements a crisis in gender occurs. People frequently start to doubt their masculinity or femininity and begin to respond in an asexual mode. With limited knowledge or facts concerning aging, the person is left with only the accumulated myths, half truths, and fears.

With a crisis in gender a person often focuses on the biological changes that are occuring. The gradual changes of aging, which can usually be accepted with minimal distress, become more acute. This is especially true with sexual function. Similar minor changes in other body systems seldom evoke the response that occurs with changes in sexual function.

One of the major tasks in helping the geriatric patient cope with changes in sexual function is to provide information concerning the developmental nature of aging. The changes in sexuality should be presented in the context of overall body changes and not as cause for alarm. The changes should be clearly identified and the person reassured that the changes are a natural part of the aging process. Changes that deviate from the norm should signal that a process is involved, which requires further investigation or treatment.

To assess appropriately the significance of sexual changes for an aging individual it is important to understand the typical changes that accompany aging.

MALE RESPONSE

In the aging male there are demonstrable changes in sexual physiology (8). Although most of these changes occur slowly, their accumulative effect is often of great concern for men as they begin to notice increased variance during sexual activity. It is important to provide appropriate information to concerned males as they age and before they confront a crisis with their sexuality. As a health care provider it is essential to acknowledge that changes do occur with aging, and that functions in all phases of the sexual response cycle are influenced. However, the problems produced by the changes are not insurmountable and with sufficient patience, knowledge, and practice most men are able to make an acceptable adaptation (12,13,22).

Desire

As they note the physiological changes that occur with aging, many men report a change in desire or libido. Sexual desire is a complex interface between the hormonal, psychological, and sociological aspects of each individual. Each component is a major contributor to the maintenance or loss of sexual desire as aging occurs.

The primary hormone associated with sexual desire is testosterone (7). Secreted initially by the adrenal cortex, testosterone levels increase dramatically during puberty as the testes assume the role of primary androgen producer. Following the second decade, testosterone levels decrease gradually with aging but the decline accelerates after the sixth decade. However, testosterone is usually produced at all ages. Similarly, libido, though diminished in the seventies, eighties, and beyond, is usually reported by most members of an aging population (2).

The use of androgen replacement therapy to help with sexual dysfunction and diminished libido remains controversial (12,17,19). Most authors agree that the use of testosterone as a mechanism for restoring or reawakening sexual interest is of limited or no value. The changes that do occur with older men exposed to androgen replacement therapy can usually be attributed to a placebo effect or to the improvement in total body economy and a renewed sense of well-being (12).

During sexual counseling sessions with the author, a number of elderly males have expressed concern about their continuing sexual desire. Most were surprised at the frequency and intensity of their sexual activity. Several expressed concern that they were abnormal or had a medical problem because of their continuing activity. These men were responding to a sociological myth of geriatric sexuality that rather blatantly conveys the message that older men should have fewer sexual feelings, except for "dirty old men" who are obviously depraved.

To help allay such fears it is important for men to understand the role sexuality plays as aging occurs. Sexual activity is socially oriented and usually involves two people (the second may be real or imaginary, as in masturbation). It is usually a time for closeness, intimacy, touching, and sharing. For the participants it is also a sociological statement, a declaration of sexual identity and an affirmation of life. Sexuality should be presented to the aging male from a lifelong perspective that acknowledges sexuality as a normal and natural part of the human experience. With this approach the aging person can see sexuality as an appropriate and viable part of the aging process. With this perspective sexual problems will be viewed like those of any other body system and patients will respond more openly to discussion or treatment.

Erection

One of the most apparent changes reported by aging males involves erection. The penis does not enlarge as rapidly nor as completely as it did during younger years. Frequently the psychogenic-type erections, those based on thoughts, memories, or sensory input other than direct stimulation, become fewer. For the aging male more direct and intense physical stimulation of the penis is required to produce an erection (12,13,22).

For each man the confrontation with decreased erectile function is a highly personal crisis with sexual identity. From this crisis a man becomes impotent to the extent that his anxiety influences his ability to achieve an erection. Therefore, difficulties with erection are usually responsive to education and counseling programs for most aging males.

When confronted with issues of erection it is important to rule out a physiological etiology as quickly as possible. The presence of morning erections or erections during the night (either by self-report or the use of a penile plethysmograph) is often helpful in determining the response capability of the patient. Once erectile capacity has been established the individual can be counseled concerning his problems with erection and an investigation into the psychological aspects of impotence can be initiated. During treatment of his impotence the patient should become familiar with the influence of culture, mythology, interpersonal relations, and personal expectations on his sexual function.

In those cases where impotence results from a physiological process, such as diabetes, alternatives should be identified and discussed. The range of alternatives is limited only by their appropriateness and acceptability to the patient. For some men the alternatives, no matter how minor a change, are simply not worth the effort. For whatever reason or secondary gain, they may choose to function in a predominately asexual fashion. At the other end of the spectrum are those willing to try anything in order to achieve an erection. These men are most likely to try a penile prothesis or related sexual device. Any man requesting an implant or penile prothesis should be carefully evaluated both physiologically and psychologically before such a definitive step is taken.

After erection occurs, most elderly men find that they can maintain their erections longer than they could in youth. These men frequently report a decreased sense of orgasmic urgency or sexual haste. For some this change has produced an improvement in their overall sexual relationship.

Ejaculation

For the aging male, as for his younger counterpart, the penis attains its greatest level of engorgement as ejaculation approaches. However, changes do occur with aging (12). The sensation of imminent ejaculation (pre-staging) experienced in youth is usually lost. The contractions for ejaculation are less forceful and the physical sensation of orgasm is frequently described as less intense and of shorter duration. The prostate gland usually increases in size with aging but decreases in contractile strength, leading to a decrease in the volume and viscosity of the seminal fluid (25).

Following orgasm the aging male experiences an extended refractory period during which he cannot achieve another erection. The refractory period becomes progressively longer with aging, extended from a few minutes during youth to days or weeks for men in their seventies and beyond. Again, it is important for aging males to understand that the changes in the refractory period are a normal part of the aging process and the sexual response cycle.

FEMALE RESPONSE

There are also demonstrable changes in sexual physiology for the aging female (12). The changes occur gradually just as they do for the male. However, for the female the onset of menopause and the cessation of reproductive capability is a dramatic indicator of the changes taking place within her body.

The attitudes of women concerning menopause can have a significant impact on their postmenopausal sexual activity. As with males, cultural stereotypes and myths abound. Some women have expressed the concern that they will lose their sexual desire with their menses whereas others have reported concern that they will not be viewed as "sexual" if their partners know they no longer menstruate.

Perhaps the most frequent response to menopause reported by women coming for sexual counseling or therapy is a concern for their gender identity. All too often menopause becomes the focal point of a life crisis, but inappropriately so. These women frequently are experiencing a reassessment of their life goals, objectives, and accomplishments. Many experience the loss of their last child leaving home and suddenly realize their life lacks satisfaction and their future is bleak. In such situations it is frequently easier to fixate on something over which the person has no control but which can be cited as the reason for their depression or anger.

To assess appropriately the impact of menopause on the sexuality of a woman it is important for her to discuss and understand menopause in the context of overall life changes. This should be an integral part of the sexual history and one regularly addressed as a woman ages.

Vaginal Lubrication

Vaginal lubrication is the biological counterpart to erection in the male. As the female ages there is a decrease in the effectiveness of the Bartholin glands, which serve as the primary supplier of vaginal lubrication. Vaginal lubrication may take longer to achieve, or may be so limited that the woman experiences painful intercourse unless a replacement lubricant is used.

In addition to the loss of vaginal lubrication the female also experiences a general decrease in the primary female hormone, estrogen. Estrogen influences breast, uterine, vaginal, and genital tissues. The lack of estrogen may make the vaginal tissues fragile, crack, and bleed (25).

The aging female may also experience estrogen deficient vaginitis and changes in the urethra, bladder, and clitoris but there is no evidence to suggest any appreciable loss in sensate focus or orgasmic potential (13,25).

The physiological changes that occur as a result of decreased female sex hormone production may lead to painful intercourse and subsequent sexual avoidance behaviors. Most of these difficulties can be corrected with the use of adequate endocrine replacement therapy (12,19). Whether all postmenopausal women require ajunctive estrogen replacement therapy remains controversial but there is general agreement that hormonal treatment should be given when lack of estrogen has produced significant sexual problems and there are no major contraindications.

For some women the use of a topical estrogen cream may be sufficient to eliminate the vaginal complications following menopause whereas others may require a tablet form, but each woman must be evaluated individually before such measures are initiated.

Desire

As has been noted earlier, the hormone associated most intimately with male libido is testosterone. Androgen is also a prerequisite for libido in the female (7). Since androgen in the female is primarily produced in the adrenal glands, its production is not adversely effected by menopause. In fact, as the estrogen and progesterone levels decrease during the female climacteric there may be an increase in libido by the unmasking of testosterone's sexually stimulating action.

Libido, however, is not solely controlled by physiological determinants but rather by a constellation of factors including opportunity for sexual expression, acceptance of personal sexuality, and understanding the role of sexuality in aging. Sexual desire and functioning during the climacteric years is highly variable and depends on this complex interplay.

ADDRESSING SEXUAL ISSUES

Concern for human sexuality has been espoused as an appropriate and essential component of the rehabilitation process (2). However, incorporating this concern into rehabilitation programming for the aged requires the resolution of several key issues. The first of these issues involves who should provide sexual counseling or education services.

A 1979 survey by the Sex and Disability Project (3) concerning providers of sex education/counseling services found that 64.2% of the respondents expected physicians to provide these services but only 11.6% had actually received such services from physicians. Similarly, the majority of the aged who have problems with sexuality will turn to their physician as their primary resource.

Unfortunately many physicians who serve a geriatric clientele do not incorporate a discussion of sexuality into their routine medical examinations. Frequently the physician will wait for the patient to raise the issue of sexuality when a problem occurs. Compounding this problem for the aged is the fact that a wide variety of allied medical, health, and rehabilitation professionals have also demonstrated a reluctance to deal with the issues of sexuality (3).

One of the primary reasons for this reluctance to deal with sexual issues is the personal stress associated with discussing sexuality. Thus, the first guideline for determining who should provide sexuality services for the aged is that the person who is to provide sexual education/counseling services should be a person comfortable with sexuality issues.

Comfort

The person providing sexual education/counseling services must be comfortable with the general topic of sexuality as well as comfortable with the specific issues of geriatric sexuality. The first step in achieving the required level of comfort is to become comfortable with one's own sexuality. Being comfortable with one's personal sexuality goes far beyond gender identity. Issues of sexual development, partner preference, and options (e.g., oral, manual, mechanical stimulation) are usually evaluated and integrated as acceptable or unacceptable to the individual. The service provider who is uncomfortable with these issues will communicate that discomfort. Patients are usually quick to pick up nonverbal cues concerning the service provider's discomfort with sexuality because so much of our sexual communication occurs on a nonverbal level. A rather unique comfort issue when dealing with geriatric sexuality is the issue of parental sexuality (15). Most people can remember those first feelings of disbelief when initially confronted with the sexuality of their parents. In developing sexual histories it is not uncommon for patients to recall early comments such as "maybe your parents did that but not mine" or "that's disgusting!" These early memories reflect the long-term impact of the primal family on an individual's attitudes, beliefs, and behaviors. These early experiences continue to influence individuals throughout their lives. These early family influences lead to much of the hesitancy many health professionals have in discussing sexuality with the elderly.

Another issue confronting the health care provider addressing sexual issues with the elderly is the myth that sexuality is for the procreation of life. For the elderly, sexuality is often an affirmation of life. Gaining insight into this rationale for sexual behavior confronts the service provider with the most basic issue of life—mortality. All too often sexual behavior is thought of in terms of continuing life (biological reproduction), whereas aging is conceptualized as a process for ending life (biological death). In this simplistic and mythical model, sexuality becomes the exclusive domain of the young and healthy. Obviously, this type of mythology needs to be excised through exposure, discussion, and education.

The fact that sexual issues are seldom addressed when working with a geriatric population is most frequently a reflection of professional discomfort rather than a lack of patient concern.

In a 1979 study of sexual function in stroke survivors (2) most geriatric patients responded readily to questions concerning their sexual function and the majority had serious questions concerning sexuality and aging. In an environment fostering acceptance and comfort between service provider and patient, the aging individual is given permission to explore sexuality to an extent never before experienced. For many people this interchange of thoughts, ideas, and information concerning sexuality provides a unique growth experience. Most grew up in a repressive era when sexuality was neither accepted nor discussed, much less explained. As adults, they were assumed to be completely knowledgeable if they were males, and coyly ignorant if female. As a service provider dealing with sexual issues, this dearth of information provides a remarkable opportunity for sexual education. Thus, the second guideline for determining who should provide the second critical dimension of sexual education/counseling services is that the sexuality service provider should be a person knowledgeable of sexual issues.

Perhaps no area in sexuality abounds with as many myths and half truths as does geriatric sexuality. These myths need to be identified, confronted, and removed through an effective educational program. People need information in order to appreciate and enjoy their sexuality. As an example, many residents recently interviewed in a long-term care facility expressed concern for the "long-term" effect of masturbation. Several attributed decreased physical stamina and mild confusion to the fact that they continued to masturbate or engage in other sexual activity. In actuality nothing could be further from the truth. It was helpful to share with these residents the conclusion of Masters and Johnson (12) that, "the most favorable prognosticator of an active and enjoyable sex life in old age is an active enjoyable sex life over a lifetime."

That changes do occur with aging is understandable but change must be maintained in proper perspective. Therefore, an appropriate knowledge of the myriad changes in sexuality that accompany aging is essential if the service provider is to function effectively.

Comfort with sexuality and an appropriate knowledge base are essential for effective change to occur. There must be a system, however, to utilize these components and to evoke the necessary change. The catalyst for change is the skill of the service provider. Thus, the third guideline for determining who should provide sexual services is that the person who is to provide sexual education/counseling services should be a person skillful as a "helping" person.

Interpersonal skills are basically tools used to help bring about change. To be effective the service provider must be able to establish rapport and have the person needing help experience warmth, genuineness, acceptance, and empathy. By the very nature of the medical model the help seeker is usually preprogrammed to trust the service provider. Trust issues are not usually difficult, therefore, to address in establishing an effective relationship.

The basic counseling skills required to address sexual issues appropriately are communications, interviewing, problem solving, and behavior management. In order to work with sexual issues it is not essential for the service provider to be an expert in each of these areas. It remains for each individual to determine the level of service he can provide.

One system that has proven to be advantageous in helping to establish the limits of involvement for sex educators/counselors is the PLISSIT model developed by J. S. Annon (1). The PLISSIT model provides four levels of intensity for addressing sexual concern: permission, limited information, specific suggestions, and intensive therapy.

Permission

Many of the sexual issues and concerns of geriatric patients can be resolved simply by someone they regard as knowledgeable reassuring them that their sexual behavior is appropriate. Often patients are simply concerned about being "normal" and safe in their behavior. The service provider gives an opportunity for frank discussion of these fears as well as reassurance that those seeking help are not alone or different in their sexual choices. This reassurance of common universality is one of the critical psychological requirements for effective change. For the aged dealing with sexual issues this insight is frequently a significant stress reducer. Patients need to be assured that they are not alone in dealing with sexual issues nor are they abnormal because of their sexual activity. Permission to discuss sexual issues is not endorsement, however, of sexual activity by the service provider. Although most service providers make no value judgments concerning an older person's sexual activities, they do have the responsibility for reality confrontation and the identification of adverse consequences for sexual behaviors that might be detrimental (3).

Limited Information

For some aging patients a general discussion of sexual concerns is not sufficient for effectively dealing with their sexual problems. In addition to acceptance and discussion they require information. One simple approach to providing the necessary information is a resource center for patients located in the office of the service provider. There are a considerable number of pamphlets and books that discuss various aspects of sexuality (3) and can be useful in resolving sexual issues for aging patients. However, it is usually advantageous for the service provider to discuss the written material with patients.

The presentation of accurate information is most helpful in addressing the multiple myths and half truths confronting geriatric patients. It provides an opportunity for the patient to reevaluate his sexual beliefs, values, and concerns from a new and expanded perspective.

Specific Suggestions

If the aging person needs more than open discussion to identify and analyze a sexual problem, or information to understand the problem, then they usually require some assistance to achieve a change in behavior. Specific suggestions can be helpful to the person experiencing difficulties with desire, orgasm, erection, or painful intercourse. To function effectively at this level it is essential for the service provider to have complete sexual information concerning the patient. A complete sex history should be completed. Based on information obtained in the history, new behavior strategies can be identified and implemented to assist the patient in coping with a sexual problem.

One problem frequently encountered with aging females is the occurrence of vaginal bleeding due to estrogen deficiency. Suggesting a topical lubricant or replacement estrogen may reduce discomfort during intercourse, but the suggestions for each woman vary according to her history and need. A comprehensive sex history is therefore essential.

Intensive Therapy

To function at the intensive therapy level requires a broad base of knowledge in both physiological and psychological aspects of human sexuality as well as special training in the techniques of sex therapy. Most service providers will have neither the skills nor time required for sex therapy, therefore most will refer their patients to certified sex therapists at this level. Because of the complex interface of emotional, social, psychological, and physiological components in human behavior, sex therapy is a sensitive and demanding activity. It is a resource to be used only after the less intense options of permission, limited information, and specific suggestions have been exhausted.

AGING, SEXUALITY, AND DISABILITY

With improved medical care more people with significant health problems are surviving to old age. For these survivors the issues of sexuality and aging are compounded by the presence of serious illness or disease. Many of these people will be referred to rehabilitation services for problems arising from their disease or illness. During their rehabilitation the issue of sexuality should not be overlooked but addressed as a significant part of their total rehabilitation program.

CARDIOVASCULAR DISORDERS

The number one health problem in America today is cardiovascular disease. One manifestation of the disease is heart attack or myocardial infarction. The survivors of heart attack frequently have concerns for returning to sexual activity and a majority alter their previous patterns of sexual activity. Decreases in sexual desire and the frequency of sexual activity are reported by nearly two-thirds of these people and 10% of male heart attack survivors report permanent impotence (10).

Residual fear of death or another coronary is common and plays a significant role in the occurrence of sexual dysfunction. Unfortunately the majority of these men never receive the education or counseling necessary for them to return to an appropriate level of sexual function (23). One reason for this lack of involvement by the allied medical health care team may be the conflicting information presented during the early years of research into sexuality and heart disease.

The initial work of Masters and Johnson (12), which reported heart rates of up to 180 beats/min during intercourse, was of significant concern to those counseling postcoronary patients. However, this work focused on healthy young males in a laboratory setting. In an attempt to establish more appropriately the implications of heart attack for sexual activity Hellerstein and Friedman (4) investigated the cardiovascular function of heart attack survivors during intercourse with their wives. The heart rate for these subjects during orgasm was between 90 to 144 beats/min with a mean for the group of 117 beats/min. The average heart rate was 98 beats/min 2 min before and after orgasm. From these findings one can surmise that sexual activity is a reasonably safe activity for most heart attack survivors if they are with a familiar partner and not in congestive failure (20).

When counseling the cardiac patient it is important to stress the benefits of following familiar sexual activities and a consistent partner (10). Recent research indicates that there are no significant differences in heart rate or blood pressure if the male varies his position from above his partner to below her or if he generally becomes more passive in his love making (14).

In summary, six recommendations can be made concerning sexuality and heart attack.

1. Sexual education, counseling, and therapy should be provided as needed to the person who has had the heart attack as well as to the person's partner.
2. Adultery, especially in unfamiliar surroundings, can be hazardous to health; sexual activity is generally safer with a familiar partner and location.
3. Sufficient time should be allowed for digestion to occur, especially after a heavy meal, before engaging in vigorous sexual activity.
4. Alcohol consumption should be limited since alcohol can reduce the cardiac output in persons with a damaged heart and increase the energy required to complete a sexual encounter successfully.
5. The person who has had a heart attack should be well rested before engaging in sexual activity because fatigue affects both performance and the capacity to respond.
6. An exercise training program can help the cardiac patient during sexual performance both physically and emotionally by providing physical stamina and confidence in the ability to engage in physical activity without incurring another heart attack.

STROKE

Although several authors have referred to the general topic of sexual functioning after stroke (2), very little has been published concerning the specific impact of stroke on sexual function. Two brief studies did suggest that sexual activity and desire decrease after stroke (6,11). The behavioral focus of these studies, however, was on the frequency of coitus. No information was presented on attitudes or physiological function and very limited information was presented on libido.

In a 1980 study of pre- and poststroke sexual interest, function, and attitudes for 35 stroke survivors no significant changes were identified in sexual interest or desire for either male or female subjects (16). The conclusion of the study concerning the impact of stroke on sexual desire is that people "who are sexually active and interested prior to a stroke will continue to experience sexual interest and desire following a stroke."

Before their strokes 75% of the males could consistently achieve erections. However, following their strokes only 46% of the males could achieve erections. The authors expressed concern for the etiology of the impotence experienced by these stroke survivors and question the role of physiology, psychology, and pharmacology in producing such dramatic changes. Similarly, 87% of the males in the stroke study could ejaculate prior to their stroke but that number dropped to 29% after stroke.

Females also demonstrated significant sexual changes following stroke. Of the sexually active females, 63% reported orgasm prior to their stroke. Following stroke, only 13% reported orgasms. All the women who were in an age range for normal menses experienced changes in their regular cycles. These changes ranged from short interruptions of two to three months to complete amenorrhea.

When questioned concerning sexual attitudes, 79% of the males and 73% of the females reported sexual function to be of importance to themselves. All of the males reported sexual function to be of importance to other men their age whereas 73% of the women felt similarly concerning other women.

The authors reached the general conclusions that the majority of stroke survivors feel sexual function is important and maintain sexual desire but "most had significant decrease in sexual function following their stroke."

Based on this conclusion there exists tremendous potential for fear, depression, anxiety, and loss of self-esteem as a sexual being. If rehabilitation is to fulfill its tasks of addressing the needs of the total person, then sexuality must be incorporated into any comprehensive program for stroke survivors.

DIABETES

Both men and women frequently experience sexual dysfunction as a complication of diabetes mellitus (5). In males the dysfunction may include impotence or ejaculatory disorders. Most investigators have reported the incidence of impotence to be approximately 50% in diabetic men (9). Neither the age of onset nor the severity of the illness seem to have a direct relationship with the occurrence of impotence (26). This raises the intriguing question of why impotence occurs with some diabetic males but not others.

After a rather thorough review of this topic, Kolodny et al. (9) stated that "despite the frequency of this disorder, the pathophysiologic mechanism resulting in loss of erective function in diabetes is unclear." With uncertain etiology, impotence in diabetic males is difficult if not impossible to treat effectively. One approach has been the use of testosterone therapy (20). However, only one researcher has reported positive results with the use of androgens and later attempts to duplicate the reported benefits of testosterone therapy have not been as successful (9).

It is important to rule out psychogenic impotence in diabetic males since impotence of this type can be much more successfully treated. Generally, the organic-type impotence occurs gradually with increasing erectile dysfunction. The men with organic dysfunction frequently describe continued sexual interest but an inability to masturbate and an absence of morning erections. The majority of men with psychogenic impotence have a sudden onset of impotence and low libido but they maintain the ability to masturbate.

Problems with ejaculation in diabetic males are reported much less frequently than problems with impotence. When ejaculatory dysfunction does occur it is usually a problem of either premature ejaculation or retrograde ejaculation. In cases of ejaculatory dysfunction, as well as impotence, it is essential to counsel both sexual partners to be sure they understand the dysfunction and develop mechanisms for coping. Studies with diabetic females have also produced significant sexual dysfunction (20). Diabetes has been found to affect orgasmic potential and reproductive capacity in females adversely. Women with diabetes have a higher incidence of uterine and ovarian atrophy in addition to a higher than average frequency of malformed infants and still births than nondiabetic women (18).

Although sexual dysfunction associated with diabetes has been well documented it is important to keep in mind that many people with diabetes will have few or no sexual changes. Each person must be evaluated as an individual and the tendency for stereotyping or generalizing should be guarded against.

SUMMARY

The available data indicate that the majority of an aging population maintain their sexual interest, desire, and function. That sexual changes do occur is undeniable but these changes should be viewed from the perspective of overall life changes associated with aging and not as a separate or isolated life issue. When sexual problems arise, the natural tendency is for the aging person to seek out help from the medical or allied health community. The response of these professionals should be a problem evaluation much as would occur for any other normal and natural process that has developed difficulties.

Sexuality is an appropriate and important consideration in geriatric rehabilitation programs. The team member(s) to address the sexual issues should be comfortable, knowledgeable, and skillful in treating the sexual concerns of an aging population.

REFERENCES

1. Annon, J. S. (1974): *The Behavioral Treatment of Sexual Problems. Vols. I and II.* Enabling Systems, Inc., Honolulu, Hawaii.

2. Bray, G. P., DeFrank, R., and Wolfe, T. L. (1981): Sexual functioning in stroke survivors. *Arch. Phys. Med. Rehabil.,* 62:286–288.
3. Chipouras, S., Cornelius, D., Daniels, S. M., and Makas, E. (1979): *Who Cares.* George Washington University, Washington, D.C.
4. Hellerstein, H., and Friedman, E. H. (1969): *Med. Aspects Human Sexual.,* 3:84.
5. Heslinga, K. (1974): *Not Made of Stone.* Charles C Thomas, Springfield, Ill.
6. Kalliomäki, J. L., Markkanen, T. K., and Mustonen, U. A. (1961): Sexual behavior after CVA: Study on patients below the age of 60 years. *Fertil. Steril.,* 12:156–158.
7. Kaplan, H. S. (1974): *The New Sex Therapy.* Brunner Mazel, New York.
8. Kinsey, A. C., Pomeroy, W. B., and Martin, C. E. (1948): *Sexual Behavior in the Human Male.* W. B. Saunders, Philadelphia.
9. Kolodny, R. C., Kahn, C. B., Goldstein, H. H., and Barnett, D. M. (1978): Sexual dysfunction in diabetic men. In: *Sexual Consequences of Disability,* edited by A. Comfort, pp. 89–98. G. F. Stickley Co., Philadelphia.
10. Mackey, F. G. (1978): Sexuality and heart disease. In: *Sexual Consequences of Disability,* edited by A. Comfort, pp. 107–120. G. F. Stickley Co., Philadelphia.
11. Malone, P. E. (1975): Preliminary investigation of changes in sexual relations following stroke. In: *Clinical Aphasiology: Proceedings of 1975 Conference.* BBK Publishers, Minneapolis.
12. Masters, W. H., and Johnson, V. E. (1966): *Human Sexual Response.* Little Brown and Co., Boston.
13. Masters, W. H., and Johnson, V. E. (1970): *Human Sexual Inadequacy.* Little Brown and Co., Boston.
14. Newman, E., and Mansfield, L. (1974): Scientific Sessions for Nurses (abstr) American Heart Association. Dallas, Tex. November 19, 1974.
15. Pfeiffer, E. (1978): Sexuality in the aging individual. In: *Sexuality and Aging,* edited by R. L. Solnick, pp. 26–32. University of Southern California Press, Los Angeles.
16. Renshaw, D. C. (1978): Stroke and sex. In: *Sexual Consequences of Disability,* edited by A. Comfort, pp. 121–132. G. F. Stickley, Co., Philadelphia.
17. Rossman, I. (1978): Sexuality and aging: An internist's perspective. In: *Sexuality and Aging,* edited by R. L. Solnick, pp. 66–77. University of Southern California Press, Los Angeles.
18. Rubin, A., and Murphy, D. P. (1958): Studies in human reproduction. III. Frequency of congenital malformation in the offspring of nondiabetic and diabetic individuals. *J. Pediatr.,* 53:579–585.
19. Rubin, I. (1970): *Sexual Life in the Later Years.* Sex Information and Education Council of the U.S. (SIECUS), New York.
20. Sandler, J., Myerson, M., and Kinder, B. N. (1980): *Human Sexuality: Current Perspectives.* Mariner Publishing Company, Tampa, Fla.
21. Solnick, R. L. (1978): Sexual responsiveness, age, and change: Facts and potential. In: *Sexuality and Aging,* edited by R. L. Solnick, pp. 33–74. University of Southern California Press, Los Angeles.
22. Solnick, R. L., and Birren, J. E. (1977): Age and male erectile responsiveness. *Arch. Sex. Behav.,* 6:1–9.
23. Tuttle, W. B., Cook, W. L., and Fitch, E. (1964): Sexual behavior in postmyocardial infarction patients. *Am. J. Cardiol.,* 13:140.
24. Van de Velde, T. H. (1962): *Ideal Marriage.* Random House, New York.
25. Weg, R. B. (1978): The physiology of sexuality in aging. In: *Sexuality and Aging,* edited by R. L. Solnick, pp. 48–65. University of Southern California Press, Los Angeles.
26. Woods, N. F. (1979): *Human Sexuality in Health and Illness.* Mosby, St. Louis.

Rehabilitation in the Aging edited by
T. F. Williams. Raven Press, New York © 1984.

Physiological Basis of Rehabilitation Therapy

Robert H. Jones

*Departments of Preventive Medicine and Medicine, University of Rochester School of
Medicine; and Medical Department and the Human Factors Laboratory,
Eastman Kodak Company, Rochester, New York 14650*

It is well known that aging is accompanied by diminution of physical capability. A few examples include a gradual decrease of vital capacity, maximum oxygen consumption (VO_2 max), and other parameters of pulmonary function; of cardiac output; and of strength. With a paucity of warning signals, the aging body "tunes" itself down to the point where sedentary physical activity becomes both the norm and essentially the capacity for exercise.

In the absence of disease, some determinants of this loss are difficult to separate and identify. On the one hand, a decrease in the number and function of cells does occur. If these changes represent the inevitable running down of the cell clock, is the timing of the event and the speed of decline partly determined by the customary demands for cellular use? Such is the central hypothesis of this chapter. Regular and appropriate exercise contributes to the longevity of the cell; both excessive and inadequate exercise tend to diminish it.

The availability of machines contributes to the phenomenon of excessive and inadequate exercise. More perniciously, we even come to think of ourselves as having many attributes of machines. Like them, we perform work; neither works well when too hot or too cold; and a brief warm up is salutary for both. We recognize that a well-lubricated machine can lie idle for years with no loss of capacity; conversely, machine use inevitably produces wear and breakdown. If we have blurred the boundary between ourselves and machines, we come to believe that longevity is ours only if we treat ourselves in the same fashion. Yet, in some respects we are entirely unmachine-like. Capacity for activity cannot be stored over the winter, and then be wheeled out on a warm day to spring into full bloom. A human idle for three or four days has lost some strength, endurance, and flexibility. In short, one key to continued physical capability rests squarely with an appropriate amount of exercise.

Illness, by definition, induces further loss of activity. This in turn leads to decreased capacity for exercise, which, if severe enough, precludes continued ability to perform some of life's basic tasks. One of the goals of rehabilitation therapy is to help the elderly in health and illness to improve performance in self-care, social, avocational, and vocational tasks.

To best help reach specific goals, a management program should be based on certain fundamental biochemical and physiologic principles. It is these principles to which this chapter attends. They have both a preventive aspect for those whose aim it is to regain former capacities, and a restorative set for those recuperating from illness. Parenthetically, the successful program also depends on attention to certain psychological and pedagogical principles not discussed here. The key, nevertheless, for all four principles is activity.

Discussion centers on the following: definitions of the various types of physical activity and some of their quantifying and qualifying characteristics; a description of the body's energy stores and how to use them for optimal performance; the impact of various factors on capacity for physical activity; the impact of physical activity on cardiovascular function; and some consequences of overactivity. In instances where the data are derived from studies of younger people, the concepts may be assumed to apply for the aging as well. However, more quantitative data in older persons are needed.

DEFINITIONS OF PHYSICAL ACTIVITY

Generally, muscular activity is divided into two broad types: dynamic (or rhythmic) and isometric (or static), depending on whether muscle length is changing during exercise (20). Coincidentally, there are other distinguishing aspects of the two types of exercise. One of considerable importance is the fact that intramuscular tension is variable in dynamic and constant in isometric exercise. As a result, cardiovascular responses to the two types differ considerably, as will be discussed later. In real life, much muscular activity is a blend of dynamic and isometric.

The cardinal intention of muscular activity is to create a force as the result of the muscle's attempt to shorten. If the effort is brief, isometric, and maximal, as in a gripping effort, the resultant force is said to represent the person's strength or maximum voluntary contraction (MVC) for the muscles used. This effort is sustained for only a few seconds, and is a measure of local muscle mechanical and biochemical capacity.

When the effort is a brief maximal dynamic exercise, as in walking, running, bicycling, or repetitive lifting, it is said to represent aerobic capacity. For testing purposes, the exercise persists for a period of only 5 to 10 min. The effort is described quantitatively in watts, VO_2 max, or in calories expended. It is dependent on the intregrity of the energy transport systems as well as local muscle status. Other terms used to measure the physical aspects of dynamic muscular effort are *work* and *power,* where work equals force X distance, and power equals force X distance/unit of time (20).

Sustained effort, either dynamic or isometric, may invoke the phenomena of endurance and fatigue. Endurance is a measure of the maximum duration of a given sustained effort. For example, grip endurance at 50% MVC may be 1 min, whereas at 100% MVC it may be only 5 sec. Endurance for dynamic exercise at 50% of aerobic capacity may be 8 hr, and for 100% of capacity only 10 to 12 min.

Fatigue occurs when these sustained efforts falter. Such loss of ability to continue a sustained effort is influenced by both physiologic and psychologic factors. The physiologic factors may represent changes in central nervous system activity (3), energy stores, accumulation of metabolic products, and local blood flow; and they may be measured or identified by changes in electromyographic (EMG) activity, heart rate, and blood lactate concentration (31,37).

FURTHER ATTRIBUTES OF STRENGTH, AEROBIC CAPACITY, AND COORDINATION

The forcefulness of maximum isometric effort is inversely related to duration of the sustained contraction. One hundred percent of MVC can be sustained for about 6 to 7 sec, 75% for 30 to 35 sec; 50% for 1 min, and 25% for about 3½ min. Fifteen percent of MVC can be sustained for a prolonged period of time (33). Such decay in peak force appears to be related to declining metabolic capacity of the muscle, induced by declining muscle blood flow as increasing muscle tension is developed (19).

Recovery of MVC after fatiguing effort also follows a time course. About 80% of MVC can be recovered after a 3-min rest, and 100% after 10 to 11 min (13). On the other hand, recovery time for isometric endurance is much longer. About 70% of prior capability is available after 10 min of rest and 90% after 40 min (13). Whether these parameters change significantly with aging warrants further study.

Thus assessment of strength alone may not be sufficient to predict the capability for performing a repetitive isometric task. One must also note work and rest times for each cycle of the effort. For example, assume that a task is to hold a 50 lb item for 30 sec, rest for 1 min, and repeat the procedure. MVC is given as 60 lb. Only 75% of this, or 45 lb, is available for a 30-sec effort. Furthermore, 1 min of rest might allow recovery of only 40 to 60% of MVC. On two accounts, therefore, this repetitive task cannot be performed.

Analysis of maximum dynamic exercise, or aerobic capacity, reveals similar limitations. Assume that a 10 to 12 min maximum effort produces a $\dot{V}O_2$ max of 50 ml/kg/min. After 30 min of sustained effort, peak consumption will have dropped to 35 ml/kg/min; after 1 hr, to 23 ml; and after 4 hr to only 15 ml/kg/min. If the intensity of exercise is increased beyond these limits, it cannot be sustained.

The state of training also influences the percent $\dot{V}O_2$ max that can be sustained. A highly trained person may be able to perform at 50% $\dot{V}O_2$ max over an 8-hr period, whereas an untrained person can sustain an 8-hr effort at only the 30% level (4). Recovery time from such efforts varies directly with both the intensity and duration of exercise, and varies between 30 sec and 90 min. Again, data are needed on the effects of age on recovery times.

Aerobic capacity and endurance are both task and muscle group specific (31). Some tasks, such as walking, involve a large muscle mass and blood supply; others utilize a much smaller mass of each, as when using the arms. Thus the aerobic capacity for walking on a treadmill may be 40% higher than that for lifting light boxes. In similar fashion, endurance for hand grip muscles is considerably less than that for the back lifting muscles. Furthermore, the lifting of 100 lb in 1 min may be carried out either by two lifts of 50 lb each or 10 lifts of 10 lb each. In the first case, the weight of the head, arms, and trunk are lifted twice; in the latter, 10 times. Thus these two tasks will require markedly different oxygen consumptions. Accordingly, when assessing the gap between capacity and demands of the task, it is best to examine the desired task directly whenever this can be safely and efficiently done. Coordination can be described as a noncortical, automatic learned behavior; involving highly coordinated, forceful, and rapid multimuscular activity; initiated, maintained, and discontinued at the will of the individual (22). Coordination, although dependent on peripheral biochemical and biomechanical factors, seems to be more clearly a process requiring precise central neurological controls. Not only are there the quantitative aspects of force, velocity, and duration, but also the qualitative aspects of precision and complexity of task. It is suggested (22) that an engram or neural pattern develops through practice, consisting of pathways of excitation, surrounded by a wall of inhibition. In this fashion, a precisely limited group of muscles is innervated; the "wall of inhibition" protects against excessive and unwanted motion.

There is a capacity for coordination just as there is for strength and dynamic exercise. The attained level of coordination through practice is even more task specific than it is for strength and aerobic capacity. It is not so much a question of becoming skilled at repetitive hand motions in general, but rather at such specific tasks as card shuffling, rug making, knitting, or playing a particular musical instrument. In addition, there are innate differences in coordinative skill from one person to another.

SOURCES OF MUSCULAR ENERGY AND IMPACT OF THEIR USE ON EXERCISE CAPACITY

The body's energy stores, although large, are not easily and readily available except in accordance with some rigid biochemical rules. When these rules are followed, the capacity for activity is significantly greater than when they are not.

About 180,000 kcal are stored in the body: 77% as fat, 22% as protein, and 1% as carbohydrate (11). The carbohydrate is the only substrate that is rapidly available. It is present in three locations: 75% as muscle glycogen, 20% as liver glycogen, and 5% as glucose in extracellular fluid. Muscle glycogen delivery is so slow that, with continuous exercise, blood-borne glucose quickly becomes the principle energy source. Free fatty acids form the major source of energy only after 3 hr or so of sustained activity (11).

In skeletal muscle, there are three pathways for energy derived from carbohydrate (26). The first is that of the phosphagens (adenosine-triphosphate and creatine phosphate). It is also called the alactic source and it is the only direct route for energy to the muscles. The other two mechanisms supply energy for resynthesis of the phosphagens. The preferred and primary resynthesis pathway is energy derived from the oxidation of food. But when the intensity and duration of exercise exceeds its delivery capability, back-up resynthesis energy is available from breakdown of muscle glycogen to lactic acid. Finally, lactate resynthesis to glycogen, a slow process, also derives its energy from oxidation of food.

The energy from phosphagens is available quickly in the muscle, but is the least abundant source per kg of body weight. Energy from muscle glycogen is delivered at one-half the rate for phosphagens, and is slightly more abundant. Oxygen and food have almost infinite availability, but delivery rates are one-quarter the rate for phosphagens.

Resynthesis time for phosphagens is 30 to 120 sec; for glycogen it is 1 to 1½ hr. Therefore, the preferred combination is phosphagen utilization (because of rapid availability and resynthesis time) and food oxidative resynthesis, which allows avoidance of lactate production and potential lactic acidosis.

With continuous exercise, phosphagens are rapidly depleted, as is glycogen: resynthesis lags behind energy needs, and this leads to lactic acidosis and exhaustion. However, with periods of intermittent exercise, oxidative resynthesis keeps pace and anaerobic glycolysis does not occur. The optimal format for maximal exercise, therefore, may approximate 15 to 20 sec of maximal effort followed by 30 sec of rest, and then repetition.

Margaria (26) portrayed the following scenario. If a person ran at maximum speed for 400 m, full recovery would take 1½ hr, and the runner could cover cumulatively only 1,200 m in 4 hr. Conversely, if the person ran only 100 m, rested 30 sec and then repeated the effort, he or she could cover 30 times the distance in 4 hr—36,000 m.

The same concept applies for the elderly. In fact, it is commonly held that one cardinal difference between youth and older people lies with the latter's wisdom in responding to the early signals of fatigue by establishing a work : rest ratio that allows them to compete successfully with youth.

If an elderly person's capacity for muscular effort can not be improved, one could at least learn appropriate work-rest cycling to optimize utilization of the available energy resources. The objective would be to determine the length of both work and rest periods to allow for total resynthesis of phosphagens and to avoid lactic acidosis.

IMPACT OF TRAINING AND DISUSE ON ISOMETRIC STRENGTH AND ENDURANCE

A maximum isometric effort for 5 to 6 sec every 2 min for a total of 30 sec of exercise per day provides the optimal stimulus for increasing strength (28). With such a program, strength increases at a rate of almost 2% per day until

75% of limiting strength is reached. Thereafter, the gains lessen progressively. More frequent and longer exercises do not alter these rates of change.

Such newfound strength can be maintained by one maximum effort every two weeks. Such exercise stimulates the muscle to produce a force that increases for one week, after which it decreases back to baseline by the 14th day (28). Alternatively, strength can be maintained by a ½ max contraction daily.

These changes in strength occur only in those muscles being exercised. Increasing strength is the only known technique for increasing isometric endurance. Such changes have no effect on dynamic aerobic capacity (28), and these responses are similar for all ages and both sexes.

Electrical and enzyme changes occur as the muscle is strengthened (21). Maximal integrated EMG activity increases; there is a suggestion of lessened EMG activity at a given muscle tension; and there is increased muscle malic dehydrogenase and succinate dehydrogenase activity.

When there is no muscle contraction, strength decreases by about 5% per day. With prolonged immobilization, muscle atrophy and degeneration also occur. Recent studies in the rat soleus (5) show that after 90 days of immobilization, recovery can occur for all functions measured, but at quite great differences in rate. Muscle weight and protein content return to control values in 14 days; ATP, glycogen, and protein concentration, in 60 days; and maximum isometric tension only after 120 days.

INFLUENCE OF TRAINING AND DISUSE ON AEROBIC CAPACITY

Exercising for 20 to 40 min sessions daily at 65 to 70% of capacity will increase aerobic capacity. Typical training programs last 8 to 12 weeks. At less than 50% maximum, little if any change will occur regardless of the frequency or duration of exercise. Maintenance of aerobic capacity, unlike strength, requires frequent exercise: about once every 2 to 3 days (12) versus once per 14 days for strength.

Possible mechanisms for an increase in $\dot{V}O_2$ max are included in the following equation: $\dot{V}O_2$ = stroke volume X heart rate X arteriovenous O_2 difference (a-v O_2 diff). In training sessions of short duration, the principal change is an increase a-v O_2 diff (25). This is thought to represent primarily increased peripheral oxygen uptake secondary to well-demonstrated muscle cellular enzyme changes (16). After longer exercise periods, stroke volume also increases, representing enhanced cardiac capacity.

Training produces increased efficiency according to some (27) in both trained and untrained muscle groups for a given individual. The trained muscles show a greater decrease in $\dot{V}O_2$, heart rate, and lactate production. It is postulated that for the trained muscles, two changes occur. First, peripherally, the muscle is now mechanically more efficient, and increased skeletal muscle mitochondrial concentration may be the mechanism explaining lowered lactate levels. Second, centrally, there is less neural activity, resulting in a reduction in the mass of muscles used. In addition, lessened sympathetic drive may be partially responsible for the decrease in heart rate. For untrained muscles, with a less pronounced decrease in these variables, it is postulated that central adaptation is the sole responsible agent.

Another change produced by training is the rate with which oxygen consumption reaches peak values at the start of exercise, and resumes baseline values during recovery (14). The initial lag is called the oxygen deficit, and the recovery delay, the oxygen debt. Before training, the initial lag and the recovery delay are large and create a curvilinear response; after training, the response more closely approaches a square wave, indicating a diminution of both oxygen deficit and debt. This can be interpreted to mean that there is more rapid delivery of oxygen to and uptake by the muscle, combined with more reliance on phosphagens and less on glycolosis—in short, greater aerobic efficiency. Such increase in efficiency has great significance particularly for those with reduced cardiac capacity. This will be discussed further below.

Analyses of hormonal and metabolic responses to training show other important changes (39). While $\dot{V}O_2$ max increases, blood glycerol, plasma-free fatty acids, blood lactate, and heart rate decrease gradually for a given absolute workload over a 7- to 9-week period. Yet, reduction in circulating catecholamines and glucagon is essentially complete at three weeks. Thus it appears that catecholamines, which are thought to stimulate glucagon production to liberate more glucose for metabolism, are less needed when one is well trained. Also, the need for these stimulants decreases at a rate that differs from other adaptive changes induced by training. This implies that reduced catechol response is not solely responsible for the training-induced drop in exercise heart rate (38).

Finally, microscopic examination of trained and untrained muscles shows changes compatible with differences in delivery and uptake of oxygen by the muscle (17). When comparing well-trained competitive female cross-country skiers with sedentary women of comparable age and weight, there were 50% more capillaries per quadriceps muscle fiber, 35% more capillaries per mm^2 of muscle tissue, and more mitochondria in fibers of the trained athletes. Similar studies for men revealed comparable findings (6).

IMPACT OF TRAINING AND DISUSE ON COORDINATION

Improvement of coordination skills would seem to depend on three factors: progression in force and the speed of motion to just under the point of failure; an increase in complexity of the task in a stepwise fashion until all the component subtasks or basic maneuvers are perfected; and practice for as many as 1 to 3 million repetitions until a perfect engram is developed (22). One important underlying component appears to be the increased capacity of the central nervous system to inhibit undesired activity as the intensity, velocity, and complexity of the effort rises. A second seems to be the development of greater peripheral ability through increased strength and/or aerobic capacity. This allows the coordinated effort to occur at a smaller percentage of maximum, thus avoiding fatigue with its attendant spread of muscular excitation (23,36).

One loses coordination skills with disuse. Supposedly this means the loss of both central and peripheral components. In terms of the peripheral contributions, since aerobic capacity is lost faster than strength, one assumption is that the duration of coordinated ability would decrease when practice is less frequent than every few days. Then, with loss of strength, the spread of unwanted muscular excitation would occur at progressively smaller workloads. The central engram probably weakens much more slowly. Yet, as disuse time increases, so does the length of warm-up needed to recall and reestablish the engram. More documentation of these phenomena is needed.

If the quality of motor performance is directly related to the speed of neuromuscular response, then decreased coordination would occur as speed is lost through disuse. Recent data suggests (10,34) that both the central component (reaction time) and, more strikingly, the peripheral component (movement time) decay with lack of use, particularly in the elderly. There are strong implications that if one keeps active, movement time will be equivalent for both young and old.

CIRCULATORY RESPONSES TO EXERCISE IN NORMALS

With isometric exercise up to 15% MVC, muscle blood flow, heart rate, and systolic blood pressure rapidly rise to a plateau and stabilize, suggesting adequate perfusion for local muscular needs (19). Above 15% MVC, heart rate and blood pressure no longer plateau, but continue to climb, with increasing steepness as one approaches sustained MVC, as if perfusion were no longer adequate. At 25% MVC, intramuscular tension within the quadriceps exceeds resting systolic blood pressure. At 70% MVC, muscle blood flow ceases, and arterial occlusion no longer affects isometric endurance. Blood flow to unused muscles varies, but is consistently increased to the skin.

Unlike the response to dynamic exercise, heart rate, blood pressure, cardiac output, a-v O_2 diff, and $\dot{V}O_2$ do not increase equally because the circulation is hyperkinetic. The a-v O_2 diff does not change, $\dot{V}O_2$ increases modestly, heart rate and cardiac output increases more, and blood pressure increases most (19).

The blood pressure response, which is equally potent for systolic and diastolic phases, increases with the duration and intensity of the isometric contraction. There is disagreement about response in relation to size of muscle mass. Earlier work suggested no correlation (9). Later work, which carefully controlled tension in muscles that stabilize the trunk and proximal extremity, supports the view that the pressor response is directly related to mass (9).

For dynamic exercises, muscle blood flow is only intermittently interrupted and appears to remain adequate for the muscle's metabolic needs. At $\dot{V}O_2$ max, flow may be double that for the same muscle group performing maximum sustained isometric exercise (19). Accordingly, the circulation is not hyperkinetic. Heart rate, systolic blood pressure, cardiac output, $\dot{V}O_2$, and a-v O_2 diff all rise proportionately. Diastolic pressure rises very little. Finally, the pressor and heart rate response to dynamic work by the arms is significantly greater than to the same amount of work performed by the legs (4).

Much work is a combination of isometric and dynamic efforts, as in carrying and in walking. Under such circumstances, the circulatory response is at least additive (19).

WORK OF THE HEART IN RESPONSE TO EXERCISE

The work of the heart can be defined in terms of myocardial oxygen consumption ($M\dot{V}O_2$), which in turn can be estimated by the product of systolic blood pressure and heart rate (29). For clinical purposes, this double product is a valid and reliable assessor of cardiac work for both isometric and dynamic exercises (7).

These parameters imply that intense sustained isometric exercise, which produces only modest increase in $\dot{V}O_2$, requires as much cardiac work as vigorous dynamic exercise. Equally important, those exercises that produce the highest heart rate and blood pressure responses induce the greatest work of the heart. Conversely, one of the more significant consequences of training is the lowering of pressor and heart rate responses and thus of cardiac work.

EFFECT OF AGE AND SEX ON EXERCISE CAPACITY

Even though one cross-sectional study shows that isometric endurance at 40% MVC did not change with aging (30), most studies show loss of strength and aerobic capacity with age (2,8,18). It is probable that these changes reflect both increasing sedentary lifestyle and the result of biological aging. For strength, peak values are found during the third and fourth decade; they decrease 10 to 20% by the seventh, and arm strength is retained better than leg strength. Aerobic capacity falls about 25% during this span of time (4,8). To the extent that regular exercising is continued, these changes may be minimized (18). Given the same initial degree of fitness for dynamic exercise, some younger and older men respond with the same changes in ability to a 4-month physical conditioning program (18).

Maximal heart rate also declines with age (4), with maxima calculated as roughly 220 minus age. Yet, at given submaximal dynamic exercise levels, the rate may remain relatively unchanged if the person stays in good condition. Resting and exercise diastolic blood pressures appear relatively stable with age; systolic pressures rise with both isometric and dynamic exercise (19).

Before puberty, strength of men and women is the same. Thereafter, the strength of women averages about 60% that for men. There is, however, variation between 40% and 85%, depending on the muscle group tested (24). There is less difference in aerobic capacity, where values for women may reach 85% of those for men (35). Reaction and movement time both increase with age (10,34), yet it would appear that vigorous exercise tends to blunt these changes.

EFFECT OF OVERUSE

Having outlined the consequences of disuse and sketched guidelines for exercises to improve strength, aerobic capacity, and endurance through patterns of proper use, it remains to recognize some causes and to weigh consequences of overuse.

Overuse problems commonly occur to several groups: those who engage in unusual spurts of activity; those who feel that therapeutically "more is better"; and those who need to be competitively the best. The first group leaps into full activity from a sedentary existence as if there has been no hiatus and therefore no loss, instead of making gradual increments to which the body could accommodate.

A second group, often recuperating from illness and having been started on an exercise program, now double or triple the exercise time or intensity in the mistaken belief that such will increase capacity. Instead, fatigue or muscle soreness may be the consequence.

A third group exerts to the limit for competitive reasons, either steadily, as in production work, or intermittently, in avocational events. The unwanted consequences are either wear and tear syndromes of soft tissues or injuries.

Less obvious are those who, unknown to themselves, have slowly gained weight or lost strength, endurance, or flexibility because of disuse. For them, the exercise now represents overuse instead of usual exercise.

One consequence of overuse is delayed muscle soreness, occurring 24 to 48 hr after vigorous exercise. This phenomenon has been studied after vigorous upper extremity weight lifting, bicycling, or step testing exercises to determine whether it appeared due to muscle spasm, muscle damage, or disruption of connective tissue elements in muscles or their attachments (1). Tests included surface EMGs, measurement of myoglobinuria, and the ratio of hydroxyproline to creatinine excretion. Myoglobinuria occurred regardless of muscle soreness and the quantity released appeared to be directly related to the intensity of exercise. No significant changes in EMG activity occurred. There was a direct relationship between symptoms and hydroxyproline excretion, especially with muscle lengthening (eccentric) exercises. This may have represented either or both increased muscular collagen synthesis or breakdown.

Studies also show a direct relation between type, duration, and frequency of exercises and musculoskeletal injuries (32). Those jogging for 45 min versus 15 min, or five days per week versus one, had significantly more leg injuries. Also those with running and jumping exercises had higher injury rates than those with fast-walking regimens.

Cardiac morbidity and mortality is associated with exercise. In one study (7), cardiac arrest from ventricular fibrillation after treadmill exertion occurred five times in over 10,000 cases (less than 0.05%), and there were no deaths. The hallmarks of these cases were severe coronary heart disease and inadequate systolic blood pressure response to exercise or exertional hypotension. If one isolated a special population with these two findings, the prevalence rose to 2%.

A review of North American cardiac rehabilitation programs (15) collected data on almost 14,000 cardiac patients who accumulated more than 1.5 million patient hr of supervised exercise (averaging 120 hr per patient). Overall death rate was 0.1%, or one fatality every 116,000 hr.

Complications were decreased in programs started since 1970, and in those that continuously monitored the exercise EKG. In these, the risk of death became essentially equal to that for postmyocardial infarct patients during the first several years after the infarct.

DIFFERENTIATING THE EFFECT OF DISEASE AND AGE ON EXERCISE

In one class of diseases, cardiovascular disease, there are now enough data comparing ventricular function in healthy and unhealthy aging populations to assess the impact of disease. Bruce and co-workers have made direct observations of exercise duration, maximum heart rate, and maximum systolic blood pressure. From these observations they have derived values for VO_2 max and other measures of cardiac function in healthy persons and patients with various combinations of hypertension, coronary heart disease, and cardiomegaly (7,8). For instance, average VO_2 max for five groups of elderly subjects—healthy, hypertensives, patients with coronary heart disease, hypertensives with coronary heart disease, and normotensives with both coronary heart disease and cardiomegaly—were roughly 33, 27, 21, 20, and 15 ml O_2 kg/min, respectively. That is, there is only half as much capacity for dynamic activity in those with both coronary heart disease and cardiomegaly, compared to healthy elderly.

In time, other studies will undoubtedly demonstrate the impact of neuromusculoskeletal diseases on exercise function to distinguish further between biologic aging and disease.

A RECAPITULATION, WITH SOME GUIDELINES FOR RESTORATIVE REGIMES

The patient should realize that, in terms of physiologic ability, one loses what is not used. All exercise programs, to be successful, must alter behavior so that exercise subsequently becomes a part of the regular daily routine.

With disuse, capability is lost by as much as 5% per day, and it is regained at about one-half that rate. Accordingly, the patient and the health team should plan that exercise programs may last several months before full capability is regained. In the case of contractures, three to four weeks of immobilization may require almost a year of exercise to regain all lost motion.

Any effort to speed the recuperative process too quickly may produce signs and symptoms of overuse. One of these is muscle soreness, which typically occurs 24 to 48 hours afterwards. One option is to decrease the next day's activities by 10 to 20%, and then slowly pick up the pace at 3- to 5-day intervals.

Training programs should clearly identify the nature of the task needing improvement: isometric strength, dynamic aerobic capacity, or coordination. The patient should know the difference in routines for these various goals. Strengthening exercises last a few minutes daily, and maintenance requires maximum effort once every 10 to 14 days. Dynamic exercises require 20 to 30 min daily and a maintenance repetition every 2 to 3 days. Coordination exercises may need 1 to 3 million repetitions before perfection is achieved.

For the most part, the results of such exercises are task and muscle group specific. That is, significant changes are found only in those muscle groups that have been trained. An isometric strengthening program does not alter aerobic capacity, and a jogging or walking program does nothing for grip strength.

One of the common needs of the ill elderly is to learn to rely on their upper extremities to assist either in transfers to the upright position or in ambulation. This changes the obligation from the lower extremities—a large mass of musculature—to a smaller one, with more limited capacity. Transfer training requires predominantly a strengthening program because of the infrequent nature of the maneuver. Ambulation training calls for an increase in strength, aerobic capacity, and endurance because of the sustained and highly repetitive nature of the task.

Rarely will one fatigue in a transfer maneuver. Yet, in crutch walking, upper extremity fatigue is common. Therefore, it is important that part of the training focus on learning to intersperse proper periods of work and rest. Sweating, sensation of muscle fatigue, and incoordination are associated with oxygen debt and can be used as markers of excess activity. When learned and avoided by proper work : rest ratios, exercise time and output can be increased significantly.

Older people differ from younger groups in several particulars. They have a higher prevalence of coronary heart and hypertensive heart disease. They more commonly have less reserve between their daily activities and capacities, and more often are called on to use their upper extremities for the activities listed above. Most of this effort is isometric, with the result that there is call for an unusual amount of cardiac work from a system with reduced cardiac capacity. The therapist should be alerted to this possibility and be aware should arrhythmias, marked blood pressure swings in either direction, pallor, complaints of chest pain, faintness, fatigue, or incoordination occur. Under certain circumstances, an immediate postexercise assessment of the double product, systolic blood pressure $\times$ heart rate, may give excellent landmark information. The most critical times in physical therapy may be when the patient's capabilities are first being tested. Thus, an elderly person, bedbound for three weeks, initially assessed for ambulatory skills by a short walk in parallel bars, may be at more risk of an untoward cardiac event than at any other time in the program.

Because conditioning programs reduce the workload on the heart for a given amount and type of activity, they may be of significant help to the cardiac patient. However, one must remember the caveat: training prepares only for the activities that have been practiced. For example, a patient with coronary heart disease was able to double his walking speed and distance before developing angina after completing an ambulation conditioning program. However, this did not prepare him for the severe upper extremity isometric load of changing a large car tire under stressful conditions. Consequently, he was not protected from a bout of coronary insufficiency.

Although the elderly cannot expect to maintain all their youthful vigor and physical aptitude, there is growing evidence that some of the lost capability is a direct result of disuse. This, at least, can be avoided.

REFERENCES

1. Abraham, W. M. (1977): Factors in delayed muscle soreness. *Med. Sci. Sports,* 9:11–20.
2. Asmussen, E., and Heeboll-Nielsen, K. (1961): Isometric muscle strength of adult men and women. Communication from the Testing and Observation Institute of the Danish National Association for Infantile Paralysis. 11:3–42.
3. Asmussen, E., and Mazin, B. (1978): A central nervous component in local muscular fatigue. *Eur. J. Appl. Physiol.,* 38:9–15.
4. Astrand, P. O., and Rodahl, K. (1970): *Textbook of Work Physiology.* McGraw-Hill, New York.
5. Booth, F. W., and Seider, M. J. (1979): Recovery of skeletal muscle after three months of hind limb immobilization in rats. *J. Appl. Physiol.,* 47:435–439.
6. Brodal, P., Ingjer, F., and Hermansen, L. (1977): Capillary supply of skeletal muscle fibers in untrained and endurance-trained men. *Am. J. Physiol.,* 232:H705–H712.
7. Bruce, R. A. (1977): Exercise testing for evaluation of ventricular function. *N. Engl. J. Med.,* 296:671–675.
8. Bruce, R. A., Fisher, L. D., Cooper, M. N., and Gey, G. O. (1974): Separation of effects of cardiovascular disease and age on ventricular function with maximal exercise. *Am. J. Cardiol.,* 34:757–763.
9. Buck, J. A., Amundsen, L. R., and Nielsen, D. H. (1980): Systolic blood pressure responses during isometric contractions of large and small muscle groups. *Med. Sci. Sports,* 12:145–147.
10. Clarkson, P. M. (1978): The effect of age and activity level on simple and choice fractionated response time. *Eur. J. Appl. Physiol.,* 40:17–25.
11. Felig, P., and Wahren, J. (1975): Fuel homeostasis in exercise. *N. Engl. J. Med.,* 293:1078–1084.
12. Fox, E. L., Bartels, R. L., Billings, C. E., O'Brien, R., Bason, R., and Mathews, D. K. (1975): Frequency and duration of interval training programs and changes in aerobic power. *J. Appl. Physiol.,* 38:481–484.
13. Funderburk, C. F., Hipskind, S. G., Welton, R. C., and Lind, A. R. (1974): Development of and recovery from fatigue induced by static effort at various tensions. *J. Appl. Physiol.,* 37:392–396.
14. Hagberg, J. M., Hickson, R. C., Ehsani, A. A., and Holloszy, J. O. (1980): Faster adjustment to and recovery from submaximal exercise in the trained state. *J. Appl. Physiol.,* 48:218–224.
15. Haskell, W. L. (1978): Cardiovascular complications during exercise training of cardiac patients. *Circulation,* 57:920–924.
16. Holloszy, J. O., and Booth, F. W. (1976): Biochemical adaptations to endurance exercise in muscle. *Annu. Rev. Physiol.,* 38:273–291.
17. Ingjer, F. and Brodal, P. (1978): Capillary supply of skeletal muscle fibers in untrained and endurance-trained women. *Eur. J. Appl. Physiol.,* 38:291–299.

18. Ismail, A. H., and Montgomery, D. L. (1979): The effect of a four-month physical fitness program on a young and an old group matched for physical fitness. *Eur. J. Appl. Physiol.,* 40:137–144.
19. Kilbom, A. (1976): Circulatory adaptation during static muscular contractions. *Scand. J. Work Environ. Health,* 2:1–13.
20. Knuttgen, H. G. (1978): Force, work, power and exercise. *Med. Sci. Sports,* 10:227–228.
21. Komi, P. V., Viitasalo, J. T., Rauramaa, R., and Vihko, V. (1978): Effect of isometric strength training on mechanical, electrical and metabolic aspects of muscle function. *Eur. J. Appl. Physiol.,* 40:45–55.
22. Kottke, F. J., Halpern, D., Easton, J. K. M., Ozel, A. T., and Burrill, C. A. (1978): Training of coordination. *Arch. Phys. Med. Rehabil.,* 59:567–572.
23. Krusen, F. H., Kottke, F. J., and Ellwood, P. M. (1971): *Handbook of Physical Medicine and Rehabilitation.* 2nd ed. Saunders, Philadelphia.
24. Laubach, L. L. (1976): Comparative muscular strength of men and women: A review of the literature. *Aviat. Space Environ. Med.,* 47:534–542.
25. Magel, J. R., McArdle, W. D., Toner, M., and Delio, D. J. (1978): Metabolic and cardiovascular adjustment to arm training. *J. Appl. Physiol.,* 45:75–79.
26. Margaria, R. (1972): The sources of muscular energy. *Sci. Am.* 226:84–91.
27. McKenzie, D. C., Fox, E. L., and Cohen, K. (1978): Specificity of metabolic and circulatory responses to arm or leg interval training. *Eur. J. Appl. Physiol.,* 39:241–248.
28. Muller, E. A. (1970): Influence of training and of inactivity on muscle strength. *Arch. Phys. Med. Rehabil.* 51:449–462.
29. Nelson, R. R., Gobel, F. L., Jorgensen, C. R., Wang, K., Wang, Y., and Taylor, H. L. (1974): Hemodynamic predictors of myocardial oxygen consumption during static and dynamic exercise. *Circulation,* 50:1179–1189.
30. Petrofsky, J. S., Burse, R. L., and Lind, A. R. (1975): Comparison of physiological responses of women and men to isometric exercise. *J. Appl. Physiol.* 38:863–868.
31. Petrofsky, J. S., and Lind, A. R. (1978): Metabolic, cardiovascular and respiratory factors in the development of fatigue in lifting tasks. *J. Appl. Physiol.,* 45:64–68.
32. Pollock, M. L., Gettman, L. R., Milesis, C. A., Bah, M. D., Durstine, L., and Johnson, R. B. (1977): Effects of frequency and duration of training on attrition and incidence of injury. *Med. Sci. Sports,* 9:31–36.
33. Rohmert, W. (1960): *Statische, Halterarbeit des Menschen.* Beuth, Vertrid, Berlin.
34. Sherwood, D. E., and Selder, D. J. (1979): Cardiorespiratory health, reaction time and aging. *Med. Sci. Sports,* 11:186–189.
35. Sidney, K. H., and Shephard, R. J. (1977): Maximum and submaximum exercise tests in men and women in the seventh, eighth, and ninth decades of life. *J. Appl. Physiol.,* 43:280–287.
36. Spano, J. F., and Burke, E. J. (1976): Effect of three levels of work intensity on performance of a fine motor skill. *Percept. Mot. Skills,* 42:63–66.
37. Viitasalo, J. H. T., and Komi, P. V. (1977): Signal characteristics of EMG during fatigue. *Eur. J. Appl. Physiol.,* 37:111–121.
38. Winder, W. W., Hagberg, J. M., Hickson, R. C., Ehsani, A. A., and McLane, J. A. (1978): Time course of sympathoadrenal adaptation to endurance exercise training in man. *J. Appl. Physiol.,* 45:370–374.
39. Winder, W. W., Hickson, R. C., Hagberg, J. M., Ehsani, A. A., and McLane, J. A. (1979): Training-induced changes in hormonal and metabolic responses to submaximal exercise. *J. Appl. Physiol.,* 46:766–771.

Rehabilitation in the Aging edited by
T. F. Williams. Raven Press, New York © 1984.

Functional Assessment in the Elderly

Gary S. Clark

*Monroe Community Hospital and the Department of Preventive, Family, and Rehabilitation
Medicine, University of Rochester School of Medicine, Rochester, New York 14642*

As age increases, the relative proportions of persons with limitations of activity
and mobility increase. Based on 1972 U.S. survey information (21), over 43%
of the 65 and over population noted significant limitation of activity (e.g., vocational, housework, hobbies, church), more than double that of the 45 to 64
age group. Similarly, almost 18% of the 65 and over age group reported significant mobility limitation, four times greater than that of the 45 to 64 age
group.

A paramount goal of medical involvement with the elderly is that of restoring
or maintaining an optimal level of function. Obviously, an individual's functional
abilities and areas of limitation must be evaluated before an appropriate plan
of care can be developed and instituted.

To assess functional status realistically, a variety of factors must be considered,
beginning with the basic areas of mobility and self-care ability. Of particular
relevance in evaluating the elderly is consideration of the impact of their social
and environmental situation, functional implications of acute or chronic disease
processes, and physical factors that may influence function, such as range of
motion, strength, endurance, and mental status. Only by combining the results
of evaluation of all of these factors will a comprehensive and accurate picture
be obtained of a particular individual's ability to live and function.

This chapter will discuss each of these factors in detail, relating how pertinent
information may be obtained by modifying the traditional history and physical
examination format. A variety of functional rating scales will also be analyzed
in terms of their usefulness and practical application.

EVALUATION OF MOBILITY AND SELF-CARE ABILITY

Most important areas of physical functioning can be included under the general
categories of mobility and self-care ability. Determination of an individual's
current mobility and self-care status is most appropriately made during questioning related to establishing the current medical status (25).

It is important to determine if any assistive devices are required, and the
degree of input required from another person for each phase of mobility and
self-care ability. The level of function can be categorized as independent, needs

supervision, needs assistance, or dependent. Independence in a particular activity means that there is no need for physical assistance or supervision from another person. Someone may be independent even though they need assistive devices (e.g., cane, brace, long-handled shoe horn) to perform an activity. Another person is involved when the individual needs supervision (someone standing by to provide reassurance, verbal cues, or instructions), needs assistance (someone physically aiding the individual in performing an activity where the individual is doing part of the activity), or is dependent (someone must do the activity essentially completely, without help from the individual).

Mobility status can be viewed on a progressive basis, beginning with bed mobility and transfer activities, up through wheelchair or ambulatory locomotion (12). Bed mobility involves moving around in bed, turning side to side, sitting up, and getting in and out of bed. Transfer activities include getting from bed to chair and back, on and off a toilet, and in and out of a bathtub or car. These activities usually involve standing up from a sitting position, pivoting or turning, then sitting down again (stand-pivot transfer). Another technique for someone unable to maintain balance or support weight on the legs is the side-slide transfer. This involves elevating the body by pushing down with the arms, and shifting laterally to the desired location. A sliding board positioned under the buttocks and bridging the gap (e.g., between chair and bed) may also be used.

The next level of mobility involves locomotion, or travel from one point to another. For an individual who is unable to ambulate, it is important to determine the reasons (e.g., stroke with hemiparesis, severe degenerative joint disease with pain) and the duration of the limitation, to aid in estimation of the potential benefits of therapeutic intervention. Such a person may use a wheelchair for locomotion, and important functional parameters include ability to propel and maneuver the wheelchair, in what environment (e.g., inside versus outside, rugs, ramps, curbs), and over what distances. Other factors involve management of the wheelchair itself, such as locking and unlocking brakes and detaching and reattaching arm rests and leg rests.

For the ambulatory individual, questions should be directed toward necessity for supervision or assistance of another person, use of assistive devices (e.g., cane, crutches, walker, brace), distances walked, and in what setting (e.g., in home, outside, in community). Specific questions should always be asked regarding the occurrence of falls, including frequency and circumstances. Ability to negotiate stairs, use of public transportation, and ability to drive are also of relevance. One practical indicator of the degree of mobility and confidence of an individual is the frequency of visits to friends, restaurants, stores, theaters, and so on.

There are several subcategories of self-care ability, or activities of daily living (ADL) as this is often termed (15). They include feeding, personal hygiene, and dressing. As with the evaluation of mobility status, it is important to determine for each area the degree of assistance necessary from another person.

Eating is the most basic of self-care functions, and most integral to an individual's self-image and survival. Eating functions involve use of a knife, spoon, and fork, as well as handling cups and glasses. The most common areas of difficulty often involve cutting food and opening containers.

Personal hygiene includes those activities associated with grooming, bathing, and toileting. Questions on grooming should include use of a toothbrush, combing hair, shaving or applying make-up, and care and use of dentures. Most people bathe in a shower or bathtub, but the elderly individual may have difficulty getting in and out of a bathtub. Another option is bathing with a sponge or washcloth while sitting in front of a sink. A useful assistive device might be a long-handled sponge to reach the back and legs. A factor that may affect which self-care tasks are actually performed is length of time necessary to complete an activity. An elderly individual might not perform bathing and dressing activities on a daily basis because of the excessive time requirements (greater than 45 to 60 min). Indeed, a recent study of elderly women found a high correlation between time required to perform various manual skills and state of dependency (30).

Maintaining bowel and bladder continence is a critical area of self-care, as this may otherwise severely limit an elderly person's potential social interaction with visitors and friends. Specific questioning should be directed toward occurrence, frequency, and patterns of incontinence, with determination whether the incontinence is due to urgency or to lack of awareness. Of particular difficulty for the elderly is nighttime voiding, because of decreased awareness and difficulty in getting to the bathroom. Post-bowel movement perineal care is also an important issue, particularly with regard to who is available and able to assist if needed.

In determining degree of function with dressing, it is important to be more specific than "Can you dress yourself?" An elderly person may have given up clothes that are difficult to manage, such as shoes and socks, clothes with buttons or zippers, and bras. Specific information should be sought, including whether street clothes are worn, and whether assistance is needed with shoes and socks, buttons, zippers, or tight-fitting underwear. Assistive equipment may include a long-handled reacher, button hook, and elastic shoelaces, among others.

There are a variety of miscellaneous activities that can also be included under ADL, basically involving fine motor coordination and hand function. Examples include writing, using a phone, handling money, opening and closing curtains or doors, setting or winding a watch, turning pages, and manipulating light switches. Another component of physical functioning, sometimes referred to as Instrumental ADL, consists of activities such as shopping, housekeeping, and cooking.

Several functional rating scales, to be discussed in a later section, are available to categorize and record the functional evaluation findings just discussed.

EVALUATION OF SOCIAL AND ENVIRONMENTAL FACTORS

It is critical to be aware of the particular environment an individual is living and functioning in, as well as what "significant other" persons are available for assistance (2). This may have profound implications for an individual's level of function, as well as the potential for improvement in functional ability with a specific therapy program. For example, a man who is independent in ambulation on level surfaces but cannot negotiate stairs may be very functional in a ground floor apartment, but might be confined indoors if he lived in a second story walk-up apartment. With an appropriate physical therapy program, he might be trained to negotiate stairs safely, thereby enabling him to be more independent. Similarly, the availability of a spouse or "significant other" who can be trained in techniques to assist with self-care activities and mobility may greatly increase that person's level of functioning.

Specifics to clarify include where the individual lives (apartment versus house, urban versus rural), whether the bedroom, bathroom, and kitchen are on the same floor, and whether there are physical barriers or hazards (e.g., narrow doorways, stairs, loose throw rugs). If there are stairs, it is important to determine whether there is a railing, the angle and number of steps, and whether there are sufficient lighting and a nonslip surface. The most common accident in the elderly at home is falling, with significant morbidity related not only to direct injury and discomfort, but also disability secondary to fear and resultant inactivity.

Immediate family members living in the home are usually more reliable for assistance than nearby friends or relatives, but their other commitments (e.g., work, school, children, illnesses) must also be taken into account. If living alone, an individual's homemaking ability must also be evaluated, including cooking, shopping, laundry, and housecleaning. Deficiencies in these areas might aggravate nutritional problems commonly seen in the elderly. Availability and utilization of community agencies should be checked, such as meals-on-wheels, homemaker services, and visiting nurse or public health nurse services.

FUNCTIONAL IMPLICATIONS OF DISEASE

In the evaluation of the elderly individual, particular attention should be paid to present illness, past medical history, and review of systems to identify injuries or disease processes that might affect function (28). Such injuries or illnesses most often involve the cardiorespiratory, neurologic, or musculoskeletal systems, as demonstrated by the leading causes of activity or mobility limitations (21): heart conditions, arthritis, lower extremity or hip impairment, cerebrovascular disease, and paralysis.

The elderly population characteristically manifests multiple and chronic disease processes, often resulting in progressive and significant functional limitations

(29). Any single disease process, and especially multiple concurrent diseases, may result in physical, psychological, nutritional, and social changes, all of which may significantly affect function. The manifestations of disease, and particularly the functional impact, are different in the elderly than in younger populations. In taking a history of present illness (or current medical status) and past medical history, it is important to determine not only what illnesses or injuries have occurred or are present, but also the duration and severity of involvement, and effect on functional abilities. One particular disease or injury may not cause any functional limitation, but combined with one or more other diseases may cause or compound disability.

There are several important principles relating to the functional impact of disease that should be emphasized. Functional limitations in an individual with an acute illness are usually transient and resolve with appropriate treatment of the underlying illness. However, chronic diseases are more often not amenable to cure, but primarily palliation or symptomatic treatment. As a result, functional impairments secondary to a chronic disease (and especially with multiple chronic diseases) are typically more permanent and progressive. In assessing functional ability and limitations, particularly in the elderly individual, it is critical to characterize accurately any illness or injuries, recent or past, in terms of the functional impact, chronicity, and amenability to treatment.

Another principle is that of determining which functional problems are a direct result of the injury or disease process, and which ones are due to secondary complications and are potentially preventable (12,14). Primary disabilities are a direct result of the pathologic process. There is no direct relationship between any particular disease and the range of disability that may result. For example, arthritic inflammation involving the interphalangeal joints of the hands may not hinder a company executive, but may be partially disabling for a typist or gardener, and completely incapacitating for a concert pianist. It is important to keep in mind that one disease process may also cause multiple disabilities. For example, a stroke may result in impairment of speech, mobility, and continence. Any one of these would significantly limit some aspect of function, but in combination they are particularly devastating.

Most secondary disabilities occur as a result of complications relating to disuse, from either excessive bedrest or relative inactivity. The multiplicity of problems resulting from disuse may cause functional limitation in and of themselves, but may also combine with the underlying illness or injury to produce significant disability. Examples of the results of disuse or inactivity include complications from stasis (e.g., urinary retention with infection, pneumonia and atelectasis, thromboembolic disease, orthostatic hypotension, joint contractures), atrophy (e.g., osteoporosis, disuse muscle weakness, decreased endurance), and pressure (e.g., decubitus ulcer formation) (19). Equally worthy of mention are the psychological effects of inactivity or bedrest, including social isolation and withdrawal, depression, and loss of motivation and confidence in ability to function.

These multiple complications of disuse, and resultant disabilities, are exaggerated or increased in frequency and severity in the elderly population. To determine how important a factor such as deconditioning is for any individual, it is essential to inquire as to their daily activity status (e.g., how much time do they spend out of bed, how much time sitting versus standing or walking, how far do they usually walk).

It is important to establish the premorbid functional status in an individual who has a major disability from an injury or illness of recent onset. This will result in a more realistic and appropriate treatment program, since it is usually difficult to improve an individual's functional ability over a premorbid status. Similarly, in someone with a progressive decline in function as a result of one or more chronic diseases, it is essential to determine the time frame of loss of function. It is easier, as a rule, to reverse those disabilities of most recent onset.

Finally, in the review of systems, there are several systems and related symptoms that should be emphasized in checking for other evidence of limitation of function from disease. These include cardiorespiratory (e.g., angina, dyspnea on exertion, claudication, easy fatigueability), neurological (e.g., weakness; incoordination; seizures; impaired sensation, perception, vision, hearing, or balance), and musculoskeletal (e.g., pain, stiffness, limitation of motion, deformity). It may also be helpful to review medications, both prescription and over-the-counter, that an individual is taking. The myriad potential side effects (especially orthostatic hypotension, sedation, and dizziness) or interactions may also affect functional ability.

To illustrate these principles, consider an elderly man who presents with severe pain in his right hip with marked limitation of mobility. Evaluation reveals moderately advanced osteoarthritis of the right hip. Initial conservative management might include prescribing anti-inflammatory drugs (e.g., aspirin, nonsteroidal anti-inflammatory drugs) and using a cane on his left side to reduce stress on his painful right hip. Further questioning of his past medical history and review of systems, however, reveals a history of fracture of his left wrist, with residual painful limited motion, and difficulty grasping objects or bearing weight. In this situation a platform crutch would be more appropriate than a cane, to allow the necessary deweighting of the right hip but avoiding painful weight-bearing on the left wrist. This case demonstrates a chronic disease amenable to symptomatic relief but not cure (osteoarthritis), with resultant functional limitation (decreased mobility secondary to pain). It also shows a prior injury (wrist fracture) with secondary complications (limited joint range and pain in gripping or weight-bearing) that were not functionally significant for this elderly man until complicated by another disease.

PHYSICAL FACTORS INFLUENCING FUNCTION

In a routine physical examination of the elderly person, giving particular attention to the neuromuscular and skeletal examination will yield valuable information on residual abilities and potential for improvement. Goals of the examination include observation of deviations from normal structure or function, evidence of secondary complications, as well as assessment of residual strengths (25,28).

Obviously the physical examination must be thorough and comprehensive, but there are several areas that should be highlighted. Skin should be closely inspected, particularly over bony prominences (e.g., sacrum, ischial tuberosities, trochanters, heels, malleoli, elbows, scapulae) for evidence of excessive pressure, friction, or maceration that may lead to skin breakdown. Peterson and Bittman (24) report a prevalence of decubitus ulcers of 43.1 per 100,000 in Denmark, with a sharp increase in incidence with advancing age. Prevention of decubitus ulcer formation is obviously preferable to the exceedingly high cost of treatment, in terms of time (of relative immobilization and/or hospitalization), dollars (estimated at $2,000 to $10,000 in 1976) (27), and associated morbidity.

With the high prevalence of diabetic and arteriosclerotic peripheral vascular disease in the elderly, it is also prudent to inspect the skin of the feet, particularly between the toes. This is often an area not well cleaned or dried, and maceration with skin breakdown and infection may eventually result in amputation.

In the cardiopulmonary examination, a check for orthostatic hypotension may prove valuable, particularly in the individual complaining of lightheadedness, dizziness, or episodes of blacking out with falling. This is vital in the patient on medications (e.g., antihypertensives including methyldopa, phenothiazines) with orthostatic side effects. Checking the resting heart rate with comparison to a postactivity heart rate may yield valuable clues to the level of endurance and tolerance of exercise. Identifying arrhythmias, murmurs, rales, or evidence of chronic obstructive pulmonary disease may help explain exercise intolerance with easy fatigueability or dyspnea.

The musculoskeletal examination must include an evaluation of the joints, particularly the knees, hips, shoulders, and hands. Evidence of arthritic involvement should be sought, including tenderness, limitation of motion (with or without pain), crepitus, ligamentous laxity, joint instability, or deformity. Joint range of motion should be checked both passively (examiner moving joint) and actively (patient moving joint under own muscle power). Limited passive range may indicate soft tissue contracture or joint destruction, whereas limited active range of motion relative to the passive range may signal muscle weakness or articular/periarticular inflammation.

Critical ranges of motion for function include: (a) shoulder abduction (90°), internal/external rotation (touch lower back and back of head, respectively); (b) forearm pronation/supination (45° each); (c) wrist flexion (45°)/extension (30°): (d) finger flexion (to within 1 inch of palm); (e) hip flexion (90°)/extension (neutral); (f) knee flexion (110°)/extension (neutral); (g) ankle dorsiflexion (neutral). Examples of functions dependent on these critical ranges include perineal care (shoulder internal rotation with wrist flexion), combing hair (shoulder abduction and external rotation, wrist flexion and finger flexion for grip), and eating (wrist flexion, pronation, and supination).

Muscle strength is best evaluated using the traditional six-grade rating system (3,18):

0 = zero   = no visible or palpable muscle contracture
1 = trace   = visible or palpable muscle contraction, but little or no actual joint movement
2 = poor   = movement of joint through full range of motion, but with gravity eliminated
3 = fair   = movement of joint through full range of motion against gravity, but without examiner resistance (or examiner easily able to move joint in direction opposite of muscle contraction)
4 = good   = movement of joint through full range of motion against moderate resistance from examiner (or examiner able to move joint in direction opposite to muscle contraction, but with some difficulty)
5 = normal = movement of joint through full range of motion against full examiner resistance (or examiner unable to move joint in direction opposite to muscle contraction)

To illustrate: a man would have poor grade wrist extensors if, with his arm resting palm down on a table, he is unable to lift his hand up off the table (against gravity), yet with palm perpendicular to table, he is able to extend his wrist (gravity eliminated).

Fair grade strength (3/5) is the critical muscle grade, because this is the minimal muscle strength necessary to perform basic functional activities, such as feeding, bathing, changing position in bed. An even higher grade of strength (in the good or 4/5 range) is usually necessary to be able to bear weight, such as for transfers or ambulation.

Factors that may alter the accuracy of muscle strength assessment include effects of pain or tenderness (e.g., patient gives way, leading to appearance of less than actual strength) and spasticity (e.g., adding involuntary to voluntary contraction, with appearance of greater than actual strength). Lack of cooperation or comprehension, as is frequently found in ill elderly persons, may also lead to inaccurate estimates of muscle strength.

A screening muscle test in an elderly individual might include checking shoulder elevators (shoulder shrug) and abductors, elbow flexors and extensors, wrist extensors, gross hand grasp as well as fingertip prehension (thumb to index finger pinch), hip and knee flexors and extensors, and ankle dorsiflexors.

In the neurologic examination, mental status should be routinely evaluated, as this may have significant bearing on an elderly individual's level of functioning and, particularly, safety. Included routinely should be a check of appearance, affect, orientation (person, place, time) and communication (receptive and expressive ability). Examples of a screening test of receptive abilities (comprehension) in an individual with aphasia poststroke might include asking the individual to point to named objects (e.g., window, watch) and to follow simple and complex commands. Expressive abilities can be checked by asking the individual to name simple objects pointed to, and by asking questions calling for simple one-word and then more complex responses. Checking reading comprehension and writing ability will indicate whether deficits extend to more than visual/verbal modalities.

Intellectual function can be evaluated by checking remote and recent memory and immediate recall, calculations (e.g., arithmetic, subtracting sevens serially from 100), and abstract thought, including similarities between groups of objects (e.g., apple and orange = fruit, hammer and screwdriver = tools), and proverb interpretation. Judgment and insight should also be considered. A standardized mental status test such as that proposed by Folstein (6) is useful for making comparisons of progress (or deterioration) over time.

Cranial nerve examination should emphasize evaluation of extraocular movements, evidence for visual field cut or extinction (with double simultaneous stimulation), and gross visual and auditory acuity. It is also important to check for dysfunction of facial muscles (causing dysarthria, drooling) or of lingual and pharyngeal muscles (causing dysphagia, aspiration).

Other areas of importance in the neurologic examination include testing of sensation (particularly proprioception), deep tendon reflexes (especially asymmetry), balance (sitting and standing), and coordination. One area frequently overlooked in evaluating the elderly is that of perceptual function (e.g., body image, right/left discrimination). A simple screen might involve having the individual draw a clock, draw a person, and point to named areas of the body.

FUNCTIONAL NEUROMUSCULAR EXAMINATION

There are a variety of maneuvers individuals can be asked to perform as part of the physical examination that will serve as very practical indicators of their functional ability. Obvious tasks to check include unsupported sitting balance (sitting on edge of bed or table), standing balance, ability to transfer from chair to a bed or another chair, and ability to ambulate for a certain distance (endurance). Observing an individual undressing for or dressing after the physical examination gives a realistic indication of function in this area. Asking a person to take a drink from a cup or glass, and to simulate eating will provide useful information on feeding skills. Manual dexterity can also be evaluated by asking an individual to pick up a coin or pen, write, and unbutton and button a shirt.

USE OF FUNCTIONAL RATING SCALES

To aid in standardized, comprehensive functional evaluation of groups of individuals, a variety of functional rating scales have been developed (1,5,13, 17,20,22,23,26). The primary clinical usefulness of these rating scales lies in the ability to assess an individual's present functional status, and monitor subsequent improvement or deterioration. These scales have also proved valuable from a research standpoint, enabling standardized serial monitoring and comparison of particular disability populations.

Most of the rating scales have been developed based on populations of chronically ill and aging persons, although some have been based on particular disabilities such as stroke, hip fracture, or arthritis. These scales generally provide a measure of overall function, but may not be sensitive enough to detect or assess very specific functional impairments.

The existence of so many scales implies that no one scale is ideal. An ideal scale would be valid and reliable, would evaluate a representative sample of activities, and would be applicable to the general population (with a wide range of impairments and levels of function). To be most useful it would provide indicators of the causes of functional deficits. Such a scale should also be reasonably brief and be simple to administer, score, and interpret. Kane and Kane recently published an excellent comprehensive review of instruments available for assessment of the elderly (16).

Two rating scales in particular appear to provide the most potentially useful information for functional evaluation of the elderly: the PULSES Profile (23) and the Barthel Index (22). The PULSES Profile (23) particularly as adapted by Granger et al. (7,9,10), provides a measure of general functional performance (Table 1). In addition to rating overall mobility and self-care ability, it also evaluates several of the other areas that have impact on function, including medical status and psychosocial factors. On this ordinal scaling, 6 is the best possible score and 24 is the worst (or most dependent) score. An individual scoring 6 is medically stable, independent in self-care and mobility, has no visual or communication impairments, is continent of bowel and bladder, and is able to fulfill usual family and financial responsibilities.

The Barthel Index (22) limits its rating to basic self-care and mobility, but is much more sensitive in terms of identifying specific difficulties within these key functional areas (Table 2). In contrast to the PULSES Profile, a higher Barthel score indicates greater functional ability. The maximum score of 100 represents an individual who is continent, independent in feeding, bathing, grooming, dressing, and toileting, and able to transfer, ambulate at least one block, and negotiate stairs.

Both of these scales heavily weigh incontinence (because of the associated time required to attend, and the social unacceptability) and the need for another person (to supervise or assist). However, they do not necessarily predict ability to live alone, since they do not evaluate homemaking skills.

Longitudinal studies evaluating groups of patients serially using both the PULSES Profile and Barthel Index have demonstrated high interscale correlation, as well as high reliability, validity, and sensitivity to changes in functional levels (4,7). Such studies have also suggested other ways these scales may prove useful. Wylie (31) and Granger et al. (7–11) have extensively studied stroke patients using the Barthel Index and PULSES Profile as a predictor of response to intensive rehabilitation involvement, as well as eventual disposition on discharge from hospital. Patients with admission Barthel scores greater than 20 showed better response to rehabilitation (with higher resultant functional levels)

TABLE 1. *PULSES Profile (adapted)*[a]

P—Physical condition: includes diseases of the viscera (cardiovascular, gastrointestinal, urologic, and endocrine) and neurologic disorders:
1. Medical problems sufficiently stable that medical or nursing monitoring is not required more often than 3-month intervals.
2. Medical or nurse monitoring is needed more often than 3-month intervals but not each week.
3. Medical problems are sufficiently unstable as to require regular medical and/or nursing attention at least weekly.
4. Medical problems require intensive medical and/or nursing attention at least daily (excluding personal care assistance only).

U—Upper limb functions: Self-care activities (drink/feed, dress upper/lower, brace/prothesis, groom, wash, perineal care) dependent mainly upon upper limb function:
1. Independent in self-care without impairment of upper limbs.
2. Independent in self-care with some impairment of upper limbs.
3. Dependent upon assistance or supervision in self-care with or without impairment of upper limbs.
4. Dependent totally in self-care with marked impairment of upper limbs.

L—Lower limb functions: Mobility (transfer chair/toilet/tub or shower, walk, stairs, wheelchair) dependent mainly upon lower limb function:
1. Independent in mobility without impairment of lower limbs.
2. Independent in mobility with some impairment in lower limbs; such as needing ambulatory aids, a brace or prosthesis, or else fully independent in a wheelchair without significant architectural or environmental barriers.
3. Dependent upon assistance or supervision in mobility with or without impairment of lower limbs, or partly independent in a wheelchair, or there are significant architectural or environmental barriers.
4. Dependent totally in mobility with marked impairment of lower limbs.

S—Sensory components: Relating to communication (speech and hearing) and vision:
1. Independent in communication and vision without impairment.
2. Independent in communication and vision with some impairment such as mild dysarthria, mild aphasia, or need for eyeglasses or hearing aid, or needing regular eye medication.
3. Dependent upon assistance, an interpreter, or supervision in communication or vision.
4. Dependent totally in communication or vision.

E—Excretory functions (bladder and bowel):
1. Complete voluntary control of bladder and bowel sphincters.
2. Control of sphincters allows normal social activities despite urgency or need for catheter, appliance, suppositories, etc. Able to care for needs without assistance.
3. Dependent upon assistance in sphincter management or else has accidents occasionally.
4. Frequent wetting or soiling from incontinence of bladder or bowel sphincters.

S—Support factors: Consider intellectual and emotional adaptability, support from family unit, and financial ability:
1. Able to fulfill usual roles and perform customary tasks.
2. Must make some modification in usual roles and performance of customary tasks.
3. Dependent upon assistance, supervision, encouragement or assistance from a public or private agency due to any of the above considerations.
4. Dependent upon long-term institutional care (chronic hospitalization, nursing home, etc) excluding time-limited hospital for specific evaluation, treatment, or active rehabilitation.

[a] PULSE total: best score is 6. Worst score is 24.
From Granger et al. (7).

TABLE 2. *Barthel Index[a] with the corresponding values for independent performance of tasks*

Index	"Can do by myself."	"Can do with help of someone else."	"Cannot do at all."
Self-care index			
1. Drinking from a cup	4	0	0
2. Eating	6	0	0
3. Dressing upper body	5	3	0
4. Dressing lower body	7	4	0
5. Putting on brace or artificial limb	0	−2	0 (not applicable)
6. Grooming	5	0	0
7. Washing or bathing	6	0	0
8. Controlling urination	10	5 (accidents	0 (incontinent)
9. Controlling bowel movements	10	5 (accidents)	0 (incontinent)
Mobility index			
10. Getting in and out of chair	15	7	0
11. Getting on and off toilet	6	3	0
12. Getting in and out of tub or shower	1	0	0
13. Walking 50 yards on the level	15	10	0
14. Walking up/down one flight of stairs	10	5	0
15. IF NOT WALKING:			
Propelling or pushing wheelchair	5	0	0 (not applicable)

[a] Barthel total: best score is 100; worst score is 0.
From Granger et al. (7).

than those with initial scores less than 20. Moreover, 84% of patients with Barthel scores greater than or equal to 60 (PULSES score less than or equal to 12) at time of discharge returned home. Of those with discharge Barthel scores less than 60 (PULSES score greater than 12), 90% required placement in a long-term care facility.

In summary, the PULSES Profile and Barthel Index may prove to be a useful adjunct clinically, primarily by providing a standardized format for functional evaluation, and by providing a sensitive monitor to detect subsequent changes in function. They may also serve as a prognosticator of the potential benefits of rehabilitation involvement and eventual disposition.

RESULTS OF FUNCTIONAL ASSESSMENT

By now it should be apparent that in evaluating an individual, it is not sufficient to determine which diseases are present. The impact of various disease processes on a particular individual's functional ability must be considered, with the knowledge that each disease may result in variable degrees of severity of multiple primary and/or secondary disabilities. This is especially true in treating the elderly with their typically multiple and chronic ailments.

Similarly, determining basic mobility and self-care ability is incomplete without consideration of what environment the individual functions in, and what resources (e.g., family, services) are available. Kane and Kane (16) repeatedly emphasize the importance and inter-relatedness of physical, mental, and social functioning for accurate assessment of the elderly person.

As stated at the outset, a paramount goal of caring for the elderly is that of restoring or maintaining an optimal level of function, in the desired environmental setting. Only by serial, comprehensive, and thorough evaluations of an individual's functional status, taking into account social, environmental, medical, and physical factors, can areas be identified that might be amenable to therapeutic input and change. Only then can an appropriate individualized management plan be devised to maintain or regain function.

REFERENCES

1. Anderson, T. P., Baldridge, M., and Ettinger, M. G. (1979): Quality of care for completed stroke without rehabilitation: Evaluation by assessing patient outcomes. *Arch. Phys. Med. Rehabil.,* 60:103–107.
2. Coe, R. M. (1976): The geriatric patient in the community. In: *Cowdy's The Care of the Geriatric Patient,* edited by F. V. Steinberg, pp. 493–503. C. V. Mosby, St. Louis.
3. Daniels, L., and Worthingham, C. (1972): *Muscle Testing: Techniques of Manual Examination.* Saunders, Philadelphia.
4. Donaldson, S. W., Wagner, C. C., and Gresham, G. E. (1973): A unified ADL evaluation form. *Arch. Phys. Med. Rehabil.,* 54:175–185.
5. Feigenson, J., Polkow, L., Meikle, R., and Ferguson, W. (1979): Burke Stroke Time-Oriented Profile (BUSTOP): An overview of patient function. *Arch. Phys. Med. Rehabil.,* 60:508–511.
6. Folstein, M. F., Folstein, S. E., and McHugh, P. R. (1975): Mini-mental state: A practical method for grading the cognitive state of patients for the clinician. *J. Psychiatr. Res.,* 12:189–198.
7. Granger, C. V., Albrecht, G. L., and Hamilton, B. B. (1979): Outcome of comprehensive medical rehabilitation: Measurement by PULSES profile and the Barthel index. *Arch. Phys. Med. Rehabil.,* 60:145–154.
8. Granger, C. V., Dewis, L. S., Peters, N. C., Sherwood, C. C., and Barrett, J. E. (1979): Stroke rehabilitation: Analysis of repeated Barthel index measures. *Arch. Phys. Med. Rehabil.,* 60:14–17.
9. Granger, C. V., and Greer, D. S. (1976): Functional status measurement and medical rehabilitation outcomes. *Arch. Phys. Med. Rehabil.,* 57:103–109.
10. Granger, C. V., Greer, D. S., Liset, E., Coulombe, J., and O'Brien, E. (1975): Measurement of outcomes of care for stroke patients. *Stroke,* 6:34–41.
11. Granger, C. V., Sherwood, C. C., and Greer, D. S. (1977): Functional status measures in a comprehensive stroke care program. *Arch. Phys. Med. Rehabil.,* 58:555–561.
12. Hirschberg, G. G., Lewis, L., and Vaughn, P. (1976): *Rehabilitation—A Manual for the Care of the Disabled and Elderly.* Lippincott, Philadelphia.
13. Huddleston, O. L., Moore, R. W., Rubin, D., Humphrey, T. L., Campbell, J. W., and Blanchette, R. (1961): Evaluation of physical disabilities by means of patient profile chart. *Arch. Phys. Med. Rehabil.,* 42:250–257.
14. Itoh, M., and Lee, M. H. M. (1982): The epidemiology of disability as related to rehabilitation medicine. In: *Krusen's Handbook of Physical Medicine and Rehabilitation,* edited by F. J. Kottke, G. K. Stillwell, and J. F. Lehman, pp. 199–217. Saunders, Philadelphia.
15. Jordan, R. I., (1968): Occupational therapy. In: *Rehabilitation and Medicine,* edited by S. Licht. Elizabeth Licht, New Haven.
16. Kane, R. A., and Kane, R. L. (1981): *Assessing the elderly: A practical guide to measurement.* Lexington Books, Massachusetts.
17. Katz, S., Ford, A. B., Moskowitz, R. W., Jackson, B. A., and Jaffe, M. W. (1967): Studies of illness in the aged. *JAMA,* 185:914–919.
18. Kendall, H. O., and Kendall, F. P. (1971): *Muscles: Testing and function.* Williams & Wilkins, Baltimore.
19. Kottke, F. J., and Anderson, E. M. (1965): Deterioration of the bedfast patient. *Public Health Rep.,* 80:437–451.

20. Lee, P., Jasani, M. K., Dick, W. C., and Buchanan, W. W. (1973): Evaluation of a functional index in rheumatoid arthritis. *Scand. J. Rheumatol.,* 2:71–77.
21. Limitation of activity and mobility due to chronic conditions. *Vital and Health Statistics.* (1972): Series 10, No. 96, pp. 11, 15–16. National Center for Health Statistics, Public Health Service, Department of Health, Education and Welfare, Washington, D.C.
22. Mahoney, F. L., and Barthel, D. W. (1965): Functional evaluation: Barthel index. *Md. State Med. J.,* 14:61–65.
23. Moskowitz, E., and McCann, C. (1957): Classification of disability in chronically ill and aging. *J. Chronic. Dis.,* 5:342–346.
24. Peterson, N. C., and Bittman, S. (1971): The epidemiology of pressure sores. *Scand. J. Plast. Reconstr. Surg.,* 5:62–66.
25. Rusk, H. A. (1977): The evaluation process. In: *Rehabilitation Medicine,* edited by H. A. Rusk, pp. 26–64. Mosby, St. Louis.
26. Schoening, H. A., Anderegg, L., Bergstrom, D., Fonda, M., Steinke, N., and Ulrich, P. (1965): Numerical scoring of self-care status of patients. *Arch. Phys. Med. Rehabil.,* 46:689–697.
27. Spence, W. R., Burk, R. D., and Rae, J. W. (1967): Gel support for prevention of decubitus ulcers. *Arch. Phys. Med. Rehabil.,* 48:283–288.
28. Stolov, W. C. (1982): Evaluation of the patient. In: *Krusen's Handbook of Physical Medicine and Rehabilitation,* edited by F. J. Kottke, G. K. Stillwell, and J. F. Lehman, pp. 1–18. Saunders, Philadelphia.
29. Tobis, J. S. (1979): Rehabilitation of the geriatric patient. In: *Clinical Geriatrics,* edited by I. Rossman, pp. 502–515. Lippincott, Philadelphia.
30. Williams, M. E., Hadler, N. M., and Earp, J. L. (1982): Manual ability as a marker of dependency in geriatric women. *J. Chron. Dis.,* 35:115–122.
31. Wylie, C. M. (1967): Guaging the response of stroke patients to rehabilitation. *J. Am. Geriatr. Soc.,* 15:797–805.

Rehabilitation in the Aging edited by
T. F. Williams. Raven Press, New York © 1984.

Development of a Rehabilitation Plan

Gary S. Clark and Grady P. Bray

Monroe Community Hospital and the Department of Preventive, Family, and Rehabilitation Medicine, University of Rochester School of Medicine, Rochester, New York 14642

This chapter will discuss the concept of rehabilitation, and describe various levels of involvement in the rehabilitation process with particular emphasis on tailoring the program to the needs of elderly individuals. Roles and functions of each of the involved health disciplines will be explained, as well as the dynamics and organization of the multidisciplinary team approach. Finally, the benefits of rehabilitation, both to the individual and society, will be explored.

THE CONCEPT

Although there are many definitions of rehabilitation, a particularly descriptive definition is: "The continuing and comprehensive team effort to restore an individual to his/her former functional and environmental status, or alternatively, to maintain or maximize remaining function" (9). For a more detailed analysis, this definition can be broken down into components of "continuing and comprehensive," "team effort," and "restore . . . to former functional and environmental status, or . . . maximize remaining function."

Rehabilitation has often been erroneously designated as the third phase in medical care (the first two phases being prevention and definitive medical or surgical treatment) (9). This implies a time relationship, with rehabilitation beginning where and when definitive treatment ends. In reality, however, rehabilitation is a continuing process with applications in all phases of medical care. One of the primary goals of rehabilitation is that of prevention: preventing deterioration of function related to aging, disease, or injury; and anticipating and avoiding complications of various disease processes, particularly those due to disuse and deconditioning. An application of this can be seen in the instruction of the amputee with severe peripheral vascular disease in proper skin care of the remaining foot, to avoid skin breakdown and infection.

Rehabilitation should become involved during definitive medical/surgical treatment, to at least prevent needless secondary deconditioning. An example might be maintaining range of motion, muscle strength and endurance in an individual confined to bed posttrauma with an extremity fracture. Rehabilitation involvement may also directly aid ongoing medical or surgical care, such as in coordinating conservative and surgical management of a decubitus ulcer.

125

Although the bulk of rehabilitation effort takes place after initial specific medical/surgical involvement, it is important to realize that rehabilitation should begin in parallel, rather than in series, with this definitive care.

Rehabilitation can be considered ongoing in another sense, that of continuing involvement with patients after initial management. For hospitalized patients this may entail coordinating ongoing health care involvement, including community services, after discharge. For individuals in the community, periodic reassessment may be indicated to ensure maintenance of functional status. There are several diagnostic categories (such as spinal cord injury and multiple sclerosis) that may require life-long rehabilitation involvement to maintain optimal function and prevent or treat complications.

Approaching the individual from a comprehensive standpoint is also a key principal of rehabilitation. This entails considering not only the medical, physical, and functional implications of disease or injury, but also psychoemotional, social, sexual, and economic/vocational factors. Although the major emphasis of rehabilitation is on medical care and reversal of functional deficits, there is also recognition of the need for input in these other areas. For a person with a catastrophic and disabling illness or injury, such as stroke or amputation, there is a well-defined sequence of psychoemotional reactions and coping mechanisms (5). It is important to be aware of the status of an individual with regard to this sequence, to facilitate appropriate supportive counseling and therapeutic intervention if needed.

Similarly, with major illness or injury associated with significant disability, there are many ramifications from a family standpoint. As an example, consider the head of the family suffering a stroke with residual hemiparesis and aphasia. This often results in considerable trauma to the family, with anxiety and confusion due to lack of accurate knowledge concerning stroke, disruption of family dynamics (leadership, decision making), and loss of the primary income-producer. This requires education of the family, counseling in how to deal with the affected family member, and advice on alternatives in insurance, equipment, supportive services, and so on. Vocational evaluation, counseling, and/or training may also be appropriate, depending on the age of the individual, severity of disability, and degree of education or training.

The next component of our definition of rehabilitation is that of "team effort." It would seem obvious that no one health discipline could accomplish the comprehensive approach to an individual and family just discussed. This requires a multidisciplinary team approach, coordinated in their efforts toward common goals. There are a variety of health care professionals involved in a comprehensive rehabilitation program, to be discussed in more detail subsequently. Briefly, however, this may include a physiatrist (physician specializing in rehabilitation medicine), rehabilitation nurse, clinical psychologist, physical therapist, occupational therapist, speech pathologist, social worker, and vocational counselor. Involvement of one or even several of these disciplines with a patient does not necessarily constitute rehabilitation per se, unless they are members of a team with common goals and coordinated efforts. In this sense, rehabilitation may be considered synergistic, in that the benefits of the combined and coordinated multidisciplinary involvement are greater than the sum of benefits from individual disciplines' involvement.

Trying to "restore an individual to his/her former functional and environmental status, or alternatively, to maintain or maximize remaining function" is the final and most important component of our definition of rehabilitation. The typical individual becoming involved in the rehabilitation process has suffered a major illness or injury with significant disability in self-care ability or mobility. Rehabilitation efforts are directed toward preventing added disability from complications, training the individual to utilize residual neuromuscular ability, and working to reverse the impairments of the illness or injury. The goals are to attain the maximum functional level and to enable the person not only to return home, but hopefully to resume former roles in the community.

This is particularly relevant to the elderly. They often live in a rather fragile environmental setting, so that a relatively minor or temporary functional impairment (e.g., acute exacerbation of a chronic illness or a fracture from a fall) may disrupt the support system sufficiently that they are unable to return home.

This ties in with the previous discussion of the "continuing and comprehensive" nature of rehabilitation. Efforts to return an elderly person to an independent living setting in the community may involve setting up community support services (e.g., meals-on-wheels, visiting nurse) and periodic reassessment to ensure maintenance of function in a safe and appropriate living situation. Continuing rehabilitation involvement, including periodic reassessment, remains important even when the individual is unable to return to an independent living situation.

THE PROCESS

To analyze the practical application of the concepts of rehabilitation to the needs of the elderly patient, a variety of factors will be considered. The functions and roles of each of the component health disciplines will be discussed, as well as the distinction between maintenance and restorative rehabilitation. Variables in the setting will also be considered.

Team Members

A rehabilitation team may include any (but usually all) of the following disciplines: physical therapy, occupational therapy, speech therapy, rehabilitation nursing, social work, clinical psychology, vocational counseling, and physiatry. Health professionals in each of these areas are highly trained specialists with expertise within their own discipline, but in a team setting they also complement and aid efforts of the other disciplines (12,19). The role of each discipline will be discussed in detail, using the example of a male individual who has suffered a stroke with resultant right hemiparesis and aphasia.

Efforts of the physical therapist (PT) are directed primarily toward improving range of motion (ROM), strength, endurance, balance, and mobility (e.g., moving around in bed, transferring in and out of a bed or chair, ambulation). Training may include the use of a variety of assistive devices as mobility aides, such as a wheelchair, cane, crutches, walker, and bracing. With the stroke patient described, the PT would train the patient to use the intact left side to compensate for the right hemiparesis, for example, in turning in bed or sitting up. The PT would also work with the patient with neuromuscular reeducation techniques to take advantage of whatever neurologic recovery had occurred on the right, particularly for weight-bearing for transfers and ambulation. Training would then progress to negotiating stairs, uneven surfaces, getting in and out of cars, and so on, as appropriate.

The main areas of concentration for the occupational therapist (OT) include activities of daily living (ADL, such as eating, bathing, grooming, dressing) as well as improving upper extremity function. With the stroke patient, the OT would test for visual, sensory, or perceptual deficits and work with the patient to compensate for these. The patient would be trained in one-handed techniques for self-care and homemaking activities. A splint might be fabricated to aid in maintaining functional position of the right hand if significant spasticity is present. The occupational therapy program complements that of PT in the areas of increasing upper extremity strength and endurance, and working on standing balance and tolerance for dressing or homemaking activities.

The speech pathologist evaluates and treats the various communication disorders (aphasia), as well as articulation disorders (dysarthria) and swallowing difficulties (dysphagia). With the stroke patient, the speech pathologist would evaluate the type and severity of aphasia, and institute appropriate therapy. Additional involvement would include advising other team members as well as the family on techniques to facilitate communication with the patient. (See also M. T. Sarno, *this volume.*)

The rehabilitation nurse complements the efforts of the therapists by encouraging the practice on the nursing unit of techniques learned in therapy, such as self-care activities and mobility. The nurse is also involved in maintaining ROM, and in developing bowel and bladder programs. With the stroke patient, the rehabilitation nurse would assist or supervise as needed with ADL, transfers, and ambulation, and would also work with the family in showing them how to assist their relative appropriately, while encouraging them to allow the patient to do as much as he is able.

The social worker functions as the discharge coordinator, as well as liaison between the rehabilitation team and the families of patients. In the case of the stroke patient, the social worker might counsel the family concerning the psychosocial, economic, and vocational implications of the stroke, and discuss available options in community agencies and services.

In addition to cognitive and personality testing, the clinical psychologist can aid the stroke patient (and family) in coping with the effects of the sudden and catastrophic event. The psychologist might provide individual or group counseling to help him cope with and adapt to his unexpectedly altered life and lifestyle. Another role of the psychologist may involve functioning as a resource to the rehabilitation team, advising in such areas as setting realistic goals for patients and dealing with staff or patient frustration, as well as suggesting appropriate intervention with patients displaying depression, denial, lack of motivation, inappropriate behavior, and so on.

Although stroke is predominantly a disease of the elderly, one-third of all stroke victims are under age 60. Many of these individuals were actively employed at the time of their stroke, and a significant proportion are interested in returning to work. For such people, as well as any individual in the working age range who becomes disabled from illness or injury, a vocational counselor provides a valuable service. Evaluation of present or predicted vocational potential, counseling as to vocational alternatives, specific education or training for a new or altered career, and assistance in obtaining or returning to work are among the services available. For the stroke patient, the vocational counselor may additionally be able to provide financial sponsorship for equipment or training to enable the individual to return to work.

The physiatrist (physician specializing in rehabilitation medicine) functions as the overall team organizer and leader. The physiatrist performs the comprehensive evaluation of the individual, determining the causes and extent of disability, predicting the potential for functional improvement, and then developing the overall rehabilitation team program. Although all health professionals are experts within their respective fields, it is the physiatrist who can, by taking into account the total needs of the individual, integrate and coordinate their talents for the maximum benefit to that individual. In the case of the stroke patient, the physiatrist evaluates the degree of disability and rehabilitation potential, and sets up the goal-oriented multidisciplinary rehabilitation program. Anticipating and preventing (or treating) complications, educating the patient and family, and coordinating subsequent health care are other responsibilities of the physiatrist.

Goals

It is important to determine whether the goals for an individual are restorative rehabilitation, in the sense of reversing disability and improving function, or maintenance, implying preservation of current level of function and preventing complications. The intensity and type of input differs greatly between these two categories. Using the example of the man who has suffered a stroke, a maintenance program would be indicated during the initial phase of his hospitalization. This entails maintaining normal range of motion of the hemiparetic limbs to avoid painful contractures, and mobilizing the patient out of bed as soon as possible, to minimize the risk of thrombophlebitis. To avoid poor nutrition secondary to difficulty in opening containers or cutting up food, or from lack of awareness of one side of the tray (due to visual field cut), the patient's eating should be supervised. Equally important are establishing bowel and bladder programs to avoid constipation, incontinence, or infection, and monitoring skin status with frequent changes of position to prevent skin breakdown. Although a therapist could reinforce or augment several of these functions, most of this maintenance or preventive care can be performed by an informed and aware nursing staff. A physiatrist could function as a consultant during this period, when the main emphasis is on neurologic work-up and medical care and stabilization. In addition to making specific recommendations for maintenance care, the physiatrist could coordinate involvement of the rehabilitation team, as the patient moves into the phase of needing restorative rehabilitation.

In this phase, the patient is essentially medically stable, and the major goal is to reverse the residual functional disability. This is the appropriate time for the various members of the rehabilitation team to become actively involved, with overall coordination and direction provided by the physiatrist. Ideally, the individual will achieve independence in self-care activities and mobility, will have adjusted psychologically and emotionally to his altered lifestyle, and will return home with the family adequately educated and prepared to encourage, supervise, or otherwise assist appropriately.

At this point, the stroke individual passes from the restorative phase back into a maintenance phase. However, this stage differs from the immediately poststroke phase since the goals now involve maintaining the level of function acquired during the restorative program. Much of this can be accomplished by a properly trained and involved family, consistently encouraging their relative to continue to do all functional tasks of which he is capable. This is not to say that functional improvement can not continue in this setting. Indeed it can and often does. The major thrust, however, is on maintaining acquired levels of function.

If there is a subsequent deterioration of function (for example, a fall with a fractured hip, or deconditioning secondary to flu-induced bedrest), a restorative rehabilitation program may once again be indicated, to regain lost function. This ties into the continuing nature of rehabilitation, with periodic follow-up evaluation or intervention as appropriate.

This concept is even more important when considering the elderly. Rudd and Margolin define maintenance therapy in a geriatric setting as "therapeutic measures which will retard deterioration in patients who are chronically ill by either slowing or arresting the process, albeit temporarily" (18). With typically multiple chronic or progressive diseases, a maintenance program to preserve optimal function is critical, and is best coordinated with a comprehensive program of medical management. Such a program may involve periodic physician visits, with frequent interim home visits (every 1 to 2 weeks) by a public health nurse. The latter may serve several purposes, including monitoring compliance with medication regimens, instructing and supervising the patient and family in specific nursing care techniques, and evaluating overall health (and functional) status in the home setting. Periodic home visits by a therapist may also prove beneficial, serving to reassess functional status, revise and reinforce home exercise and activity programs, and in general to provide encouragement to the individual and family in keeping active.

This type of organized health surveillance system can also help to identify if and when the individual requires more intensive care, most often as a result of an acute exacerbation of an illness or an injury (24). A restorative rehabilitation program may then be instituted, reverting back to the maintenance program once optimal functional and health status is achieved. It is not uncommon for the elderly to require short periods of restorative care at varying intervals (for functional "retuning") with interim maintenance programs to maintain a particular level of function. Related benefits of a maintenance rehabilitation program include improved quality of life, less frequent hospitalization, and less depression due to added socialization and psychological support (18).

Setting

There are a variety of settings in which rehabilitation involvement may occur, related primarily to the factors of goals (restorative versus maintenance) and intensity of involvement indicated, and which team members are necessary to implement the specific program.

The initial contact with rehabilitation for many elderly individuals is during hospitalization for treatment of an acute illness or injury that has resulted in deterioration of function. Examples might include a person requiring surgical repair of a fractured hip suffered in a fall, someone deconditioned secondary to prolonged bedrest during treatment of an acute infectious disease, or an individual poststroke. In most general hospitals, a restorative therapy program would be started, often limited to one discipline. Although PT is almost always available, OT and speech therapy are much less frequently available.

Although this limited program is sufficient for the majority of hospitalized patients, a person with severe and multiple functional deficits (such as after a severe stroke) would benefit most from a comprehensive and intensive restorative program, with multiple therapy involvement. In such a case, transfer to a rehabilitation unit may be indicated and most appropriate. The rehabilitation unit, which may be a free-standing center or part of a general hospital, represents the practical application of the concept of rehabilitation previously discussed. A full complement of team members, representing all the disciplines previously discussed, provides a comprehensive, goal-directed, and coordinated team approach. The program is tailored to accomplish specific goals, based on the potential, motivation and needs of the individual and family. In addition to availability of all disciplines, involvement in individual therapies is usually much more intense than that available in hospitals without specific rehabilitation units. This is true both in terms of greater frequency of attending therapy (usually twice daily) and more comprehensive and individualized therapy programs. Another factor is that team members on the rehabilitation unit have more training and experience in dealing with the multiple and severely disabled individual. Continuity of care is accomplished by organized disposition planning with the individual and family, including home modifications, equipment, community services, ongoing medical care, and rehabilitation follow-up evaluation. The organization and functions of a sample rehabilitation unit will be discussed in further detail in a subsequent section.

From a rehabilitation program as an inpatient, an individual, on discharge home, can be phased into a less intense program as necessary. This can occur either on an outpatient basis at a local hospital or rehabilitation facility, or via community services in the home. Although such involvement is usually primarily maintenance in nature, a limited restorative program may also be provided.

Disciplines offering outpatient services are usually limited to the therapy areas, in particular PT and to a lesser extent OT and speech therapy. Although individuals may be seen daily for a limited period of time, frequency of visits usually range from several times per week to once a month or less. The therapist will usually instruct the individual and family members in a home exercise and activity program to continue during interim periods between visits, with reevaluation, reinforcement, and revision of the home program during therapy sessions. Psychological counseling and vocational evaluation and training services may also be available on an ambulatory basis.

A concept applied successfully in Great Britain to facilitate transition of geriatric patients from hospital to home is that of the day hospital (3). Transportation is provided for elderly individuals from their home to the day hospital, where a variety of programs and services can be provided. These include physician, nursing and therapy involvement, socialization, and lunch. These programs have resulted in earlier discharge home, with less frequent subsequent readmission, and less frequent institutionalization.

Depending on the region, a variety of community services can be provided in the home setting, including PT, OT, speech therapy, nursing, and homemaker or home health aide (17). Usually the community health or visiting health nurse will evaluate the home situation, with provision of services as appropriate. The nurse usually visits from once to several times per week, checking vital signs, medication and diet compliance, skin or wound care, and so on. The home health aide, visiting for up to several hours on a daily basis, can be instructed to provide certain types of nursing care (e.g., wound dressings), as well as assistance to the individual for self-care activities, mobility, and meal preparation. Frequency of therapist visits depends on the needs of the individual and goals of the home program. Although daily or several times per week visits may be possible for a short period of time for a limited restorative program, once every one to two weeks visits are more common. With this latter maintenance type of program, a home health aide or family member might be instructed in a specific activity and exercise program to be carried out on a daily basis. The therapist would then reevaluate and revise the program as appropriate during the weekly or biweekly visit.

An example of a restorative program continuing after discharge home might be an amputee undergoing further gait training with prosthesis, trying to progress from a walker or crutches to a cane. The advantages of an outpatient setting include the availability of a variety of sophisticated equipment that can be used to augment the therapy program. Examples may include exercise apparatus for strengthening upper or lower extremities, and therapeutic modalities, such as diathermy, to aid in stretching out contractures. In contrast, advantages of a therapy program in the home include working with the individuals in the actual environment in which they will be functioning. This may be particularly useful in working on stairs, rugs, or uneven surfaces outdoors, as well as making suggestions for structural modifications or equipment purchases.

A maintenance program for the same amputee individual, after training is complete, might involve periodic reevaluations to check for complications (e.g., joint contractures, skin breakdown) and to revise and reinforce home exercise and activity programs. This can again be accomplished either on an outpatient basis or with a visiting therapist in the home. Once the individual and family members become well versed in the maintenance program, professional involvement can be phased out progressively, with reinvolvement only on an as-needed basis. This implies the individual and family are reliable, and understand what circumstances require professional intervention. They should also know how to contact the appropriate agencies or individuals.

Although it is most common for such outpatient or home therapy programs to be set up after hospitalization for an acute event, this is not a prerequisite. Indeed, a limited restorative or basic maintenance therapy program (outpatient or in-home) may be prescribed by a physician to avoid hospitalization for an individual. Examples might include an elderly person who becomes deconditioned secondary to a bout of influenza (short restorative program), or someone with gouty arthritis resulting in significant joint destruction and secondary pain and limitation of motion (maintenance program in conjunction with anti-inflammatory/analgesic drugs).

Another setting that must be considered in dealing with the elderly is that of the long-term care facility. Most long-term care facilities (proprietary or boarding home, health-related or intermediate level, skilled nursing or nursing home) offer some form of therapeutic program for their residents. This most often consists of physical therapy, perhaps in conjunction with recreational therapy and the nursing staff. Occupational and speech therapy are available much less commonly and to a limited population. A good maintenance program (to maintain strength, endurance, mobility, and current level of function) would ideally be coordinated between a trained and attentive nursing staff, and recreational and physical therapy. Limited restorative therapy programs may be indicated to reverse deterioration of function from an acute exacerbation of an illness, or to try to improve function to a level that would permit an individual to move to a lower level of care (ideally back into the community with relatives, friends, or community services).

Timing

Ideally, the patient hospitalized with an illness or injury that significantly interferes with function should be referred for rehabilitation evaluation as early as possible. This is particulary true with major or catastrophic illness or injury and in any elderly patient in whom reserves are limited and the adverse effects of deconditioning appear rapidly. Early rehabilitation involvement maximizes effectiveness of rehabilitation input, enabling the therapist to concentrate on improving range of motion, strength, and function, rather than diverting time and effort trying to reverse complications. Even in the intensive care unit with a medically unstable patient, the therapist can work with the nursing staff on maintaining range of motion, avoiding skin breakdown, and preserving muscle strength and endurance. As the patient stabilizes, the therapy program can progress to working on mobility and self-care ability.

For the patient with multiple and severe functional deficits, referral to a rehabilitation unit for a comprehensive, intensive therapy program should also occur early. This allows arrangements to be made for transfer when most appropriate, resulting in greater time, personnel, and cost efficiency, and maximum benefit to the patient.

The majority of the elderly do not reside in long-term care facilities or hospitals, but are living in the community. They often have few or no family support systems, having lost their spouse and siblings, and their children having moved away. In this situation, an individual's ability to cope with multiple illnesses and still function independently may be precarious. A relatively minor exacerbation of a chronic illness may prove sufficient to disrupt the balance. Prompt involvement in the community health support services system may avoid hospitalization. More importantly, it may prevent the significant secondary deterioration of function that would necessitate institutional placement. Most commonly, the family physician, relatives, or neighbors are the first to become aware of the deteriorating home situation. It is crucial that they be aware of the availability of various community services, and know how to get them involved.

TEAM STRUCTURE AND DYNAMICS

The structure of a sample rehabilitation unit will be analyzed, including discussion of the team functions relating to achieving goal-oriented and coordinated patient care. Issues of team dynamics will also be explored, including leadership, membership, and communication.

Team Functions

For the elderly who must enter a hospital-based rehabilitation program, the experience can be extremely stressful. The patient entering a rehabilitation service is coming to a new environment and frequently has feelings of abandonment by the support network of family, friends, or even previous medical personnel with which a nurturing relationship had been established. This sense of abandonment occurs despite the fact that it is the patient who physically leaves the support network and not the opposite. This fear of abandonment and isolation is primal but endures for a lifetime. Because of this need for a support system the rehabilitation team can expedite the patient's adaptation to the rehabilitation service by providing a nuclear support group with which the patient can identify.

Most geriatric patients experience a period of disorientation when they are initially admitted to a rehabilitation service. It is important for the team to be aware of this transient confusion and reorientation rather than to label inappropriately the person as demented or psychotically disoriented. To facilitate the patient's adaptation to the rehabilitation unit the team should provide consistent structure to the patients' environment and activities. Written schedules of daily activities and an ongoing reality orientation program are helpful for the new patient (22). During the first critical days after admission, it is also beneficial to limit the number of staff members working with the patient. This gives the patient an opportunity to establish a relationship with specific team members and develop a sense of continuity with the rehabilitation team.

As the patient becomes more secure and established, increasing amounts of information concerning the rehabilitation process and team functions can be presented. Patients are often curious about the meetings and functions of their rehabilitation team and in most cases feel reassured that the team meets regularly to discuss the patient's progress.

Case Conference

Within one week of admission, members of the patient's team will meet to develop a comprehensive rehabilitation plan. Prior to this meeting (or case conference) each team member will have assessed the patient and, working in conjunction with the patient, will have developed individual goals by discipline for the patient's rehabilitation (20). Each discipline reviews its findings and goals with the entire team. Based on these evaluations, team goals are identified and a comprehensive rehabilitation plan is established. It is important to incorporate into the plan the patient's goals and self-assessment since the patient is a partner with the team in the rehabilitation process. It is the responsibility of the physician to record the overall patient care plan for the rehabilitation team, based on the case conference.

The case conference is also important because it establishes a format, based on the patient's problems, for subsequent meetings throughout the patient's rehabilitation. The patient's problems also play a role in determining the composition of the rehabilitation team. From the more active members of the patient's team, one person is selected to be the patient's case recorder or discussion leader. The discussion leader will be responsible for documenting in the medical record all subsequent team meetings concerning their patient.

The first review during the case conference is a physician summary of the patient's history and physical exam. This review allows each team member to have a more appropriate awareness of the patient's overall physical status and medical problems. The physician also presents an initial problem list that can be modified as additional information is presented and discussed.

Following the medical presentation, a social history that reviews family relationships, education, vocational background, and financial resources is presented. The social worker also presents information concerning the patient's premorbid activities, socialization, and avocational interests.

The patient's functional status is reviewed by the occupational therapist. This evaluation usually includes a summary of the patient's ADLs, sensory testing, upper extremity strength, range of motion and function, as well as any perceptual difficulties. The rehabilitation nurse also reviews the patient's self-care function and presents issues that might overlap any of the disciplines.

The physical therapist reports primarily on mobility, lower extremity function, ambulation, and transfers. Language difficulties are reviewed by the speech pathologist, and both intellectual and emotional issues are addressed by the psychologist.

After each discipline has reported the results of their evaluations, goals for the patient's comprehensive rehabilitation are identified. These goals become the criteria for assessing the patient's progress, and a length of stay that should enable the patient to achieve these goals is estimated.

Within a few days of the case conference, a family conference is scheduled for the patient, the patient's family, and the rehabilitation team to discuss the patient's progress and current status, review the rehabilitation goals, and consider potential discharge plans. Discharge planning is an essential component of the rehabilitation program and should be an integral part of all plans from the time of admission (3).

Weekly Team Meetings

Once each week every patient on the rehabilitation service is reviewed by the team. During these meetings, goals from the previous week are reviewed and the patient's progress is assessed. It is the responsibility of the team member designated as discussion leader to record the information presented by each member of the patient's team. This information is recorded in the patient's chart under a heading of *team meeting*. The format for reporting the results of the team meeting includes the following.

Medical

A physician review of the patient's medical status with emphasis on any significant changes that might affect the patient's rehabilitation program. Precautions or new directions for the patient during rehabilitation are presented to the staff.

Continence

Continence is often a major factor in determining discharge plans. Because of its significance, a separate section is allocated for discussion of the patient's bowel and bladder status. Bowel and bladder management plans are developed, monitored, and documented in this section of the patient's record.

Communication

A section is allocated for documentation of speech or language difficulties. In this section the speech pathologist will review, document, and monitor patient progress as well as identify how the team can facilitate the patient's improvement with language difficulties.

ADL

The ADL section is subdivided into categories of feeding, grooming, bathing, and dressing. Nursing and occupational therapy usually present most of the information recorded under this section. It is important that the patient's activities be reported very specifically so significant changes can be documented and continuing problems can be both identified and programmed for resolution during the patient's rehabilitation stay.

Mobility

Mobility has also been subdivided into its more significant components: bed mobility, transfers, wheelchair function, and ambulation. During the patient's rehabilitation there will often be a natural shift in focus from limited, simple tasks to very complex, almost unlimited tasks associated with unsupervised mobility. Again specific documentation is essential to establish the patient's progress and determine future directions for the rehabilitation plan.

Neuromuscular

The neuromuscular section is where changes in muscle tone, strength, and function are recorded. It is also a section used to denote significant neurological changes that might affect the patient's rehabilitation program.

Cognitive-Emotional

The patient's psychological status is usually recorded under this section. Changes in intellectual function, mood, and affect are typically addressed and documented.

Social-Disposition

The impact of the patient's problems on the family and social environment is documented under this section. It is also an area where discharge plans and estimated length of stay are developed.

Goals

After the patient's progress and status have been thoroughly discussed and reviewed, the team identifies its goals for the patient's rehabilitation during the coming weeks. Goals are established for each discipline and documented under the appropriate heading, including medical, nursing, occupational therapy, physical therapy, speech, psychology, and social work.

Goal setting should be target specific. Thereby, each discipline establishes exactly what they hope to accomplish during the coming week. Care should be taken not to express goals in so nebulous a way as to make accountability impossible. Studies in team goal setting in rehabilitation have indicated that attainment of goals is enhanced when goals are expressed in measurable terms (21). For example, a nonspecific goal of "increased ambulation" is replaced with a specific goal of "increase this patient's ambulation distance from 75 feet to 200 feet." Similarly, a medical goal of "monitor" is replaced with "patient's medical status will be reviewed three times during the coming week through direct contact between patient and physician."

As a rule, several members of the rehabilitation team will visit the patient's home to assess the environment with regard to architectural barriers. Based on this assessment, recommendations can be made for modifications in the home as well as the need for adaptive devices. Additionally, the patient's rehabilitation program can be better tailored to facilitate a return home.

Toward the end of their rehabilitation program, patients are encouraged to return home on therapeutic weekend passes. This helps the patient and family to identify practical problems at home that can be addressed prior to actual discharge.

Within two weeks of discharge another meeting is scheduled for the patient, family, and rehabilitation team. This final family meeting is a time to review the patient's progress, current rehabilitative status, and discharge plans. Discharge planning has been an integral part of the patient's rehabilitation from admission, when an estimated length of stay was presented to the family. As the estimate was replaced by reality the family was regularly informed of any changes by the social worker, so they could have a time frame and appropriately plan for discharge.

This final family conference is also a time when the need for continuing therapy as well as arrangements for equipment, community services, and medical and rehabilitation follow-up can be discussed.

Team Dynamics

Although there are many issues in geriatric rehabilitation that do involve the patient directly in the rehabilitation process, there are some that influence the process but do not involve the patient. Many of these issues center around the dynamics of the team as a group. These issues include team leadership, membership, and communications.

Leadership

Leadership is the most critical issue in the function of a multidisciplinary rehabilitation team. Without appropriate leadership, the team fragments into independent, discordant units struggling to gain a sense of control, structure, and balance. Within the rehabilitation team, as within all task-oriented groups, there is an inherent need for order and structure. The fulfillment of this need provides security and enables the group to direct its energy toward the accomplishment of productive tasks. Otherwise, the group focuses its energy on the establishment of order and structure. This results in a constant internal focus with little energy, time, or productivity for patient rehabilitation.

Leadership exists in all productive groups. Unfortunately, the qualities necessary for leadership are not always found in those people who must direct others. For the rehabilitation team to function most effectively the physician should be the leader. By law and custom the physician is the person responsible for overall team supervision, and is ultimately accountable for the patient's care (13,14). However, the dynamics of leadership do not always acknowledge the legal status of the person leading the team. Leadership by virtue of status or position is quickly lost in practical settings unless the leader has and appropriately uses power.

Power does not mean the leader functions as an autocratic dictator, for rehabilitation is a team effort embracing the concept that no one individual can meet the complex needs of rehabilitation patients (23). Rather, power is the ability to elicit the maximum function from each team member for the enhancement of the patient's rehabilitation.

It is difficult to identify a single leadership style most appropriate for a rehabilitation team. Unfortunately, leadership styles are usually presented in a continuum from autocratic (dictatorial) through democratic to laissez-faire (indifferent). It is important to stress the fallacy of labeling a given leadership style solely in terms of absolutes such as these (15).

The autocratic leader is not necessarily a demagog who relies on coercive tactics to ensure compliance. Autocracy also embraces positive concepts such as the acceptance of responsibility, the ability to make decisions, and accountability for success or failure.

Because of social and cultural bias it is more acceptable to be labeled a democratic leader, but is this the best approach to use in a medical situation where a variety of professionals may have divergent views on the most pressing needs of an aging patient? Potential drawbacks of this leadership style may include the inability to reach a decision, as well as the inappropriate exercise of group control.

The label of laissez-faire is also an offensive one for it implies a lack of control and competency. Yet, this leadership style allows for individual initiative, creativity, and motivation.

What general conclusions can then be drawn concerning leadership and leadership style? First and foremost, leadership for a rehabilitation team is not an issue of absolutes but of practical necessities. In addition, the style of leadership directly affects the functions of the team and ultimately the service to the patient. Finally, it is important to stress that leadership is a dynamic process, changing with the needs of the team and patient. Generally, as the patient functions with greater safety and independence, the rehabilitation team leader will be able to expand the functions of leadership to a greater number of team members. Similarly, as a team matures, greater responsibility and authority can be delegated to team members by the leader.

Membership

Rehabilitation is a process involving many disciplines. Each discipline brings to the team a unique and valuable perspective that can enhance the function of the team (15). Therefore, no single discipline is of greater or lesser importance on the rehabilitation team. Similarly, each team member as a representative of a discipline has a right to express an opinion concerning issues before the team. Care should be taken to ensure that each person is afforded the opportunity to express concerns, feelings, findings, and contributions for the patient's rehabilitation.

Rehabilitation teams are also interdependent and cooperative, with members crossing traditional disciplinary boundaries to address the complex issues involved in comprehensive rehabilitation. This demands that team members be aware of their own abilities, limitations, and how their activities affect the programming of other team members. Team members must not only respect one another but they must also be able to confront one another, to disagree when necessary, and to monitor each other's functions to ensure the highest quality of care for their patients (8).

To function at this level requires that team members be mature and secure in their knowledge, position, and value as a team member. The key to harmonious membership lies in mutual respect and a basic acceptance of each discipline's right to participate in the rehabilitation process.

Communications

Communication barriers have been identified as a primary obstacle to interpersonal collaboration (7). If these barriers are to be removed, the team must maintain a commitment to information sharing. The rehabilitation team, as a component in an evolutionary process, must have ready access to essential information as well as an active system of information feedback and dispersal.

Barriers to communication, such as vested interests, differences in philosophy or interpersonal conflicts, should be quickly identified, confronted, and eliminated. To accomplish this task, the systems for communication must be readily available to all team members and regularly used.

Effective communication must not only exist within the team but should also extend outward to embrace the patient and family. Coordination of information presented will avoid confusion due to conflicting messages. The converse should also apply. The team should encourage and be receptive to input from the patient and family.

A communications system of this nature allows the free exchange of information. This strengthens the team's ability to develop the most appropriate rehabilitation program. It also acknowledges the roles of the patient and family in the rehabilitation process.

BENEFITS OF REHABILITATION

In this era of escalating inflation and high health care costs, questions of cost-effectiveness are increasingly raised. In light of the apparent high costs involved with rehabilitation efforts, and the increases in the elderly population, these questions are particularly relevant. Unfortunately, the literature is sparse with regard to studies evaluating cost-effectiveness of rehabilitation intervention. This is true with specific disease or disability categories, as well as the general population of elderly and/or disabled individuals.

However, analysis of data from a variety of sources may prove enlightening. Dow et al. (4) studied the effects of developing a rehabilitation program in a general hospital on discharge patterns for stroke patients. Comparing patients with strokes of equal severity, they found the percentage of those returning home increased from 13 to 58%, with no similar trend at other area hospitals during a comparable period. Similarly, Anderson et al. (1) compared outcomes of patients poststroke with and without rehabilitation. Of those not receiving rehabilitation, 42% were institutionalized, compared to only 18% of the rehabilitated group.

The importance of these significant differences becomes even clearer when Kottke's data on relative costs of different levels of institutionalization are considered (10). He conservatively estimated the costs of institutional maintenance care of a totally dependent individual as approximately $8,300 per year, in 1972. By solely improving this individual's level of function to the point that he was able to feed himself, the annual institutional costs decreased by $2,300 to $6,000. If that individual became partly independent (to the point of independent ambulation and limited self-care) the annual costs decreased to $4,600. If he achieved complete independence, but still needed room and board, the annual cost decreased further to $2,400. If the individual had an interested and involved family, he probably would have been cared for adequately at home when he reached either of the latter two functional levels, thereby eliminating all institutional costs. Even if rehabilitation intervention only results in a limited functional improvement, this still represented a sizeable reduction in maintenance costs. Kottke estimated that the savings in these types of maintenance costs through rehabilitation efforts run into the billions of dollars annually.

In addition to trying to regain an optimal functional level and enable the individual to return to live in the community, rehabilitation efforts are also directed toward maintaining the acquired functional and environmental status. This is accomplished primarily by educating and training families of patients (2), as well as detailed disposition planning with coordination of equipment, services, and follow-up. Lehman et al. (11) demonstrated that the improvements achieved by a group of stroke patients during rehabilitation were well maintained over a period of up to four years after discharge.

Emphasizing the critical nature of appropriate disposition planning, Brocklehurst (3) found that in cases of elderly hospitalized individuals returning to previous living situations, 21% of such returns were viewed as unwelcome by their relatives. The frequent hospital readmissions resulting from inadequate discharge planning has more than just monetary implications. Rosin and Boyd (16) identified 70% of geriatric patients admitted to a hospital as having developed a complication occurring after admission. One-half of these complications were incidental, unrelated to the illness. The most common complications included respiratory infections, falls, drug reactions, and decubitus ulcers.

Aside from the monetary implications of rehabilitation in the elderly, there are important considerations relating to quality of life. As self-care functional ability deteriorates, psychological and social adjustment problems increase. A major goal of the rehabilitation team, with the comprehensive approach considering medical, functional, psychoemotional, socioeconomic, sexual, and vocational factors, is to help the individual live a useful and happy life.

To summarize the benefits of rehabilitation, consider the following statement by Krusen, as modified by Kottke: "As modern medicine is adding years to life, rehabilitation becomes increasingly essential to add meaningful life to these years" (10).

REFERENCES

1. Anderson, T. P., Baldridge, M., and Ettinger, M. G. (1979): Quality of care for completed stroke without rehabilitation: Evaluation by assessing patient outcomes. *Arch. Phys. Med. Rehabil.,* 60:103–107.
2. Bray, G. P. (1980): Team strategies for family involvement in rehabilitation. *J. Rehabil.,* 46:20–23.
3. Brocklehurst, J. C. (1978): Geriatric services and the day hospital. In: *Textbook of Geriatric Medicine and Gerontology,* edited by J. C. Brocklehurst, pp. 747–762. Churchill Livingstone, New York.
4. Dow, R. S., Dick, H. L., and Crowell, F. A. (1974): Failures and successes in a stroke program. *Stroke,* 5:40–47.
5. Fordyce, W. E. (1982): Psychological assessment and management. In: *Krusens' Handbook of Physical Medicine and Rehabilitation,* edited by F. J. Kottke, G. K. Stillwell, and J. F. Lehman, pp. 124–150. W. B. Saunders, Philadelphia.
6. Gullickson, G., and Licht, S. (1968): Definition and philosophy of rehabilitation medicine. In: *Rehabilitation and Medicine,* edited by S. Licht, pp. 1–14. Elizabeth Licht, New Haven, Conn.
7. Haselkorn, F. (1958): Some dynamic aspects of interprofessional practice in rehabilitation. *Soc. Casework,* 37:396–400.
8. Hawke, W. A., and Auerbach, A. (1975): Multi-discipline experience: A fresh approach to aid the multi-handicapped child. *J. Rehabil.,* 41:22–24.

 9. Hirschberg, G. G., Lewis, L., and Vaughan, P. (1976): Levels and places of rehabilitation. In: *Rehabilitation—A Manual for the Care of the Disabled and Elderly,* edited by G. G. Hirschberg, L. Lewis, and P. Vaughan, pp. 143–155. Lippincott, Philadelphia.
10. Kottke, F. J. (1974): Historia obscura hemiplegiae. *Arch. Phys. Med. Rehabil.,* 55:4–13.
11. Lehman, J. F., DeLateur, B. J., Fowler, R. S., Warren, C. G., Arnhold, R., Schertzer, G., Hurka, R., Whitmore, J. J., Masock, A. J., and Chambers, K. H. (1975): Stroke: Does rehabilitation affect outcome. *Arch. Phys. Med. Rehab.,* 56:375–382.
12. Licht, S. (ed) (1968): *Rehabilitation and Medicine.* Elizabeth Licht, New Haven, Conn.
13. Matheson, L. N. (1975): The interdisciplinary team in cardiac rehabilitation. *Rehabil. Lit.,* 36:366–375.
14. McCoin, J. M. (1973): A quest for dynamic leadership in the mental health rehabilitation team. *Clin. Soc. Work J.,* 1:32–37.
15. Napier, R. W., and Gershenfeld, M. K. (1973): *Groups: Theory and Experience.* Houghton Mifflin Co., Boston.
16. Rosin, A. J., and Boyd, R. V. (1966): Complications of illness in geriatric hospital patients. *J. Chronic Dis.,* 19:307–313.
17. Rossman, I. (1979): Environments of geriatric care. In: *Clinical Geriatrics,* edited by I. Rossman, pp. 668–680. Lippincott, Philadelphia.
18. Rudd, J. L., and Margolin, R. J. (eds) (1968): *Maintenance Therapy for the Geriatric Patient.* Charles C Thomas, Springfield, Ill.
19. Rusk, H. A. (1977): *Rehabilitation Medicine.* C. V. Mosby, St. Louis.
20. Saper, B. (1974): Patients as partners in a team approach. *Am. J. Nurs.,* 74:1844–1847.
21. Schmitt, N., et al. (1980): *Goal Setting by Nurses and Patients in a Rehabilitation Environment.* Presentation, American Congress of Rehabilitation Medicine, Washington, D.C., October, 1980.
22. Stryker-Gordon, R. (1977): *Administration of Rehabilitative Care in the Long-Term Care Facility.* American College of Nursing Home Administrators, Bethesda, Md.
23. Wagner, R. J. (1977): Rehabilitation team practice. *Rehabil. Counsel. Bull.,* 20:206–217.
24. Williams, T. F., Hill, J. G., Fairbanks, M. E., and Knox, K. G. (1973): Appropriate placement of the chronically ill and aged. *JAMA,* 226:1332–1335.

Rehabilitation in the Aging edited by
T. F. Williams. Raven Press, New York © 1984.

Rehabilitation of the Patient with Stroke

Charles J. Gibson and Bruce M. Caplan

Rehabilitation Division, Department of Preventive, Family, and Rehabilitation Medicine, University of Rochester, School of Medicine and Dentistry, Rochester, New York 14642

The various categories of cerebral vascular accident (stroke) constitute the third leading cause of death in the United States, trailing only heart disease and cancer. Stroke is also a leading cause of physical and emotional morbidity. Deaths attributed to stroke have been slowly declining in recent years, and the incidence of stroke in the United States may also be diminishing (15). However, with over 200,000 new episodes of completed stroke occurring in this country each year, two-thirds of them affecting people age 65 and over, stroke will remain a frequent adversary for the physician who cares for an aged population.

Hypertension is the major risk factor for stroke, and indeed, if the incidence of stroke is declining, this may be partially attributed to better medical treatment of hypertension. Other significant risk factors include a history of transient ischemic attacks, diabetes mellitus, and coronary artery disease or cardiac arrhythmias. There is relatively little difference in incidence rates between men and women, although some surveys show men to be at slightly greater risk (19).

The rehabilitation of stroke patients presents an enormous challenge to both health professionals and the community. The condition is common and the functional consequences often serious. But in view of the enhanced longevity of poststroke patients (more than half survive seven years) and the proven benefits and cost-effectiveness of rehabilitative therapy (20), the widespread availability of such programs is clearly desirable.

Rehabilitation produces its best results when initiated as soon as possible. A rehabilitation program should be instituted within 48 hours of hospital admission, and the intensity of the program increased as the patient's medical condition stabilizes. In addition to minimizing possible complications (which rehabilitation staffs clearly have a vested interest in preventing), this helps to forestall the possibility of patients developing inefficient compensatory behaviors which later have to be unlearned.

EARLY CARE

Several aspects of early care may significantly affect the rate of progress and even the ultimate rehabilitation achievement. Two essential responsibilities are the maintenance of joint range of motion and prevention of pressure sores. Range of motion of the affected extremity should begin no later than the second or third day in the hospital. This can be performed by physical therapists, occupational therapists, or nurses, the quality of the individual professional being more important than the professional degree. In the early flaccid stage, each joint in an affected extremity should be carried through the complete range of motion daily with three to five repetitions. With increasing spasticity, the program may need to be carried out twice daily, perhaps with an increased number of repetitions. Any muscle that does not have the ability to achieve full range of motion against gravity actively must receive passive range of motion.

A foot board is frequently used to prevent foot drop, although it is not always easy to position the patient's foot properly against the board, and skin breakdown on soles of the feet may occur if excessive pressure is allowed. Foot drop can be prevented in most instances by attention to the necessary passive joint range of motion. Resting splints for the wrist and fingers may be useful for maintaining the hand in the functional position. It must be emphasized that passive joint range of motion should be given gently by experienced personnel. Otherwise, soft tissue injury can occur from overzealous stretching, which may produce superimposed disability, slowing the rate of recovery and possibly producing pain when the patient becomes active.

Pressure sores can usually be prevented if adequate nursing staff is available. Such nurses must be well versed in skin care of the paralyzed and/or cognitively impaired patient. Pressure sores may develop over any bony prominence, but in stroke patients they are most likely to occur over the occiput, sacrum, greater trochanters, and malleoli. A variety of mattresses and bed surfaces have been developed with the aim of aiding in the prevention of sores, but the crucial factor in prevention is good nursing care. Ideally, the patient should be turned in bed every 2 hr. One must exercise care when turning a patient onto the affected side, as this may create pain in the shoulder area. Uncooperative patients may refuse to stay in the position in which they have been placed, often returning to the supine position and thereby increasing the likelihood of a sacral pressure sore.

While the patient is still in bed, the nurses should attempt to support flaccid extremities in a neutral position and prevent prolonged overstretching of weakened muscles. In particular, the affected shoulder should be abducted for at least some periods of time when the patient is supine, and the affected hip can be kept in the neutral position with pillows, rolled towels, or sand bags placed against the lateral side of the thigh and calf. The affected hand may easily become edematous if not elevated intermittently.

Cognitively impaired patients are particularly prone to complications from sensory deprivation, especially if hospitalized in a private room. Such patients should be placed with their uninvolved side nearest the entrance to the room so that they can receive sensory input from the surrounding ward or hall. Radios or television sets may also provide needed stimulation. When the patient's mental status permits, the staff should attempt, gently, to keep the patient oriented to time and place.

Some patients with stroke have difficulty swallowing. These patients often do very poorly with liquids, and they are likely to be better able to eat solid foods of smooth texture (e.g., puddings). When these foods can be swallowed easily, the patient can advance to finely chopped foods even though they may still have difficulty swallowing liquids.

As soon as they are medically stable, patients should be gotten out of bed, even if they are only able to sit in a chair at bedside for a period of 15 min. However, care must be taken to support the affected extremities. In such cases, the impaired arm should be supported on a pillow or by use of a sling. The foot must not be allowed to remain in the plantar flexed position for extended periods of time.

EVALUATION OF REHABILITATION POTENTIAL

When evaluating the rehabilitation potential of a stroke patient, the physician must estimate the probable functional outcome and discharge disposition in order to decide whether a full rehabilitation program will be of significant benefit. The standard goals of rehabilitation for stroke patients include preventing complications, compensating for the physical and intellectual loss and minimizing the social and economic loss.

Prevention of complications has been considered in the preceding section. Compensation for the physical and intellectual loss refers to maximization of the patient's independence in mobility and self-care skills, and improvement in communication and cognitive/perceptual skills. Minimizing the social loss refers primarily to reintegration of the patient into the family and community. Conservation of the patient's and family's economic resources can best be achieved if the patient can be kept out of a nursing home or other long-term care facility. This is also cost-effective to the community, as most long-term nursing home residents eventually become dependent on public support. Therefore, a major rehabilitation goal should be to return as many patients as possible to private living situations.

One might question the cost-effectiveness of intensive rehabilitation services provided to patients whose inevitable destination is a nursing home. But improved function is certainly of value to long-term care patients in nursing homes, and reasonably good rehabilitation services are available in many of the better staffed facilities. In such cases it is advantageous for the patient to have early discharge from the acute hospital and receive rehabilitation services in the setting where the patient will be living.

In evaluating a patient for rehabilitation, one must consider the following items:

1. The patient's functional ability before the stroke.
2. The patient's social situation and options for returning to the community.

3. The patient's ability to cooperate with nurses and therapists.
4. The patient's capacity to learn new material.
5. Age of the patient.
6. Bowel and bladder (in)continence.

The importance of most of the items is self-evident. No patient is too old for rehabilitation, but one cannot ignore the impact of chronological age on the patient's motivation for and ability to participate in an active program. Persistent incontinence of bowel and/or bladder is usually regarded as a pessimistic prognostic indicator (13). This area will be covered more extensively in a later section.

Physicians should also keep in mind that rehabilitation is primarily a learning and training process, and thus proper rehabilitation candidates must have the potential to absorb and retain new skills. A brief mental status assessment (with special emphasis on memory functions) is therefore crucial. In evaluating aphasic patients, one must judge the extent to which their language difficulty will hinder their progress in rehabilitation. Some patients with aphasia suffer only minor comprehension problems, others understand very little, and still others can be helped to understand task instructions through the use of pantomime and gesture.

Evaluation of the patient's physical potential is more important for designing the rehabilitation program than for making a decision about whether or not rehabilitation is appropriate. Muscle strength, sensation, visual fields, joint range of motion and spasticity should all be assessed.

A good comprehensive rehabilitation program can improve a patient's functional status beyond that which would occur through spontaneous recovery (20), but it is difficult accurately to predict functional outcome before the patient has undergone at least some rehabilitation training. Most spontaneous recovery occurs within the first 4 to 6 months following onset (2,24), although patients may continue to improve functionally after that time through continued practice, e.g., mobility and self-care. It must be emphasized that rehabilitation requires a truly coordinated effort throughout the waking hours, in which the whole exceeds the sum of the individual contributions. The rehabilitation process suffers if therapy is doled out in isolated sessions; optimal results cannot occur if the lessons learned in therapy are not implemented elsewhere. However, when all of the professional disciplines, together with the patient and family, can agree upon common goals and a course of action, and are able to communicate frequently about progress and technique, then the patient may expect to make the kind of progress to which he is entitled.

PSYCHOLOGICAL CHANGES

The psychological changes which may be observed in the poststroke individual can be roughly divided into alterations in intellect, and alterations in personality and emotional behavior (4,18). Although particular examples of the former frequently follow involvement of specific brain regions (e.g., visuospatial deficit consequent to compromise of the right parietal lobe), the latter, while occasionally having some lateralizing or localizing significance (14,28), are more apt to reflect the patient's manner of coping with the illness and its consequences.

Comprehensive neuropsychological evaluation can provide vital information about the extent of impairment or preservation of particular mental functions in individual patients. Furthermore, such information may yield helpful suggestions for the design of remedial interventions (8). An adequate assessment should include tests of attention span, memory, language, various perceptual abilities, and higher cognitive functions such as problem solving and abstract thinking.

Common neuropsychological deficits manifested by patients with right hemisphere lesions include spatial disorientation, constructional apraxia, and a variety of visual-perceptual disorders. Frequent sequelae of left hemisphere injury include aphasia (see pp 151–152), alexia (reading difficulty), and ideomotor apraxia (inability to perform well-learned complex acts on command; e.g., "Show me how you would light a match.").

Some behavioral consequences of stroke may appear following damage to any area of the brain. Reduction of attention span is especially common, particularly in the first few weeks after onset. Some patients may appear lethargic, drowsy and inattentive, while others exhibit rapid and impulsive attentional shifts. In both instances the result is the same—inability to sustain concentration on a therapeutic task. Impulsive patients tend to ignore the functional limitations imposed by their deficits and to neglect important safety factors (e.g., failing to lock the brakes before arising from the wheelchair, walking without the necessary supportive device or physical assistance). For such patients prolonged effort will only serve further to impair their performance, resulting in the rehearsal of erroneous and inefficient techniques. A series of brief (10–15 min) one-to-one therapy sessions may be indicated initially. Lethargy tends to lessen as the patient stabilizes, but impulsivity may be a persistent problem. Self-instructional methods, which have been shown to reduce impulsive behavior in hyperactive children (22), may prove useful with poststroke patients as well.

Recent memory is often impaired to some degree, particularly with left hemisphere lesions that may affect the integrity of verbal encoding processes. Thus, new learning may be difficult which would clearly hinder the patient's progress in rehabilitation and might even dictate the delay of such a program. Mnemonic devices, imagery-based techniques or notebooks may be suitable memory aids for some patients (16,21).

It is important that the essential findings of intellectual assessments be transmitted to the patient's family, for they may have been puzzled and distressed by the behavioral sequelae of the stroke. For example, many patients with right hemisphere lesions fail to attend adequately to the left side of space, a condition known as unilateral neglect (29). This problem differs from homonymous hemianopsia in which an absolute field cut is present. Patients with a pronounced degree of neglect may bump into walls or other obstacles while walking or maneuvering their wheelchairs. Food on the left side of the tray may go uneaten, and the reduced food intake may be interpreted as a sign of depression. If approached from the "bad" side, a "neglecter" may fail to respond, and this may be variously misinterpreted. When reading, patients with subtler degrees of neglect may not see words on the left side of the page. Surprisingly, many remain unaware of these omissions, even when the flow of printed text is thereby disturbed and the sentence becomes meaningless. Patients may be taught to compensate for their inattention by the use of scanning exercises which require exaggerated head and eye movements toward the neglected side. Prominent visual anchors located on the extreme left side may be helpful (12).

The devastating impact of stroke almost invariably elicits a profound emotional response. Depression is clearly justified and is apparent in most patients who can appreciate the magnitude of their illness. However, flattening of affect, euphoric indifference, and rapid shifting of emotional state are also observed. Emotionally labile patients can be extremely sensitive to the moods and actions of people around them, and they often respond in exaggerated ways to minor incidents (so-called "emotional incontinence").

The reaction of each patient is shaped to some extent by the nature of their premorbid personality and by their characteristic manner of coping with stress. Nonetheless, patterns of adjustment are complexly determined and prediction is hazardous. Although an aggressive forceful individual may view stroke as an adversary to be conquered, the same patient, feeling a loss of prowess and self-esteem, might adopt a passive attitude and submit to the prospect of chronic disability.

The patient's emotional response to the illness determines, in large measure, their level of motivation for rehabilitation. Patients who are depressed are not ideal candidates for rehabilitation, but most patients are not depressed all of the time. Furthermore, progress in therapy can be an effective antidepressant. Nonetheless, the problem of maintaining motivation for the arduous and often lengthy process of rehabilitation is a constant one. It is advisable to focus on the achievement of a series of small manageable goals, thus providing continuing experiences of success for the patient. It is also useful to remind the patient of the progress that has been made since the start of therapy, and to encourage comparison of the current functional level to that of the week or two (not six months!) ago. Emotional support, the presence of concerned family and friends, and an active therapeutic environment all contribute to enhanced motivation. Judicious use of antidepressant medication may be useful in some difficult situations.

It is extremely important that family members understand the reasons for the behavioral changes that they will observe in the patient. Certain disturbing behaviors may be transient, treatable, or permanent, and the family should be given the prognosis for each of these behaviors as soon as consensus is reached by the treating team. While formal family counseling may only be indicated in some cases, it is the rare family that does not need opportunities to air their anger, grief, and frustration in the presence of experienced and empathic rehabilitation specialists. Stroke causes physical damage to individuals, but it induces psychological stress in entire families, and this can effectively subvert much of the rehabilitation effort.

COMMUNICATION DISORDERS

Impairment of language function is perhaps the most devastating and frustrating consequence of stroke. Depending upon the locus and extent of brain damage, any or all linguistic processes may be affected.

Poor articulation (dysarthria) may follow from involvement of either the central (cortical or subcortical) or peripheral nervous system (3). It is important to distinguish this condition from the aphasias, which are characterized by breakdown of the more unique symbolic and representational functions of human language (10,27).

Various syndromes of aphasia have been described and correlated with particular brain loci. Patients with damage to the anterior portion of the language-dominant hemisphere (usually the left) often exhibit the syndrome of Broca's aphasia, in which speech is slow and labored, but comprehension of spoken language is relatively well preserved. Lesions in the posterior temporal region may give rise to Wernicke's aphasia in which speech is fluent and well articulated but characterized by numerous neologisms, paraphasic errors, and stereotypes. Comprehension of spoken language is typically defective. Broca's and Wernicke's aphasias are sometimes called "nonfluent" and "fluent" aphasias, respectively, in reference to the quality of speech output. Reading and writing are usually impaired in both syndromes, although in different ways and to different degrees.

Patients with global aphasia, are those who can neither produce nor understand language. Lesions in such cases tend to be massive, and the prognosis is therefore poor. For some stroke patients the only linguistic deficit is difficulty retrieving single words, especially on demand. These patients can often describe the function of an item while failing to name it (anomic aphasia). Aphasic syndromes following thalamic (5) and other subcortical lesions (23) have been reported with increasing frequency in recent years.

A careful evaluation by a speech pathologist will yield a profile of the patient's linguistic strengths and weaknesses and can provide suggestions for treatment approaches. For dysarthric patients, who are often more easily understood when they speak slowly, therapy may consist largely of reinforcing reductions in the rate of speech. Patients with primarily expressive difficulties may benefit from extensive rote repetition. Several innovative techniques which may be useful for some patients with impaired expression have been introduced in recent years, including various visual symbol systems and therapies that incorporate rhythmic or melodic elements as aides to fluency. Patients with defective language comprehension may find it easier to understand pantomime or gestural communication.

In all cases, the goal of the speech therapist should be to discover the most effective means by which each patient can communicate with the staff and family. Here again, a highly individualized approach is indicated. (See also M. T. Sarno, *this volume.*)

The prognosis in aphasia is a function of several factors. The best results can be expected from patients who are relatively young, have small infarcts, are well educated, and are either left-handed or have close left-handed relatives. This last factor is related to the higher incidence in sinistrals of anomalies of cerebral dominance for language. In this group, language functions tend to be more widely distributed in the dominant hemisphere (and are sometimes bilaterally represented) than is the case in the typical right-handed person. This increases the likelihood that some cortical language areas will escape involvement and thus be able to support some degree of poststroke linguistic function.

Family members should be given a nontechnical understanding of the nature of the patient's language difficulties, as well as suggestions for communicating with the patient most effectively (e.g., use of gestures, drawings). Relatives and friends, who usually spend more time with patients than do therapists, can often provide useful reports of the patient's language performance in situations more natural than the therapeutic milieu. The importance of emotional support for patient and family alike in dealing with this frustrating and disabling condition cannot be overestimated.

UPPER EXTREMITY FUNCTION

In many patients with stroke, the upper extremity is more severely compromised than the lower. Although most people will understandably mourn the loss of this function, it is possible for a person to be quite independent with only one functional upper extremity.

It is extremely important to maintain full joint range of motion in the upper extremity, beginning very early in the hospitalization. There is a significant tendency for stroke patients to develop a painful shoulder on the affected side (6). Once established, this shoulder pain can be difficult to cure. Shoulder pain may have a variety of etiologies, and the physician must ascertain whether the patient had a preexisting shoulder problem. Failure to maintain full range of motion may lead to tight muscles that become painful when stretched. Care must be taken by all staff members when moving or lifting a stroke patient, as traction or twisting of the shoulder may produce injury and lead to a chronic pain condition. Also, the pull of gravity on paralyzed muscles located over the shoulder joint may result in some degree of subluxation of the shoulder joint. This frequently occurs in conjunction with a painful shoulder, but since significant subluxation also occurs in patients with normal sensation and no shoulder pain, the cause and effect relationship between subluxation and pain remains unclear. Subluxation can usually be easily detected on physical examination, and X-rays are seldom of significant benefit in clarifying the etiology of the pain. The hemiplegic shoulder should be supported by a sling, pillow, or wheelchair arm board. Constant use of the sling should be discouraged because the patient's shoulder is then kept in an adducted and internally rotated position. The use of a pillow or arm board has the advantage of allowing a small amount of abduction and placement in neutral rotation.

If a painful shoulder does develop, it is usually advisable to attempt aggressively to maintain joint range of motion. Preheating with hot packs or ultrasound may prove helpful, but since different tissues are heated by different modalities, the physician and therapist should not immediately abandon preheating if one modality does not seem helpful. If the patient has a localized area of considerable tenderness, injection with a mixture of local anesthetic and corticosteroid may provide some relief. Some investigators have felt that rotator cuff tears play an important part in the development of shoulder pain but, again, deterioration of the rotator cuff is quite common in older patients with no complaints of pain. If the patient has persistent shoulder pain which is refractory to physical therapy, local injections, and systemic anti-inflammatory agents, a more passive method of treatment may be indicated (7). In this approach, the range of motion program is reduced so that the patient keeps just enough abduction and rotation ability for hygiene and dressing purposes. The shoulder is not ranged into the severely painful area if at all possible. This method has been shown to be effective in some patients who have extensive paralysis of the upper extremity. However, it may not be the method of choice for someone with a potentially functional upper extremity.

A few patients may develop a full-blown shoulder-hand syndrome in which the painful shoulder is accompanied by a hand that has some degree of swelling, often some vasomotor instability, coolness, and pain on passive range of wrists and fingers. Good results have been reported by treatment of this condition with a 2- or 3-week course of oral corticosteroids, accompanied by an active therapy program (11). It is usually extremely helpful if the swelling of the hand can be reduced, and joint range of motion of the wrist and fingers must be aggressively maintained.

When upper extremity voluntary movement is compromised by spasticity, several measures may be taken. The only drugs currently available that have an effect on spasticity are diazepam, dantrolene sodium, and baclofen. Baclofen is currently not recommended for treatment of spasticity resulting from stroke, and thus the clinician should restrict use to diazepam and/or dantrolene. Dantrolene has occasionally been reported to produce serious liver damage, and therefore routine monitoring of liver function tests is necessary. If spasticity cannot be reduced from the use of medications, and if aggressive passive range of motion is not helpful for more than a short time, the physician may consider isolated motor point blocks in some of the most spastic muscles. Such blocks should be performed only by physicians who are skilled in this technique. Finally, biofeedback can be useful in strengthening some muscles that are weak but capable of voluntary isolated control (1). If such muscles can be strengthened sufficiently, they may be able to overcome some of the offending spasticity.

For the person with impairment of one upper extremity, a wide variety of adaptive equipment that may facilitate eating, dressing, and grooming is available. The need for such equipment should be carefully evaluated by an occupational therapist and prescribed on a highly individual basis. Excessive prescription of adaptive equipment may well prove wasteful or may have the unfortunate consequence of sustaining the patient's dependence. Judicious selection of a few pieces of adaptive equipment, however, can make a significant difference in the patient's ability to function at home. It must be stressed that the presence of a single sound upper extremity is fully compatible with independence in self-care and in many household tasks. Furthermore, patients can be taught a few simple methods by which even the most severely paralyzed upper extremity can be made useful as a passive assist or stabilizing extremity.

Training in kitchen and homemaking tasks is usually more complicated than that for basic self-care skills, and thus such instruction must come later in the rehabilitation process. However, even if the patient is unable to walk, many chores can still be performed when wheelchair mobility is adequate. Training is usually conducted by the occupational therapist, using a model kitchen or apartment if available. More adaptive equipment may be required in the kitchen than for self-care activities, but again the therapist should recommend only those pieces of equipment that the patient actually needs and can utilize. Many light housekeeping activities can be performed from a wheelchair, but if the patient has significant residual paralysis, heavy homemaking tasks will require the assistance of another person. Sometimes rearrangement of furniture or appliances or even structural modifications may be necessary to allow independent function.

Kitchen and homemaking skills may be important for many reasons. Obviously, for the person living alone such skills are essential. Also reacquisition of such skills may be of great psychological importance, especially if the person's premorbid role was that of homemaker. Finally, the ability to do these tasks may become of extreme practical importance for the patient should the spouse fall ill. Not all homemaking skills need to be taught during the inpatient rehabilitation phase; training often can continue either at home or on an outpatient basis.

MOBILITY

The ability to walk sometimes seems to be the exclusive goal of the patient, family, and health professional. This sort of tunnel vision is unfortunate, as it is perfectly possible for a nonambulating stroke patient to function nearly independently at home from a wheelchair.

Patients with an impaired lower extremity are initially mobilized by instruction in transfer techniques (usually leading with the uninvolved side) and by standing in the parallel bars. A patient's strength in the supine position is often not a good indicator of his ability to support his weight in the standing position.

Balance is obviously important, and the ability of the patient to sit unaided on the edge of the bed is an encouraging early sign. If the patient has a relatively sound unaffected side, two requirements are necessary for ambulation (25): standing balance, including single limb balance on the unaffected side, and the ability to advance the paretic leg without compromising standing balance.

These minimal skills are not sufficient for a normal gait, but they may allow for limited indoor mobility. Although spasticity, particularly in the extensor pattern, may help support the patient during standing and walking, it can also interfere with the same functions. Because the severity of spasticity will probably fluctuate, it should be frequently reevaluated by the physician and therapist. Treatment of spasticity is essentially the same as outlined in the preceding section.

Patients may begin walking in the parallel bars, but they should advance to the use of a mobile walking aid as soon as possible so as not to become dependent on a fixed support. Since the patient usually has a significant impairment of one upper extremity, a four-legged hemi-walker or quad cane controlled by the intact hand is preferable to the conventional two-handed walker. If the patient can walk adequately with a quad cane, he may progress to a straight cane and, finally, to unassisted ambulation. However, at any given time the patient should use whatever assistive device is necessary to allow him to walk efficiently and safely. It should not be thought that a straight cane is "better" than a quad cane or hemi-walker. The use of a long-leg brace (knee-ankle-foot orthosis or KAFO) is rarely indicated for a hemiplegic patient because a locked knee will actually hamper walking even further. If a patient has a great deal of medial-lateral instability of the knee, a long-leg brace with an unlocked knee may occasionally be useful. However, the vast majority of hemiplegic patients will require only a short-leg brace (ankle-foot orthosis or AFO) (26). The short-leg brace can help correct foot drop and provide for correct foot placement at heel strike. It can also be useful in stabilizing the knee. Most physicians and therapists prefer a plastic short-leg brace for the patient with weak ankle dorsiflexion and only mild spasticity. If significant spasticity is present, a double-upright metal brace may be more useful in controlling the action of the foot during swing phase and in positioning the foot correctly for heel strike. For patients with weak ankle dorsiflexion, biofeedback treatment may help strengthen these muscles, possibly eliminating the need for an orthosis (1). The technology of brace making has improved considerably during recent years, and further improvements are anticipated. Decisions regarding bracing are best made by a physician (usually physiatrist or orthopedist) in consultation with the physical therapist.

Hemiplegic patients who are ambulatory on a level surface can usually be taught to go up and down stairs safely. Firmly attached railings on both sides are highly recommended, but if only one railing is feasible, it should be located on the side of the unaffected hand when going down stairs. The patient should be taught to lead with the unaffected foot when going up stairs and with the affected foot when going down stairs, a sequence that can be easily remembered by the phrase, "up with good and down with the bad."

The inability of some patients to ambulate usually results from impairment of balance (with or without sensory loss) or from some preexisting physical impairment of the neurologically unaffected side. For such patients, a wheelchair may still allow considerable independence. The wheelchair is usually most effectively propelled by using the uninvolved arm, along with the unaffected leg for both pulling and steering. Wheelchairs that can be propelled and steered using the unaffected arm alone are usually too complicated for the stroke patient to learn to use effectively.

BOWEL AND BLADDER CARE

Incontinence of bowel and bladder are not uncommon during the first week or two following stroke, but few patients with good long-term rehabilitation potential will suffer prolonged incontinence. Prolonged bowel incontinence is thought to be a particularly discouraging prognostic sign, probably because of the extent of the cerebral lesion necessary to create this condition. However, for the patient who has bowel incontinence with diarrhea, the physician must satisfy himself that this is not the result of either a fecal impaction or of a local disturbance as in diabetic neuropathy. Even if the patient does not have substantial rehabilitation potential, a bowel training program should be instituted for the purpose of simplifying nursing care. Incontinent patients will usually respond to a program of alternate day administration of a bisacodyl suppository, accompanied by judicious use of stool softeners and bulk-forming preparations.

Urinary tract incontinence does not usually carry the same prognostic weight as does bowel incontinence because multiple causes exist other than the stroke for this difficulty. As always, an accurate history of the patient's bladder habits prior to the stroke is useful in determining the nature of the patient's problem and in formulating a management plan. An enlarged prostate gland may cause a man to have a large capacity bladder with small, frequent voids of an overflow type. In women, the presence of a cystocele or other anatomic abnormality of the lower urinary tract may be related to problems with urinary incontinence. For male patients who seem to be voiding well, but without voluntary control, the application of an external urinary collecting device is often indicated. If the male patient has difficulty in voiding, a program of intermittent catheterizations at 6-hr intervals has been shown to be quite useful. Men who have difficulty in voiding on the basis of an enlarged prostate gland may be difficult to catheterize, but the use of a small straight catheter (such as #10 French) can usually overcome this difficulty. If the personnel required for an intermittent catheterization program are not available, an indwelling Foley catheter may be required. However, this can lead to complications such as urethritis, prostatitis, and/or epididymitis. Unless there is a significant anatomical obstruction, severe lower motor neuron lesion, or mental confusion, voluntary control of voiding will return although this sometimes takes as long as two or three months. (See also R. L. Davis, *this volume.*)

Unlike men, women rarely present with urinary retention poststroke, but the occasional problem patient can be managed either by intermittent catheterization or by an indwelling Foley catheter. Urinary incontinence in women must be handled either by catheterization or by the use of ample incontinence padding. Again, this problem should be transient in an alert patient unless there is some other anatomical lesion. The persistently incontinent patient, male or female, should have a complete evaluation performed by a qualified urologist.

VOCATIONAL REHABILITATION

The issue of vocational rehabilitation is usually not a consideration in elderly stroke patients. However, for any patient who was employed at the time of the stroke, the prospect of vocational rehabilitation should be seriously considered. For those with a significant degree of deficit, decisions may need to be delayed for several months. In fact, a premature decision can prove unwise. As in all other medical conditions, the unaffected skills of the patient must be carefully measured against the demands of the particular job.

DISCHARGE PLANNING

Effective discharge planning begins with determination by the staff, patient, and family of what the patient and family can and should do alone, what aid will need to be supplied, and what services can be provided by community agencies. It is extremely helpful if the hospital has a skilled discharge coordinator (e.g., social worker or public health nurse), because a thorough knowledge of community resources (such as Public Health Department, Visiting Nurse Service, Meals-On-Wheels, and Division of Vocational Rehabilitation), the services they provide, and their criteria for eligibility will enable the health team to match the requirements of the patient and family with the most suitable agencies. If continuing therapy is indicated, factors such as availability, cost, and transportation may determine whether this will be done at a hospital outpatient department or in the home by a visiting professional. A comprehensive home care organization can provide needed services and can also lend expertise to the assessment of the patient's needs. The services of a home health aid may be valuable in many situations.

The process of resocialization is particularly vexing for many stroke patients and their families (17). Although real physical difficulties are a limiting factor, it is frequently self-consciousness about impaired mobility, speech problems, or other sequelae of stroke that primarily prevents stroke patients from resuming their previous social activities. A community stroke group may serve an important function for such patients by providing recreational, social, and educational opportunities, as well as a place where solutions to mutual problems can be shared.

Resumption of driving often represents a final step, both symbolic and real, toward independence and reintegration into the community. Although the presence of significant visual field defects or visual-perceptual problems obviously present major barriers to the resumption of driving, the degree of paralysis on the affected side is usually less important. If possible, the patient's driving potential should be evaluated by a rehabilitation professional who is experienced in driver education with physically disabled persons.

Lastly, a word needs to be said about the term *stroke victim*. Many rehabilitation specialists now feel that the use of this term, with its pessimistic connotations, is antithetical to, and may actually retard, the rehabilitation effort (9). Rehabilitation professionals can encourage a positive perspective, more appropriate to the discipline, by substituting less pejorative terms.

REFERENCES

1. Baker, M. P. (1979): Biofeedback in specific muscle retraining. In: *Biofeedback—Principles and Practice for Clinicians,* edited by J. V. Basmajian, pp. 81–91. Williams & Wilkins, Baltimore.
2. Bard, G., and Hirschberg, G. G. (1965): Recovery of voluntary motion in upper extremity following hemiplegia. *Arch. Phys. Med. Rehabil.,* 46:567–572.
3. Benson, D. F. (1979): *Aphasia, Alexia, and Agraphia.* Churchill Livingstone, New York.
4. Benton, A. L. (1970): *Behavioral Change in Cerebrovascular Disease.* Harper & Row, New York.
5. Brown, J. W. (1979): Thalamic mechanisms in language. In: *Handbook of Behavioral Neurobiology—Neuropsychology,* edited by M. S. Gazzaniga, pp. 215–238. Plenum Press, New York.
6. Caillet, R. (1980): *The Shoulder in Hemiplegia.* F. A. Davis Co., Philadelphia.
7. Caldwell, C. B., Wilson, D. J., and Brown, R. M. (1969): Evaluation and treatment of the upper extremity in the hemiplegic stroke patient. *Clin. Orthop.,* 63:69–93.
8. Caplan, B. (1982): Neuropsychology in rehabilitation: Its role in evaluation and intervention. *Arch. Phys. Med. Rehab.,* 63:362–366.
9. Corcoran, P. J. (1977): Pejorative terms and attitudinal barriers. *Arch. Phys. Med. Rehabil.,* 58:500.
10. Darley, F. L. (1982): *Aphasia.* W. B. Saunders Company, Philadelphia.
11. Davis, S. W., Petrillo, C. R., Eichberg, R. D., and Chu, D. S. (1977): Shoulder-hand syndrome in a hemiplegic population: A 5-year retrospective study. *Arch. Phys. Med. Rehabil.,* 58:353–356.
12. Diller, L., and Weinberg, J. M. (1977): Hemi-inattention in rehabilitation: The evolution of a rational remediation program. In: *Advances in Neurology: Hemi-inattention and Hemisphere Specialization,* edited by E. A. Weinstein and R. P. Friedland, pp. 63–80. Raven Press, New York.
13. Feigenson, J. S., McDowell, F. H., Meese, P., McCarthy, M. L., and Greenberg, S. D. (1977): Factors influencing outcome and length of stay in a stroke rehabilitation unit. *Stroke,* 8:651–656.
14. Gainotti, G. (1972): Emotional behavior and hemispheric side of lesion. *Cortex,* 8:41–55.
15. Garraway, W. M., Whisnant, J. P., Furlan, A. J., Phillips, L. H. II, Kurland, L. T., O'Fallon, W. M. (1979): The declining incidence of stroke. *N. Engl. J. Med.,* 300:449–452.
16. Gasparrini, B., and Satz, P. (1979): Treatment for memory problems in left hemisphere CVA patients. *J. Clin. Neuropsych.,* 1:137–150.
17. Gresham, G. E., Fitzpatrick, T. E., Wolf, P. A., McNamara, P. M., Kannel, W. M., and Dawber, T. R. (1975): Residual disability in survivors of stroke: The Framingham study. *N. Engl. J. Med.,* 293:954–956.
18. Heilman, K. M. (1974): Neuropsychologic changes in the stroke patient. *Geriatrics,* 29(1):153–160.
19. Kurtzke, J. F. (1980): Epidemiology of cerebrovascular disease. In: *Cerebrovascular Survey Report,* edited by R. G. Siekert, pp. 135–176. Whiting Press, Rochester, Minn.
20. Lehmann, J. F., DeLateur, B. J., Fowler, R. S., Jr., Warren, C. G., Arnhold, R., Schertzer, G., Hurka, R., Whitmore, J. J., Masock, A. J., and Chambers, K. H. (1975): Stroke: Does rehabilitation affect outcome? *Arch. Phys. Med. Rehabil.,* 56:375–382.

21. Lewinsohn, P. M., Danaher, B. G., Kikel, S. (1977): Visual imagery as mnemonic aid for brain-injured persons. *J. Consult. Clin. Psychol.,* 45:717–723.
22. Meichenbaum, D. H., and Goodman, J. (1971): Training impulsive children to talk to themselves: Means of developing self-control. *J. Abnorm. Psychol.,* 77:115–126.
23. Naeser, M. A., Alexander, M. P., Helm-Estabrooks, N., Levine, H. A., Laughlin, S. A., and Geschwind, N. (1982): Aphasia with predominantly subcortical lesion sites. *Arch. Neurol.,* 39:2–14.
24. Newman, M. (1972): The process of recovery after hemiplegia. *Stroke,* 3:702–710.
25. Perry, J. (1969): The mechanics of walking in hemiplegia. *Clin. Orthop.,* 63:23–31.
26. Perry, J. (1969): Lower-extremity bracing in hemiplegia. *Clin. Orthop.,* 63:32–38.
27. Sarno, M. T. (1981): *Acquired Aphasia.* Academic Press, New York.
28. Valenstein, E., and Heilman, K. M. (1979): Emotional disorders resulting from lesions of the central nervous system. In: *Clinical Neuropsychology,* edited by K. M. Heilman, and E. Valenstein, pp. 413–438, Oxford University Press, New York.
29. Weinstein, E. A., and Friedland, R. P. (1977): *Advances in Neurology: Hemi-inattention and Hemisphere Specialization.* Raven Press, New York.

Rehabilitation in the Aging edited by
T. F. Williams. Raven Press, New York © 1984.

Communication Disorders in the Elderly

Martha Taylor Sarno

Speech Pathology Services, New York University Medical Center, Institute of Rehabilitation Medicine, New York, New York 10016

Communication in humans comprises all of the behaviors used to transmit information—gestures, pantomime, sounds, words—and the processes of hearing and understanding whereby we interpret visible (reading) and oral symbols.

Speech is one of the most human of characteristics and speech behavior varies greatly among normal speakers. An individual's personality, intelligence, dialect, and social and educational experiences all contribute to the broad range of differences that characterize each normal speaker (35). These characteristics are equally important in older and younger persons.

LANGUAGE

Languages differ in their linguistic characteristics but are essentially composed of three systems: a system of sounds called phonology, a system of grammar also known as syntax, and a semantic or meaning system. The smallest units of speech, called phonemes, generally divide into consonants and vowels and are the basic units from which words and sentences are constructed. The rules that determine how words are organized into sentences are called the grammar or syntax of a language. Word order is controlled both by grammar and the meanings of words. The variations of intonation and stress, called prosody, sometimes convey subtleties of changes in meaning that may express emotion or carry important grammatical information. An example of this in English is the rising inflection of the voice at the end of a question.

Language incorporates the physiologic production of units of speech (the motor speech system) into patterns and combinations governed by apparently innate rules of grammar and meaning, and modified by cognitive and affective factors. It is the highest expression of human cerebral function.

SPEECH PRODUCTION

During speech we change the size and shape of the vocal tract and thereby determine the characteristics of the sound wave by (a) vibrating the vocal cords, which converts air into audible sound (phonation); (b) moving the tongue, lips, and pharyngeal wall; and (c) differentiating sounds by closing the nasopharynx

161

with the soft palate in order to prevent air from escaping through the nasal cavity.

The size and shape of the vocal tract is changed most extensively by movements of the tongue and lips, which interrupt and modify the air stream. The result of articulation during speech is referred to as intelligibility. The perception of speech depends not only on the precision of articulation but also the loudness of a speaker's voice, the anticipation of an utterance, familiarity with the subject matter, and even background noise. Other essential acoustic characteristics of speech include rate, phonation, resonance, pitch, rhythm, and stress patterns (35).

COMMUNICATION FUNCTION IN THE HEALTHY ELDERLY

There is evidence suggesting that there are changes in communication function that take place throughout the life span (30). Yet until recently the speech pathology literature reflected an essentially indifferent attitude toward the effects of age on communication function, except for a limited repertoire of studies addressed exclusively to hearing impairments in the elderly. Recent work makes it clear that there are certain changes in communication functions that are common among healthy aging persons that are not associated with structural or neurological changes resulting from disease.

In the normal aging person certain changes in the acoustic characteristics of the voice have been identified. There is, for example, a shift to the lower frequencies in vocal pitch among aging persons (16,20). Ryan and Burk (33) found that when judgments of tape recorded speech samples of older people were made by trained listeners, voice tremor, laryngeal tension, air loss, imprecise consonant production, and slow rate of articulation were strong predictors of perceived age.

In addition to changes noted in the motor speech performance of healthy older people, certain observations have been made with respect to language function, i.e., the use of the vocabulary (lexicon), grammar (syntax), and meaning system (semantics) of a given language. An important observation that has been reported is that the elderly display a greater variability in linguistic performance than younger adults. Changes in emotional state, cognitive deficits, memory loss, and social expectation all contribute to this variability in performance. Obler points out that language changes in the healthy older person consist primarily of a decrease in speech comprehension (29). This finding might be accounted for by deficiencies in attentional systems, which has been identified as one of the greatest changes associated with aging (17). The healthy elderly also manifest a reduction in the availability of words. While word recognition remains unchanged, the active use of vocabulary (i.e., object naming) may decrease. Goodglass (18) reports that healthy aging persons do not make errors of sound substitution as do aphasic speakers but rather tend to make semantic errors, often using words that are only peripherally related to the target word.

They also tend to use longer, more complex sentences (with respect to syntax) than younger people to say the same things. In addition the melody (prosody) of language of many older persons is frequently disturbed (29). For those older people with sensorineural hearing losses there is often an associated decrease in the precision of speech resulting from auditory diminution.

COMMUNICATION DISORDERS IN THE ELDERLY

In 1965, in recognition of the special needs of the communication-impaired elderly population, the American Speech-Language-Hearing Association established a standing committee on Communication Problems of the Aging. Thus began an ongoing program of public education and professional training geared toward drawing attention to the many communication problems manifest in the elderly (1–3). It is estimated that 3 to 4% of those over the age of 65 are disabled by speech and language disorders (6).

Among those unhealthy aged who manifest communication disorders, the majority are those who have suffered strokes with residual verbal impairments. Tumors and degenerative diseases, as well as the effects of laryngectomy on the use of speech for communication, also account for a large part of the elderly population with communication disabilities. In addition, certain language disorders are associated with dementia in the elderly, particularly among institutionalized patients.

Many tests that were designed to help identify and quantify communication disorders have been published. Measures of language performance both in speech and writing and of motor speech performance are an integral part of the armamentarium of diagnostic skills that the qualified and specialized speech-language pathologist[1] brings to the management of verbal impairment in the elderly. The tests help to define the presence and degree of impairment in each of the modalities comprising communication (e.g., gestures, speech). For those interested in more information regarding the rationale and implementation of tests of communication function reviews can be found by Darley (13) and by Sarno and Hook (43).

The psychological impact of communication impairment in brain damaged patients cannot be overstated. The magnitude of the emotional consequences is the result, in part, of the intimate relationship between personality, self-image, and verbal skills. Our society places a high value on communication skills, particularly speech. In fact, communication skills are often considered reflective of intelligence and provide the basis for academic and vocational alternatives.

---

[1] The American Speech-Language-Hearing Association (1801 Rockville Pike, Rockville, Maryland) certifies individual speech pathologists and accredits clinical service programs through its Clinical Certification Program and Professional Services Board (PSB). The Council of Professional Standards has defined a rigorous set of standards for staff, physical facilities, ethics, and procedures for programs providing speech pathology and audiology services. PSB accreditation should be viewed as an appropriate standard for speech pathology services in rehabilitation medicine programs.

As a result, a patient with a communication disorder may sometimes fear that he is demented (40).

Aphasia

Aphasia is defined as an acquired language disorder characterized by disturbances in any or all linguistic systems: phonology, vocabulary, syntax, and semantics. It is the most common communication disorder among the elderly. Speech and language functions are mediated by the left hemisphere in about 93% of the general population, and aphasia occurs in about 40% of those who sustain strokes in the left hemisphere (36).

There is a wide range of differences among aphasic disorders, encompassing differences in severity as well as type. There are those aphasic patients who retain the ability to use only a few words whereas others may retain a larger vocabulary but have difficulty with uncommon words or grammar. Detailed descriptions of the classification and nature of aphasia may be found in several texts (19,42).

In general, aphasiologists characterize aphasia as either fluent or nonfluent according to a judgment of the flow of uninterrupted strings of words produced and the normality of speech rate. This method of classifying aphasia type corroborates localization studies reporting that anterior (pre-Rolandic) lesions are identified with nonfluent aphasia and that posterior (post-Rolandic) lesions with fluent types of aphasia (5). In addition to the fluent and nonfluent categorization, patients who are severely impaired with deficits embracing all modalities and little preserved functional speech are classified as having global aphasia.

Fluent aphasia, sometimes referred to as mixed aphasia, Wernicke's aphasia, or sensory aphasia, is generally associated with lesions in the vicinity of the posterior portion of the first temporal gyrus of the left hemisphere. It is characterized by fluently articulated speech with the melody and rate of speech generally normal in all respects. Auditory comprehension is impaired and word and sound substitutions (paraphasia), characteristic of this type of aphasia, are sometimes of such magnitude and frequency that speech is virtually meaningless jargon (e.g., "trefilision" instead of "television"). The fluent aphasic patient is likely to have no physical disability (hemiplegia) although he may suffer some mild weakness or sensory deficit on the right side. His speech is generally vague with preserved syntax but lacking high information words such as nouns and verbs. Many fluent aphasic patients circumlocute, that is, they tend to talk around a subject (e.g., "I had that thing you drink for breakfast" instead of "I had coffee for breakfast"). This is probably the result of being restricted to the less substantive parts of speech such as prepositions and articles. They may also appear to lack awareness of specific communication deficits although they may evidence some general appreciation of difficulty in communication.

Nonfluent aphasia is variously called predominantly expressive aphasia, Broca's aphasia, or motor aphasia. It is generally characterized by awkward articulation, limited vocabulary, a hesitant and slow output of speech, and restricted use of grammatical forms with relative preservation of auditory comprehension. The nonfluent aphasic syndrome is generally associated with anterior left hemisphere lesions, usually involving the third frontal convolution. The majority of nonfluent aphasic patients have right hemiplegia. Their residual vocabulary is generally limited to a repertoire of high information words (i.e., nouns, verbs, adverbs, and adjectives) and an absence of the functors (i.e., prepositions, conjunctions, and articles). Nonfluent aphasic patients are usually acutely aware of errors and frustrated by their failure to communicate normally.

Global aphasia, which is sometimes referred to as total aphasia (27), is characterized by an "evenness" of severe dysfunction across all language modalities and a severely limited residual use of all communication modes for oral/aural interactions (23,45,47,54). Global aphasia has been cited by several investigators as the most common type of aphasia in patients referred for speech rehabilitation services (31,38,39,47,53). Several investigators interested in localizing aphasic deficits have identified massive and sometimes bilateral lesions with global aphasia (22,23,25,54).

There is a wide range of residuals and combinations of symptoms in the broad category of severe impairment referred to as global aphasia. The range of severity within global aphasia is broad, ranging from mutism to the use of greetings or single word responses. There is also a large variety of concomitant symptoms coexisting with global aphasia: levels of alertness, activation, and initiation vary greatly from patient to patient. Visual field deficits, confusion, limb apraxia, disorientation, and many other neuropsychological deficits may also be manifest in different global aphasic patients. In these respects, the category of global aphasia does not designate a specific syndrome but rather a degree of severity with probably several syndromes subsumed (46).

Dysarthria

The second most common communication disorder affecting the elderly population is dysarthria, a speech disorder resulting from infracortical pathology. In the stroke patient, dysarthria is due to lesions in the brain stem where the nuclei innervating the speech musculature are located. Dysarthric patients usually have difficulty in the mechanical aspects of speech production. This means that the rate, voice quality, phonation, loudness, and articulation of speech may be impaired. In some instances the extent of impairment is almost imperceptible, whereas in the more severe cases patients may be rendered mute (anarthria) as the result of extensive limitations of movement and incoordination of the speech musculature.

Darley et al. (14) identified five types of dysarthria: flaccid dysarthria (in bulbar palsy), spastic dysarthria (in pseudo-bulbar palsy), ataxic dysarthria (in cerebellar disorders), hypo-kinetic dysarthria (in Parkinsonism), and hyper-kinetic dysarthria (in dystonia and chorea).

Characteristically, the bulbar palsy patient manifests hypernasality, misarticulation, and breathiness. Many patients in this category are unintelligible. Patients with pseudo-bulbar palsy, on the other hand, are usually imprecise in articulation with monotonous pitch, monotonous loudness, and reduced control over the rhythm of speech yet remain intelligible despite their symptoms. The ataxic speaker generally makes errors primarily related to the timing of speech and may give equal stress to each syllable. There is rarely a severe impairment of intelligibility.

Parkinson's disease is more prevalent in the elderly than in younger age groups. One of the frequent motor consequences of Parkinson's disease is dysarthria. The dysarthria associated with the disease is characterized by uncontrolled rate of speech (propulsive rate), reduced loudness, monotonous stress, and imprecise articulation. These dysarthric symptoms are particularly disabling in parkinsonian patients and may make it difficult for the patient to communicate by telephone or participate in conversations (37).

Laryngectomy

The number of laryngectomized patients has increased substantially in recent years. Many older patients have required removal of the larynx as a result of cancer. Absence of the larynx makes it impossible for an individual to speak despite the integrity of the structures of articulation. Patients who have had laryngectomies often seek the services of the speech pathologist for training in esophageal speech or fitting with an artificial larynx. The problems presented by the laryngectomee are complicated and challenging, encompassing both physiological and psychological changes that require management.

Language in Dementia in the Elderly

The elderly patient with dementia often manifests communication disorders that help to establish the diagnosis. Obler and Albert (30) identified two types of dementia, cortical and subcortical, which can be distinguished on clinical neurobehavioral grounds. The subcortical dementia syndrome is found in patients with a variety of neurological illnesses in which prominent pathological changes are seen in subcortical structures (e.g., progressive supranuclear palsy). These patients usually manifest emotional or personality changes, memory disorder, defective ability to use information, impairment of judgment, and a striking slowness in the rate of information processing. In subcortical dementia, vocabulary and general facility with language are thought to be perserved.

In the cortical dementias, aphasia, agnosia, and apraxia are present in varying combinations along with some of the same signs and symptoms identified with subcortical dementia (29). Alzheimer's disease is the commonest type of dementia in the elderly. The communication function of patients with Alzheimer's disease is particularly impaired in the semantic aspects of speech. In the advanced case, vocabulary loss, comprehension impairment, disorganized syntax, and word and sound substitutions are pronounced. Obler (29) pointed out that the difference between the Alzheimer's disease patient with dementia and the patient with Wernicke's aphasia is that the latter intends to communicate a particular idea but has not the available vocabulary for its expression. The Alzheimer's disease patient, on the other hand, has not only lost the specific linguistic components of the utterance but also its general intention.

RECOVERY AND REHABILITATION

Aphasia

In the aphasia literature there has been a greater concern with pathophysiology, localization and classification than with recovery and rehabilitation.

Many variables have been cited as important in the evolution of aphasia, whether a patient is treated or not. Age, etiology, size and site of lesion, type and severity of aphasia, time since onset, and educational level have been thoroughly elaborated by various authors (11,12,39,42,52). There is general agreement among investigators on certain issues: that aphasia secondary to trauma leads to a better outcome than poststroke aphasia, that severity of aphasia correlates with degree of recovery, and that comprehension improves before expression.

Age has been reported as both a decisive and a weak factor in studies of recovery from aphasia. Sarno and Levita (44), Culton (7,8), Sarno et al. (47), Rose et al. (32), Messerli et al. (26), Kertesz and McCabe (23), and Basso et al. (4) reported that age was not a significant correlate of improvement in their investigations. In contrast to these reports, others have found a relationship between recovery in aphasia and age (34,52).

Although age is considered an important variable it is of interest that to date only one study has addressed itself exclusively to the influence of chronological age per se in the elderly poststroke aphasic population (41). This study examined 63 patients with aphasia secondary to left hemisphere strokes who ranged in age from 51 to 77 years of age (mean, 61.4). Only right-handed English speakers who were alert, attentive, and able to cope with testing were selected for study. Those with aphasia associated with dementia or with hearing impairments that interfered with functional hearing were excluded. Table 1 shows the age, sex, and educational characteristics of the patients according to aphasia type. The aphasic groups were essentially equivalent in terms of these variables.

All of the aphasic patients were receiving speech therapy in a comprehensive rehabilitation medicine setting for the entire study period. Improvement was measured by comparing test results obtained at a mean of 6 weeks poststroke (range, 4 to 13 weeks) with follow-up test results obtained on an average of 24 weeks poststroke (range, 16 to 24 weeks).

The primary result of the study was the lack of an age effect on recovery

TABLE 1. *Characteristics of total group*

Group	Age (years)		Sex		Education (years)		Employment		Severity Index (percent)[a]	
	Median	Range	M	F	Median	Range	Active	Inactive	Median	Range
Global (N = 29)	61.0	52–77	19	10	14.0	8–19	22	7	15.4	1–28
Fluent (N = 16)	60.5	51–73	10	6	15.5	12–20	13	3	33.2	20–72
Nonfluent (N = 18)	59.5	51–72	12	6	13.5	10–20	13	5	40.1	16–79
Total (N = 63)	60.0	51–77	41	22	14.0	8–20	48	15	26.2	1–79

[a] Functional Communication Profile/overall intake score. On this rating scale, 100% represents an estimated premorbid normal communication effectiveness.

in poststroke aphasic patients over 50. There was no age difference in recovery between the most improved and least improved groups of patients. There were also no differences in recovery between the 10 oldest and 10 youngest patients. The characteristics of the oldest and youngest groups are shown in Table 2.

In a recent study that addressed itself to exploring the influence of time on recovery (45), a group of 34 poststroke aphasic patients receiving speech therapy was selected from a pool of 1,730 consecutive admissions and systematically examined during the first poststroke year. One of the most important findings was that the patients showed persistent improvement during the period 4 to 52 weeks poststroke regardless of type or severity of aphasia. There were marked differences, however, in recovery rates during the year related to type and severity (see Fig. 1).

In the global aphasic group the greatest improvement was noted in the latter part of the first poststroke year. Gains were particularly notable in auditory comprehension. Despite progress, global aphasics remained considerably more impaired than the other groups. In fact, the entire group of aphasics, regardless of type, made the greatest gains after six months. The results of this study pointed up the importance of time since onset as a variable influencing recovery (45).

The course of recovery in the aphasic patient is characterized by an evolution of emotional adaptive reactions that are in some ways inseparable from the linguistic evolution. Personal accounts by patients who have recovered sufficiently to write of their experiences describe the great loneliness and frightening sense of loss experienced by aphasic patients (9,28).

There are some parallels between the recovery course in aphasia and the model that Kubler-Ross (24) offers for understanding individuals responding to knowledge of impending death (42). In the period immediately following the onset of symptoms, the recovery stage is usually characterized by either a marked denial syndrome or the classic features of severe depression. Not all patients evolve beyond the first recovery stage. Generally, the fluent patient is more likely to manifest a denial syndrome and the nonfluent patient a depression. When symptoms of denial predominate, they may be manifested in various ways. The patient may make unrealistic plans based on complete recovery, underestimate the permanence of disability, or appear overly self-confident and optimistic regarding the potential outcome. This person may set deadline dates for recovery, stalling for time while the underlying depression resolves. Health care professionals are generally poorly equipped to deal with denial mechanisms, tending to express anger at the patient's "unrealistic attitude" instead of interpreting these symptoms as a natural consequence of the disability. The worker generally feels frustrated because therapeutic efforts to bring the patient closer to reality are failing. Some patients eventually find denial an unsatisfactory means of handling depression as the chronic state of disability continues.

The speech therapy process serves an important purpose during the depression stage. Directly addressing a patient's linguistic deficits and channeling his atten-

TABLE 2. *Characteristics of 10 oldest and 10 youngest patients*

Group	Age (years)		Sex		Education (years)		Employment		Type		
	Median	Range	M	F	Median	Range	Active	Inactive	Global	Fluent	Nonfluent
10 Oldest	72.0	69–77	6	4	16	8–20	5	5	5	3	2
10 Youngest	53.5	51–54	7	3	16	10–20	10	0	3	4	3

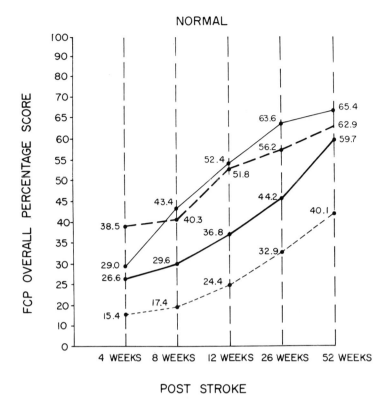

FIG. 1. Functional Communication Profile (FCP) overall scores, based on mean scores by groups. *Dashed line,* global; *solid line,* fluent; *bold dashed line,* nonfluent; *bold solid line,* total group. (From Sarno, ref. 48, and Taylor, ref. 49.)

tion and energy toward constructive ends can sometimes bring about a noticeable reduction in the depressive reaction. Speech therapy in this instance may act as an equivalent for work, which has long been considered an antidote for depression. As the patient adapts and sees evidence of recovery, the depression tends to reduce.

In the second stage, the patient's anger, originally directed toward himself, is now outwardly directed. Some patients may act out through physical means or through confrontations with members of the family or staff. During this stage, the patient presents particularly difficult management problems, which may be especially evident to those who share a more intimate relationship with the patient in his daily life. The inevitable angry reactions to a patient who is hostile demand that staff members understand this stage as a natural part of the recovery course.

The third and last stage is a period of adaptation that continues for the remainder of the patient's life. It is in this stage that the patient mobilizes and brings to bear all of his strength and begins to compensate for losses.

Aphasia rehabilitation is a process of patient management in the broadest sense. Since the impact of aphasia, mild or severe, affects all aspects of life in significant ways, effective aphasia rehabilitation must combine social, psychological, linguistic, and all other therapies into a cohesive regimen. It is difficult to imagine that any speech therapy technique could represent a total answer to a condition as catastrophic and complex as aphasia (42).

The holistic approach to therapeutic intervention traditionally practiced in the rehabilitation medicine setting seems essential to the goal of maximizing a patient's residual verbal abilities. Effective aphasia rehabilitation is a total management process in which speech therapy (i.e., the application of remediation techniques) is essential and important but not exclusively responsible for optimal outcome.

Taking the stages of recovery into account and attempting to maximize the characteristics and needs according to the particular recovery stage, the speech pathologist who is attuned to the psychological evolution of recovery applies an armamentarium of therapeutic approaches. For example, group therapy, a technique frequently employed in the management of patients with chronic aphasia, serves its best function after the acute and spontaneous recovery periods. At this time, the patient is generally more aware of his deficits, less preoccupied with symptoms, and more capable of interacting with others. Patients can gain support from others by sharing feelings with those who have gone through the same experience. Knowledge that one is not alone helps to reduce depression and loneliness.

Group speech therapy, stroke clubs, and other social groups have been mentioned by many authors as important for support and stimulation in aphasic adults (6,15,21).

> Older people, whether at home or in an extended care facility, often suffer from social neglect to the point that a sort of verbal "atrophy of disuse" sets in. Family and community resources to promote sociability, stimulation, motivation and practice are among the most powerful therapeutic agents available to use. They were potent stimuli in our learning to speak in childhood; they can be equally helpful in relearning speech. They greatly extend the effectiveness of our clinical skills (6).

Dysarthria

A variety of treatment techniques are employed in the rehabilitation of the patient with dysarthria. The specific techniques selected for a given dysarthric patient depend on what parts of the motor speech system are impaired. In practice, speech pathologists generally work primarily on the articulation of speech rather than pitch, volume, rhythm, voice quality, or rate. For this purpose, exercises that focus on particular classes of sounds requiring certain basic movement patterns are selected. For example, a patient with difficulty elevating the tongue tip may be impaired in the production of the *t, d, l,* and *n* sounds. In this instance, the speech pathologist would first work with the patient in front of a mirror on isolated, voluntary tongue movements from a rest position toward a position of tongue tip contact with the upper alveolar ridge. Exercises repeating these movements in alternating, rapid fashion might be practiced. Eventually the sounds are practiced embedded in syllables, words, and finally sentences.

Many elderly patients with dysarthria show improvement with speech therapy, especially if the dysarthria is associated with a nonprogressive disease (10). Because Parkinson's disease is generally progressive, speech therapy with these patients may be of little more than supportive benefit (37).

It is sometimes appropriate to consider an alternate or augmentative communication device for the patient with anarthria or severe dysarthria. The requirements for using these devices, however, are generally more rigorous than might be thought on casual consideration. Patients must have reasonably intact cognitive function, no significant language deficits, and good auditory comprehension in order to make practical use of such devices. A large body of information and technology and many sophisticated devices are now available. The wide range of options and their technical characteristics require that patients with anarthria be considered on an individual basis by a team of specialists expert in the prescription and implementation of such devices (50,51).

Laryngectomy

Not all laryngectomized patients are able to learn the techniques of esophageal speech. This alternate method of speech requires that the patient take air into the esophagus and then expel it forcefully, with sound being produced by vibration of residual laryngeal structures. Articulation is provided as usual by the lips, tongue, and other oral structures. Some patients who cannot master this method are dependent on writing for expression. Others may be candidates for an artificial larynx.

Many laryngectomized patients derive much needed emotional support from the many clubs affiliated with the International Association of Laryngectomees and the Lost Chord Clubs sponsored by the American Cancer Society.

CONCLUSION

Rehabilitation of the patient with communication disorders secondary to brain damage is an extremely complex process involving the recuperation of our most human behavior. Recovery of these high-order skills cannot be viewed as being solely concerned with the mechanics of sound production, precision of movements, or the form of language execution. Current thinking in speech pathology is directing more emphasis toward a humanistic approach to the rehabilitation of the brain damaged patient with communication impairment. This philosophy is nowhere more crucial than in one's therapeutic posture toward the elderly, who are almost a lost segment in Western society. They need the technical assistance medical service has to offer, but even more the knowledge that their problems warrant society's attention and efforts.

This view encourages a greater participation by all members of the rehabilitation team, particularly those in closest daily contact with the patient. Although the speech pathologist, as the person with special expertise in this area, must remain responsible for the design and selection of therapeutic interventions that are appropriate for a given patient at a given time, all members of the team play an important role in the recovery and rehabilitation process.

REFERENCES

1. ASHA Committee on Communication Problems of the Aging (1975): *Resource Materials for Communication Problems of Older Persons.* American Speech and Hearing Association, Washington, D.C.
2. ASHA Committee on Communication Problems of the Aging (1980): *Agencies and Organizations in the Area of Aging.* American Speech and Hearing Association, Washington, D.C.
3. ASHA Committee on Communication Problems of the Aging (1980): *Recognizing Communication Problems Among the Aging.* American Speech and Hearing Association, Washington, D.C.
4. Basso, A., Capitani, E., and Vignolo, L. (1979): Influence of rehabilitation on language skills in aphasic patients. *Arch Neurol.,* 36:190–196.
5. Benson, D. F. (1967): Fluency in aphasia: Correlation with radioactive scan localization. *Cortex,* 8:373–394.
6. Bloomer, H. H. (1980): Speaking of aging. *ASHA,* 22:458–459.
7. Culton, G. (1969): Spontaneous recovery from aphasia. *J. Speech Hear. Res.,* 12:825–832.
8. Culton, G. (1971): Reaction to age as a factor in chronic aphasia in stroke patients. *J. Speech Hear. Disord.,* 36:563–564.
9. Dahlberg, C. C., and Jaffee, J. (1977): *Stroke: A Physician's Personal Account.* Norton, New York.
10. Darley, F. L. (1963): Speech problems in the aging. *Postgrad. Med.,* 33:294–300.
11. Darley, F. (1972): The efficacy of language rehabilitation in aphasia. *J. Speech Hear. Disord.,* 37:3–21.
12. Darley, F. L. (1975): Treatment of acquired aphasia. In: *Advances in Neurology. Vol. 7,* edited by W. J. Friedlander, pp. 111–145. Raven Press, New York.
13. Darley, F. (1979): *Evaluation of Appraisal Techniques in Speech and Language Pathology.* Addison-Wesley, Reading, Mass.
14. Darley, F. L., Aronson, A. E., and Brown, J. R. (1975): *Motor Speech Disorders.* Lea & Febiger, Philadelphia.
15. DeBrisay, O. T., and Stuart, C. K. (1964): Recovery of communication in the elderly, with special reference to hemiplegic patients: Interim report on program. *J. Am. Geriatr. Soc.,* 12:687–693.
16. Endres, W., Bambach, W., and Flosser, F. (1971): Voice spectograms as a function of age, voice disguise, and voice imitation. *J. Acoust. Soc. Am.,* 49:1842–1848.
17. Geschwind, N. (1980): Language and communication in the elderly: A clinical and therapeutic overview. In: *Language and Communication in the Elderly: Clinical, Therapeutic, and Experimental Aspects,* edited by L. K. Obler and M. L. Albert, pp. 205–209. Heath, Lexington, Mass.
18. Goodglass, H. (1980): Naming disorders in aphasia and aging. In: *Language and Communication in the Elderly: Clinical, Therapeutic, and Experimental Aspects,* edited by L. K. Obler and M. L. Albert, pp. 37–45. Heath, Lexington, Mass.
19. Goodglass, H., and Kaplan, E. (1976): *The Assessment of Aphasia and Related Disorders.* Lea & Febiger, Philadelphia.
20. Hollien, H., and Shipp, T. (1972): Speaking fundamental frequency and chronological age in males. *J. Speech Hear. Res.,* 15:155–159.

21. Hudson, A. (1960): Communication problems of the geriatric patient. *J. Speech Hear. Dis.,* 25:238–248.
22. Kertesz, A. (1979): *Aphasia and Associated Disorders: Taxonomy, Localization and Recovery.* Grune & Stratton, New York.
23. Kertesz, A., and McCabe, P. (1977): Recovery patterns and prognosis in aphasia. *Brain,* 100:1–18.
24. Kubler-Ross, E. (1969): *On Death and Dying.* Macmillan, New York.
25. Mazzocchi, F., and Vignolo, L. A. (1979): Localisation of lesions in aphasia: Clinical-CT scan correlation in stroke patients. *Cortex,* 15:627–654.
26. Messerli, P., Tissot, A., and Rodriguez, J. (1976): Recovery from aphasia: Some factors of prognosis. In: *Recovery from Aphasia,* edited by Y. Lebrun and R. Hoops, pp. 124–135. Swets & Zeitlinger, Amsterdam.
27. Mohr, J. R., Sidman, M., Stoddard, L. T., Leicester, J., and Rosenberg, P. B. (1973): Evolution of the deficit in total aphasia. *Neurology,* 23:1302–1312.
28. Moss, C. S. (1972): *Recovery with Aphasia: The Aftermath of My stroke.* University of Illinois Press, Urbana, Ill.
29. Obler, L. K. (1980): Narrative discourse style in the elderly. In: *Language and Communication in the Elderly: Clinical, Therapeutic, and Experimental Aspects,* edited by L. K. Obler and M. L. Albert, pp. 75–90. Heath, Lexington, Mass.
30. Obler, L. K., and Albert, M. L. (1980): Language and aging: A neurobehavioral analysis. In: *Aging: Communication Processes and Disorders,* edited by D. Beasley and G. Davis, pp. 107–121. Grune & Stratton, New York.
31. Prins, R., Snow, C., and Wagenaar, E. (1978): Recovery from aphasia: Spontaneous speech versus language comprehension. *Brain Lang.,* 6:192–211.
32. Rose, C., Boby, V., and Capildeo, R. (1976): A retrospective survey of speech disorders following stroke, with particular reference to the value of speech therapy. In: *Recovery from Aphasia,* edited by Y. Lebrun and R. Hoops, pp. 189–197. Swets & Zeitlinger, Amsterdam.
33. Ryan, W., and Burk, K. (1974): Perceptual and acoustic correlates of aging in the speech of males. *J. Commun. Disord.,* 7:181–192.
34. Sands, E., Sarno, M. T., and Shankweiler, D. (1969): Long term assessment of language function in aphasia due to stroke. *Arch Phys. Med.,* 50:203–207.
35. Sarno, J. E., and Sarno, M. T. (1969): The diagnosis of speech disorders in brain damaged adults. *Med. Clin. North Am.,* 53:561–573.
36. Sarno, J. E., and Sarno, M. T. (1979): *Stroke: A Guide for Patients and Their Families.* McGraw-Hill, New York.
37. Sarno, M. T. (1968): Speech impairment in Parkinson's Disease. *Arch Phys. Med.,* 49:269–275.
38. Sarno, M. T. (1970): A survey of 100 aphasic medicare patients in a speech pathology program. *J. Am. Geriatr. Soc.,* 18:471–480.
39. Sarno, M. T. (1976): The status of research in recovery from aphasia. In: *Recovery in Aphasics,* edited by Y. Lebrun and R. Hoops, pp. 13–30. Swets & Zeitlinger, Amsterdam.
40. Sarno, M. T. (1979): Rehabilitation of the client with communication impairment. In: *Current Perspectives in Rehabilitation Nursing. Vol. 1,* edited by R. Murray and J. C. Kijek, pp. 193–199. Mosby, St. Louis.
41. Sarno, M. T. (1980): Language rehabilitation outcome in the elderly aphasic patient. In: *Language and Communication in the Elderly: Clinical, Therapeutic, and Experimental Aspects,* edited by L. K. Obler and M. L. Albert, pp. 191–204. Heath, Lexington, Mass.
42. Sarno, M. T. (1980): Aphasia rehabilitation. In: *Aphasia: Assessment and Treatment,* edited by M. T. Sarno and O. Hook, pp. 61–76. Masson, New York.
43. Sarno, M. T., and Hook, O. (eds.) (1980): *Aphasia: Assessment and Treatment.* Masson, New York.
44. Sarno, M. T., and Levita, E. (1971): Natural course of recovery in severe aphasia. *Arch Phys. Med.,* 52:175–179.
45. Sarno, M. T., and Levita, E. (1979): Recovery in aphasia during the first year post stroke. *Stroke,* 10:633–670.
46. Sarno, M. T., and Levita, E. (1981): Some observations on the nature of recovery in global aphasia after stroke. *Brain Lang.,* 13:1–12.

47. Sarno, M. T., Silverman, M., and Levita, E. (1970): Psychosocial factors and recovery in geriatric patients with severe aphasia. *J. Am. Geriatr. Soc.,* 18:405–409.
48. Sarno, M. T. (1969): *The Functional Communication Profile: Manual of Directions.* Institute of Rehabilitation Medicine, New York University Medical Center, New York.
49. Taylor, M. L. (1965): A measurement of functional communication in aphasia. *Arch. Phys. Med.,* 46:101–107.
50. Vanderheiden, G. (1978): *Non-vocal Communication Resource Book.* University Park Press, Baltimore.
51. Vanderheiden, G., and Harris-Vanderheiden, D. (1976): Communication aids for the nonvocal severely handicapped. In: *Communication Assessment and Intervention Strategies,* edited by L. Lloyd. Unversity Park Press, Baltimore.
52. Vignolo, L. (1964): Evolution of aphasia and language: A retrospective study. *Cortex,* 1:344–367.
53. Vignolo, L. A. (1973): Afasia. In: *Enciclopedia Medica Italiana, Vol. 1,* pp. 845–870. Edison, Scientifiche, Firenze.
54. Yarnell, P., Monroe, P., and Sobel, L. (1976): Aphasia outcome in stroke: A clinical neuroradiological correlation. *Stroke,* 7:514–522.

Rehabilitation in the Aging edited by
T. F. Williams. Raven Press, New York © 1984.

Rehabilitation Aspects of Arthritis in the Elderly

John Baum

*Monroe Community Hospital and the Department of Medicine, University of Rochester,
School of Medicine and Dentistry, Rochester, New York 14603*

Arthritic and rheumatic disorders in the elderly have similarities and differences from these same conditions in the younger age group. In general, although older persons may not respond as quickly to physical therapy as part of a total program, their degree of improvement with time can be just as good. In some ways, because they may not have the same constraints of returning to employment as a younger person has, they are more compliant and more understanding of the time that it takes to return to full function.

In the management and rehabilitation of patients with arthritic problems, the medical and physical treatment modalities are so closely interrelated that they must always be considered together. An active program of physical therapy should *always* be part of the treatment of the older patient with any rheumatic disease. Treating only with medication is to half treat these individuals.

In this chapter the major arthritic rheumatic diseases of the elderly patients will be described as well as the standard medical and rehabilitative therapeutic measures.

OSTEOARTHRITIS

Although there are a number of types of arthritis that will appear in the aged, the one most commonly associated with the aging process (although not necessarily the most disabling) is osteoarthritis. Although it is difficult to give precise information about the frequency of this condition, the best available information is probably that from the National Center for Health Statistics. The following data are obtained from one of their recent publications (2). From age 55 to 64 the frequency of severe to moderate osteoarthritis in the knees was about the same in both sexes (about 1.0% of the population). However, in the age group from 65 to 74 there was a striking increase in this condition in women when compared to men (6.6 versus 2.0%). Involvement of the hips was twice as frequent in the 55 to 64 age group in women as in men (1.6 versus 0.7%). This reversed itself in the older men, however, the figure being twice as frequent in men as it was in women (2.3 versus 1.2%). Severe to moderate sacroilitis was much more frequent in the 55 to 64 age men (2.7 versus 0.3%), whereas it was about the same in the 65 to 74 age group in both men and women. Thus, as they age, women have greater problems in their hips followed by a substantial problem with their knees.

The higher frequency of osteoarthritis in women in the older age group has long been known and has been attributed to a number of factors. Among them is the increased body weight of the older women and the increased angulation of the knee joint. The combination of these two factors, and possibly others, leads to this problem occurring in almost 7% of women over age 65.

The higher frequency of sacroiliitis in younger men might be associated in some cases with the sacroiliitis related to ankylosing spondylitis.

Most of the information obtained in this survey was from X-ray film examination, so that the figures do not necessarily indicate symptomatic disease. However, two-thirds of the people who were reported to have moderate osteoarthritis of the knees did have pain on most days during a one-month period. Thus there was a moderately good relationship between the X-ray findings and symptoms in disease of the knee.

Osteoarthritis of the hips seen on roentgenograms is less likely to be correlated with clinical symptoms, since only 28% of those individuals with moderate or worse osteoarthritis reported having pain in their hip or hips over the one-month period. About half the individuals with sacroiliitis also did not report having ever been treated for any kind of joint problems.

Limitation of activity due to arthritis is fairly consistent from age 25 to 64. From about age 65 on, however, the difficulties appear to double and even triple in frequency. The degree of restriction steadily increases with age so that patients who stated that they were "quite a bit" restricted increased from 1% at age 24 to 34 to 2% at age 35 to 44, to around 5% from age 45 to 54, 6% from age 55 to 64, and 9% from age 65 to 74.

Osteoarthritis can be primary or secondary. Primary osteoarthritis affects specific joints: the distal interphalangeal joints (Heberden's nodes), the proximal interphalangeal joints (Bouchard's nodes), and another joint in the hand that often is not realized to have a major involvement with osteoarthritis, the first metacarpal joint (at the base of the thumb). Also frequently involved are the hips, the knees, and the first metatarsal phalangeal joint of the feet. Secondary osteoarthritis can follow traumatic or several types of metabolic arthritis.

CLINICAL CHARACTERISTICS OF OSTEOARTHRITIS IN THE ELDERLY

Although osteoarthritis involving the hands with Heberden's and Bouchard's nodes is capable of producing deformity, the patient often retains a high degree of function. The major difference in the appearance of the hands of a patient with osteoarthritis as compared to rheumatoid arthritis is the site of involvement. Rheumatoid arthritis in the adult rarely involves the distal interphalangeal joints. The pattern of disease with distal interphalangeal joints and proximal interphalangeal joints (Heberden's and Bouchard's nodes) is quite different from the usual metacarpal phalangeal joint and wrist involvement of the patient with rheumatoid arthritis. In addition, the patient with osteoarthritis often will show "jack straw fingers." This results from lateral deviation of the fingers with overlapping, whereas in the patient with rheumatoid arthritis the ulnar deviation occurs at the metacarpal phalangeal joint.

Osteoarthritis of the hip is sometimes difficult to diagnose. The pain usually presents around the greater trochanter (where it can be confused with trochanteric bursitis) but can appear in other sites as well. Pain can appear in the groin, the front of the thigh, the area around the knee, and occasionally is noted close to the sacroiliac joints as well. Usually it appears in several of these sites but when pain is present over the greater trochanter plus other sites it points to the hip joint.

The finding of osteophytes on the X-ray film is frequently taken as an indication of the presence of osteoarthritis. This appears to be true in hip disease although not with the osteophytes seen around the knees which are more an indication of aging. The presence of osteophytes correlates with progressive lesions in the hip joint. There is also a high correlation with subchondral osteolytic lesions in the hip, which are seen as cysts on the X-ray film (6).

The development of osteoarthritis of the hips with advancing age has, on the basis of recent studies, been linked with other primary diseases occurring at a younger age. In fact it has been stated that it may, in most cases, be secondary to mild congenital subluxation and slipped capital epiphysis, i.e., diseases of childhood. Murray and Duncan (23) found that osteoarthritis of the hip may be found in young men who have been active in sports during their school days.

Another possible cause of the degenerative changes in the hips is discrepancies in leg length. Osteoarthritis of the hip, when it appears unilaterally, is claimed to have a high association with increased leg length even when present to only a slight degree on that side (12). Thus osteoarthritis of the hip can be associated with factors other than aging.

Low back pain is another complaint that can become frequent in the elderly. It is often hard to diagnose properly and can sometimes require lengthy workups before the correct diagnosis is made. The etiologies of low back pain range from the self-limited "lumbosacral strain," degenerative disc disease, spondylolisthesis, and fractures, to neoplastic metasteses.

Diagnostic studies should include (besides routine blood studies) erythrocyte sedimentation rate, calcium, phosphorus, alkaline phosphatase, liver enzymes, thyroid tests, serum protein immunoelectrophoresis, and careful roentgenographic evaluation. Occasionally bone scans will add needed information (13) by ruling out infection and/or inflammatory arthritis.

These tests need careful interpretation since the X-ray film examination can be of less value in the older patient. Osteoarthritic changes may conceal the developing erosions of rheumatoid arthritis. The osteophytes of degenerative joint disease of the spine on casual inspection can be mistaken for the syndesmophytes of ankylosing spondylitis. The edge of an erosion of a bone by a tophus can be mistaken for an osteophyte. Back pain may appear to be caused by degenerative disease suggested by osteophytes on the X-ray film. However, osteophytes of the spine, as seen on the X-ray film, may have little relationship to clinical symptoms.

Somewhat similar changes can be caused by a specific disease known as diffuse idiopathic skeletal hyperostosis. This latter condition can be distinguished by the appearance of osteophytes mostly on the right side. The treatment is no different than that for osteoarthritis involving the spine. However its recognition is important since it is limited to the spine.

Patients with degenerative arthritis of the spine can develop narrowing of the spinal canal (spinal stenosis). These changes usually take place at L3–4 and L4–5. In these cases, low back pain (often relieved by leaning forward) is a major complaint; however, there is frequently pain in the buttocks, over the trochanters, and radiation down the back of one or both legs similar to the distribution seen with disc herniation. These patients may complain of night pain. The diagnosis is made by a high index of suspicion and proven by myelography or CT scan.

As noted above osteoarthritis in the knee seems to be related more to excess body weight and is seen more frequently in women probably because of the different carrying angle at the knee. Osteophytes around the knee (when seen on the X-ray film) correlate best with aging and therefore do not necessarily indicate the presence of clinical osteoarthritis (15).

CHONDROMALACIA PATELLAE

This condition is a degeneration of the cartilage on the posterior surface of the patella. Although this is usually a disease of the young, it can occur in elderly patients. The patients typically complain of knee pain and will point directly to the patella as the site of their pain. The symptoms are aggravated by using stairs, especially when going down, because the quadriceps are then tightened for stability and the patella is pulled back against the femur. Joint effusions are rare in this condition. The diagnosis can be made by rubbing the patella over the femur and reproducing the pain.

CRYSTAL SYNOVITIS AND CHONDROCALCINOSIS

There is a group of diseases in which there are varying degrees of arthritis but which are all characterized by the findings of crystals in the joint. On this basis the diseases that are included under crystal synovitis are gout, where the offending material is uric acid, and pseudogout, which, although generally characterized by calcium pyrophosphate dihydrate, has recently been found to be induced by hydroxyapatite as well. The disease most related to the aged is calcium pyrophosphate dihydrate crystal deposition (CPPD) disease. When the crystals are in the joint, they can activate the inflammatory response. When the crystals are in the articular cartilage, the condition is then chondrocalcinosis. At this stage the calcification is found in the joint cartilage by X-ray examination. Diagnosis is best made, however, by examination of the synovial fluid for the characteristic crystals.

Chondrocalcinosis is definitely related to the aging process and the appearance of this material is relatively common when surveys are done of elderly populations. For example, in one recent study of 58 subjects with a mean age of 82.6 years, 28% were found to have chondrocalcinosis (10). The knee is the most commonly involved joint and was usually bilaterally involved. Wrists were the next most involved joint, with a few showing chondrocalcinosis in the hip and symphysis pubis. When the patients with chondrocalcinosis were compared with those who did not have the disease, a significantly higher frequency of various deformities of the knees, increased wrist complaints, and wrist involvement in the chondrocalcinosis group were noted.

There are several clinical states that are associated with the chondrocalcinosis. One is pseudogout, where acute attacks occur, usually in the knee, which can last anywhere from a day to several weeks when untreated. Some patients show a syndrome with multiple joint involvement (usually wrists and knees). The intensity of the arthritis does not appear to be as acute as with a single joint.

In a number of patients with chondrocalcinosis there is progressive degeneration of the joints, principally the knees with the development of osteoarthritis. The specific areas involved are different from those with primary arthritis. These patients occasionally will show true episodes of pseudogout as well.

Probably most of the patients in whom chondrocalcinosis can be found have no symptoms.

There are a number of diseases that have been described in association with pseudogout. These are hyperparathyroidism, hypophosphatasia, neurotropic joint disease, and hemachromatosis. As with true gout, attacks often appear to follow surgery and it has been proposed by O'Duffy (25) that this is due to a fall in serum calcium causing "crystal shedding" with the appearance of the crystals in the joints.

In general, the differentiation of this disease from primary osteoarthritis is based on the following features described by McCarty (20). The first is uncommon sites. The major areas included in this condition (which are not seen in osteoarthritis) are involvement of the wrists, elbows, shoulder, and metacarpalphalangeal joints.

The next is the nature of the lesion. This is especially true when there is narrowing of the patellar-femoral joint space, an area rarely involved in primary osteoarthritis. These patients also have prominent and numerous subchondral cysts. There appears to be greater and more progressive severity of joint degeneration with the crystal deposition. Osteophyte formation is variable and inconstant.

Gout, the original type of crystal synovitis, can be seen in the elderly but it is unusual for primary attacks to appear in the older age groups. The disease is usually well established by the time the patient is over 60.

LABORATORY TESTS

Most laboratory tests are of little help in the diagnosis of degenerative joint disease. Their major value is to eliminate the possibility that inflammatory disease is present. The two most valuable tests are the sedimentation rate and the rheumatoid factor. If the sedimentation rate is normal, the possibility of inflammatory disease being present is low. However, it must be remembered that in the elderly, especially in those over 70, the sedimentation rate is frequently increased for unknown reasons above what are normal levels in a younger age group.

Rheumatoid factor is also present to a greater degree in the elderly and the presence of rheumatoid factor in a patient with arthritis should not be considered to make the diagnosis of rheumatoid arthritis. Titering the rheumatoid factor will be helpful since patients with rheumatoid arthritis are more likely to have high titers.

The presence of a normochromic normocytic anemia can be an indicator of chronic inflammation and is often found, for example, in patients with rheumatoid arthritis.

Synovial fluid analysis should be performed when an effusion is present in a joint and a clear-cut diagnosis cannot be made. In an elderly patient, examination of the fluid for crystals of uric acid or calcium pyrophosphate dihydrate should be part of the routine examination of the fluid. If the patient has fever, the fluid should be cultured (as well as obtaining a blood culture). A white blood count and differential of the synovial fluid will help in the diagnosis of an inflammatory state. The synovial fluid glucose and protein are rarely of value. Testing the viscosity of the fluid by direct handling of a drop of fluid between the thumb and forefinger will help diagnose an inflammatory state. A thin fluid usually indicates inflammation.

TREATMENT OF DEGENERATIVE JOINT DISEASE

The treatment of degenerative joint disease should make use of all modalities. The best way to look at it is to treat the patient as though it was an active inflammatory disease because, in this situation, the physician's therapeutic regimen involves the use of drugs, physical therapy, and, perhaps eventually, surgery. All of these have their role in the treatment of degenerative diseases as well.

Unfortunately there is little that can be done to reverse the disease once the diagnosis is made (regardless of the etiology). Reassurance as to the correct diagnosis is important. Many individuals are acquainted with the effects of rheumatoid arthritis and the patient who has degenerative arthritis can be helped by making the correct diagnosis and prognosis and informing the patient. The patient also should be reassured that the hip pain is not due to inflammatory disease and is unlikely to spread to the hands and feet and cause the degree of destructive change seen in rheumatoid arthritis.

Symptoms in the elderly are frequently associated with obesity. Weight loss is a part of the therapy for a number of patients. The use of diet plans supplied by the physician can be beneficial but I have found my greatest success is by sending the patient to one of the organizations that specialize in group therapy. They have a higher degree of success with inducing and maintaining weight loss.

Exercise programs should always be used. More and more local YMCAs and clubs for the elderly have active exercise programs and these will often benefit the patient with arthritis. General tuning up exercises to maintain muscle function are just as vital as exercises to strengthen specific muscle groups around an involved joint.

The classic physical modalities should not be neglected. Local application of heat can be beneficial, especially when used before exercise. However, it has been shown that occasionally patients respond better to applications of cold to a joint. The analgesia provided by the cold is probably the major reason for this preference.

It is gratifying how often the simple use of a cane will increase the patient's ability to ambulate. A valuable trick for the patients with mild to moderate arthritic changes in a knee or a hip is to teach them to use a cane properly. It does not help just to tell the patient to use a cane; he must be taught how to use it efficiently. Since elderly people often feel that it is a sign of weakness or age, the use of a cane can be encouraged by having the patient purchase something attractive. Men seem to go in for walking sticks or cudgels whereas women seem to be attracted to thin canes with decorative handles.

Therapy is difficult for chondromalacia patellae. Having the patient strengthen the quadriceps muscle and use crutches and analgesic agents will provide partial relief.

Drug therapy consists primarily of the use of analgesic anti-inflammatory drugs. Aspirin is still a standby because of its effectiveness. The irritating effect of aspirin on gastric mucosa is a major drawback. However, this can often be avoided by the use of enteric-coated aspirin. In recent studies, we have shown that in a group of elderly patients, enteric-coated aspirin provided the same or higher serum salicylate levels than did regular aspirin (26). The use of enteric-coated aspirin obviates many of the gastrointestinal problems that are drawbacks to the regular use of aspirin (28).

If the patient does not respond well to, or has side effects from, aspirin then any one of the nonsteroidal anti-inflammatory drugs on the market have been found to be effective in the treatment of degenerative joint disease. The dosages can be high or low depending on the response of the patient and a particular drug should not be abandoned until dosages that are often as high as those used for rheumatoid arthritis have been tried by the patient.

For additional pain relief, pure analgesic agents (in addition to aspirin or nonsteroidal anti-inflammatory drugs) such as acetaminophen or codeine can be used.

Surgical intervention provides the greatest benefit to a patient with hip involvement because of the high level of success of hip surgery today. A patient who has continuous pain and cannot comfortably be relieved by the above modalities to the point of normal function should be referred to an orthopedic surgeon for evaluation for prosthetic replacement. (See also C. M. Harris, *this volume.*)

Knee prostheses have not been shown to be as trouble free or as effective as hip prostheses. However, in some patients they are effective in returning the patient to almost normal activity.

An X-ray film examination in addition to a measurement of the range of motion at the hip joint is necessary to determine whether surgical intervention is necessary. The marked beneficial effect of a hip prosthesis has enabled many people who cannot be treated with the usual therapeutic measures of analgesics and physical therapy to regain almost completely normal function.

For those patients who do not wish surgery or whose surgery is delayed, physical therapy and the use of a cane or canes as well as analgesic agents may relieve many of their symptoms.

TREATMENT OF CRYSTAL SYNOVITIS

If gout has been diagnosed earlier, then even into old age the patient should continue with therapy to reduce uric acid levels. In the older patient with decreased renal function, the xanthine oxidase inhibitors such as xyloprim may be easier to use. However, if the patient has been well treated up to this point, then either this drug or those that increase uric acid excretion, such as probenecid or anturane, are equally as effective.

In the elderly patient with established gout, if the disease has been treated over a long time period, then attacks of acute gout should be infrequent or should practically never occur. If the patient has not been faithful with his prophylaxis and the uric acid has been allowed to build up, then intermittent acute attacks can appear. The effectiveness of colchicine is often blighted by the appearance of diarrhea, and if diarrhea appears when close to the effective dosage, the patient probably should be treated for acute attacks with nonsteroidal anti-inflammatory agents. Diarrhea in the older age group will be more of a problem and more likely to disturb the patient.

Although it has been claimed occasionally that colchicine (particularly intravenously) is an effective agent for pseudogout, it appears that the best therapy is aspiration of the joint and treatment with a nonsteroidal anti-inflammatory agent.

No other specific rehabilitative measures are usually needed for these types of acute arthritis. Once the acute condition has resolved the patient should be encouraged to resume normal activity.

RHEUMATOID ARTHRITIS AND ITS CLINICAL PRESENTATION IN THE AGED

The United States Health Survey (2) did not give specific information about the frequency of rheumatoid arthritis per se. This diagnosis would be difficult without careful examination of the X-ray films for evidence of typical erosions in addition to the presence of rheumatoid factor. However, there was information on significant swelling of joints and tenderness in the various age groups. The joint that is more frequently involved in rheumatoid disease (especially with swelling and tenderness) is the wrist and some information might be obtained on the frequency of rheumatoid arthritis by looking at wrist involvement. The percentage of the population showing this type of joint involvement was 0.5% of men and 1.2% of women. What is also interesting about this data is that the distribution by sex is consistent with the known involvement by sex of rheumatoid arthritis. The highest frequency of involvement for this joint was from age 45 to 64 (1.3 and 1.6%), which is again consistent with the age group that is known to have the highest frequency of inflammatory arthritis. In the 65 to 74 age group the frequency of wrist disease was 0.9%. This compares with a 3% involvement of the knees, much of which is probably due to osteoarthritis.

The distribution of rheumatic diseases was looked at in patients in a general practice in England (8). During the survey about 5% of the patients were seen for rheumatic diseases. About 45% were over 50, with the distribution of women slightly in excess. When these patients were examined by a rheumatologist they found three diagnostic groups accounting for 92% of the patients: 60% had "monarticular rheumatism," 24% had degenerative joint disease, and 8% had inflammatory arthritis. Thus it seems that, in the elderly, there is an approximate 10 to 1 ratio of osteoarthritis to rheumatoid arthritis.

Rheumatoid arthritis starting after age 50 was reported to occur in a frequency of 5.7 to 30% in a review of a number of series (22). When rheumatoid arthritis has its onset in the aged, the prognosis is said to be slightly worse than the prognosis in young patients (5). This is not a universal opinion.

In a study from the Mayo Clinic (5), 2.1% of the patients seen had the onset of rheumatoid arthritis after age 65. The most frequent joints were the wrists, followed by the metacarpal phalangeal joints and knees. These joints appeared in more than 50% of the patients.

In two-thirds of these elderly patients the onset of the arthritis was insidious whereas in a quarter the onset was found to be abrupt. The disease acted almost like a systemic illness and a quarter of the patients had weight loss with the onset of the arthritis. Morning stiffness, a particularly prominent feature of the disease in the elderly, was found in all patients, and in a third of the patients lasted more than 2 hr.

Shoulder involvement was found in almost half of the patients and is thus more prominent than in younger patients.

Laboratory features were somewhat different from those noted in younger patients. The erythrocyte sedimentation rates in 58% of the elderly patients were more than 60 mm/hr (Westergren method). However, an unexpected feature of the laboratory findings in these patients was less anemia since 55% had hemoglobin values of more than 12 g.

Rheumatoid arthritis can start in the very old. I have seen two men, both 90 years old, with the onset of rheumatoid arthritis. Onset of rheumatoid arthritis in an older person does not lead to the same degree of disability as onset in a younger one. The disease itself is not as relentlessly progressive and, of course, with this there is less disability. The marked inflammation of the joints seen in the younger patients is rarer in the elderly. Laboratory examination shows a lower frequency of rheumatoid factor. On X-ray film examination, again correlating with the lower intensity of the disease, fewer erosions are noted. Of course, in older persons in whom the disease began at an early age, the extent of disability may be great.

Shoulder involvement seems to be common in the elderly. Patients who present with shoulder involvement occasionally are diagnosed as having bilateral shoulder/hand syndrome, but this may actually be the onset of their rheumatoid arthritis. Thus, if shoulder/hand syndrome should appear in an elderly patient, a bilateral presentation instead of just one shoulder should make the physician suspicious of the presence of rheumatoid arthritis.

MEDICAL TREATMENT OF RHEUMATOID ARTHRITIS

The basic therapy for the treatment of rheumatoid arthritis is aspirin. It is useful for its analgesic, but more importantly its anti-inflammatory, properties. There are a number of forms in which aspirin can be given. Recent studies have shown that less gastric irritation is found when enteric-coated aspirin is used when compared to both regular and buffered aspirin. In the experience of at least one group (28) and in my experience (26), salicylate levels are the same with enteric-coated aspirin as with the other forms.

Aspirin should be used with caution in the elderly. When trying to achieve maximum therapeutic levels sometimes a small increase in the number of tablets will cause large changes in the salicylate level. Acidosis can easily be produced in that case. For the adult, salicylate levels of about 20 mg/dl should be maintained.

In some patients some of the side effects, such as tinnitus, appear before a good therapeutic level or dosage is reached. In these patients and in patients who do not appear to get good response at an adequate level, one of the newer nonsteroidal anti-inflammatory drugs will be beneficial. These drugs have not proved dramatically superior to aspirin but they appear to cause fewer side effects and occasionally the patient will describe a better response. They also have the advantage, especially with the older patients, that fewer capsules or tablets are generally required than with aspirin. Some, for example, Naproxen, Sulindac, and Diflusinal, can be effective on only a twice a day dosage. Piroxicam can be used once a day. Of interest are some of the others that were initially recommended to be used three to four times a day can sometimes be given by giving the total dose on a twice a day basis (e.g., Tolmetin).

In patients with rheumatoid arthritis, in whom a major complaint is morning stiffness, the long acting nonsteroidal anti-inflammatory drugs are occasionally more effective than aspirin. However, the use of enteric-coated aspirin, with its delay in absorption of 3 to 8 hr, can sometimes permit the patient to get maximum effect early in the morning when the medication is given at bedtime.

Occasionally the patient will require additional analgesia to "take the edge off the pain." Then a drug such as acetaminophen or codeine is added to the regimen of nonsteroidal anti-inflammatory agents. Because they are not anti-inflammatory these drugs do not have the irritating effect on the gastric mucosa that seems to be a particular characteristic of most nonsteroidal anti-inflammatory drugs.

For the patient who appears to be having fairly continuous activity not well controlled by the short acting drugs, the long acting agents useful in the treatment of rheumatoid arthritis should be used. The most widely and best known agent is gold. This is used in the form of gold compounds such as gold sodium thiomalate and aurothioglucose. Gold is a valuable agent and seems to induce some degree of remission in about 60% of the patients in whom it is given. That is, with the use of this drug there appears to be decreased activity in the involved joints and fewer new joints appearing during the course of the disease. Because of the possible effects of gold on the bone marrow and the kidneys, the patient should be followed carefully. Gold is probably just as efficacious in the older patient as it is in the younger patient. An oral form of gold, auranofin, will soon be available.

Another drug, which is less used in the United States and more frequently used in Europe, is the antimalarial, hydroxychloroquine. With short-term use the greatest problem appears to be with gastrointestinal upset. Recent reviews have indicated that the reported eye problems are probably not as severe or as much of a threat as originally stated and the drug probably could be given for several years at a time before it is stopped to allow the hydroxychloroquine to leave the body. It is not as effective as gold but it has the advantage of being an oral agent.

Recently penicillamine has been proposed in the treatment of rheumatoid arthritis. Its effectiveness appears to be found in about 60% of patients, although, as with gold, about 30% will have side effects. The advantage of penicillamine is that it can be given orally and, with care, its side effects can be caught early. As with gold, once the medication is stopped most of the side effects will disappear.

REHABILITATION OF THE OLDER PATIENT WITH RHEUMATOID ARTHRITIS

The rehabilitation of 101 severely disabled persons with rheumatoid arthritis was studied for 5 years (18). There was emphasis on programs of group exercises and activities of daily living. Of the 101, 20% were 65 and over whereas half were in the age group of 50 to 64. Although there were varying degrees of improvement, the most important point to note was that there was no clustering of improvement according to age. Elderly patients with severe rheumatoid arthritis were just as responsive to the rehabilitation program as were younger patients. Ehrlich et al. (9) have reported a greater responsiveness to therapy in the elderly patient.

Most of the elderly patients seen with rheumatoid arthritis will have developed the disease during their younger years. Although a number might still continue to show active involvement, most will be suffering from the long-term effects of joint destruction. That is, destructive and degenerative changes can be more prominent than the problems due to active inflammation of the joint. In general, therefore, the physician is dealing with somewhat similar rehabilitation problems to those seen in degenerative joint disease with two major differences. Much of the destructive effect of rheumatoid arthritis involves the small joints and this damage to the small joints of the hands and wrists may require active surgical intervention before rehabilitation can be started. Distortion and fusion of carpal bones and the destruction and subluxation of the interphalangeal joints make rehabilitation a long and sometimes discouraging process. Active involvement of the hand surgeon in the early stages of rehabilitation is valuable. Reconstructive procedures can then be followed by vigorous physical therapy with a greater restoration of function than when muscle strengthening or splinting is done without this evaluation and operation, if justified. If fusion of joints is performed and reeducation of muscles is minimally required, it might become a case of simple adaptation to the activities of daily living. If prostheses are inserted to replace the finger joints, then active rehabilitation to restore function is needed.

Rehabilitation of the patient with active inflammatory disease is wasteful unless the inflammation and the pain and disability derived from this are well controlled by the use of the drugs prescribed above.

The physician must be aware throughout the rehabilitation process of changes in the status of the inflammatory disease as well as the effects of the degenerative processes. The patient might need more anti-inflammatory medication or, on the other hand, might need heavier doses of pure analgesic medications such as acetaminophen and codeine to control pain while they are undergoing therapeutic exercises. These drugs, given just before the exercise period, are then used to the patient's greatest benefit.

Knowledge of the way in which rheumatoid arthritis affects the patient is important. Morning stiffness can be markedly disabling in the patient with rheumatoid arthritis and if this cannot be controlled with heavy or well-timed doses of anti-inflammatory drugs or by small doses of nighttime steroids, then exercise programs should be delayed until later in the day when the patient gets over the morning stiffness. Afternoon fatigue in these patients, however, is also a problem and the onset of fatigue must be known for the individual patient to again make sure that active therapy then is scheduled between the end of morning stiffness and the onset of fatigue.

SYSTEMIC LUPUS ERYTHEMATOSUS

Recently systemic lupus erythematosus in the elderly was reviewed by Baker et al. (1). About 12% of lupus appears beyond age 50 and because of the age at which it presents, it can go unrecognized and undiagnosed. This group showed that this late onset lupus presents a more benign course and, therefore, medical therapy should not be pushed too vigorously. The most common presenting manifestations were pleuritis and/or pericarditis. Other manifestations seen in the elderly were arthritis and rash. Skin involvement appeared to be less common in the older age group. Neuropsychiatric symptoms and peripheral neuropathy appeared in the elderly but were less common than in the younger age group.

The most prominent feature in many of the patients was nonspecific constitutional symptoms such as fever, fatigue, malaise, anorexia, and weight loss. A third of the patients received no steroid therapy at all and less than half required high dose therapy. Death occurred from sepsis and almost half of those who were on corticosteroids died. This should be recognized as a possible complication of steroid therapy. The usual tests for antinuclear antibody were found positive in all of the patients.

Rehabilitation of this patient requires maintenance of muscle strength by regular exercise. Since joint involvement is minimal, special attention is not required to maintain range of motion.

MULTIPLE MYELOMA

A disease prevalent in the elderly is multiple myeloma. In a review of over 800 cases from the Mayo Clinic (19), 65% of the men with this diagnosis were 60 and over, whereas 58% of the women were in this age category. There are several features of multiple myeloma that relate to arthritis and arthritis symptoms. Bone pain was present at the time of diagnosis in most of the patients. In this age group osteoarthritis of the spine is often present, thus, when elderly patients come in with back pain myeloma should be part of the differential diagnosis. The distinguishing features by which a diagnosis can be made with a relatively high degree of certainty is to perform several simple laboratory tests. For example the sedimentation rate was 50 mm/hr and over by the Westergren method in 76% of the patients. Anemia is also present in a high frequency. Therefore, patients presenting with back pain who have anemia and a striking elevation of the sedimentation rate should be considered to have myeloma until the disease has been ruled out. The X-ray film can be diagnostic but may just show osteoporosis. Because of pain these patients can become debilitated rapidly. Control of back pain with analgesics and a simple program of exercise to maintain normal activity and the activities of daily living are an important part of the therapeutic regimen for this group of patients. Support corsets may also be helpful.

POLYMYALGIA RHEUMATICA

The inflammatory rheumatic disease most characteristic of the patient over 60 years of age is polymyalgia rheumatica. The mean age of those involved is between 65 and 70. This condition is somewhat more common in women than in men. The symptoms are more likely to be severe in the older patient. Although this is not a common condition its frequency in the population seems to be equivalent to that of gout patients.

Polymyalgia is a syndrome characterized by stiffness and pain of the muscles of the shoulder and pelvic girdle without evidence of arthritis in these joints. The patients clearly describe difficulty in getting out of bed in the morning or rising from a chair during the day. Because of the stiffness they even find it difficult to lower themselves into a chair and fall as they try to sit. Although pain can be a significant feature of this syndrome, the patients' strongest complaints are reserved for the stiffness.

Most patients state that the symptoms came on suddenly. Although arthritis is not generally considered to be a part of this condition, occasionally effusions have been found in the knees.

Many of the patients lose their appetite and weight loss can be substantial. Although the patients have difficulty in moving their shoulders and hips when asked, passive joint motion is usually found to be normal.

The most striking feature of the laboratory examination in these patients is the marked elevation of the erythrocyte sedimentation rate. By the Westergren method mean values of 60 mm/hr are found and values above 100 mm/hr are not uncommon. As with many diseases there are exceptions; rarely a normal erythrocyte sedimentation rate has been reported.

Hypochromic normocytic anemia is usually present with hemoglobin values around 12 g/100 ml. A major differential point from rheumatoid arthritis is the absence of rheumatoid factor in these patients.

Although electromyography might be thought to be positive in a condition where muscular symptoms are so prominent, they are found to be normal and the serum enzyme elevations usually associated with muscle disease are found to be within the normal range. X-ray film examination may show osteoporosis, depending on the duration of the disease, but there are no changes characteristic of this condition (23).

A major concern in patients with polymyalgia rheumatica is the possible development of giant cell arteritis. Depending on the series reported, giant cell arteritis has been found in 15 to 78% of cases of polymyalgia. Those patients who develop giant cell arteritis usually show symptoms related to this arterial disease. Headache is the most common and is usually localized by the patient to the temporal area of the head (overlying the temporal arteries). Examination will often reveal marked tenderness in this area. Because of possible involvement of the arteries supplying vessels to the eye the patient may also complain of visual changes ranging from blurring to permanent blindness.

The diagnosis is best made by biopsy of the temporal arteries (16). Therapy of polymyalgia rheumatica is usually with oral corticosteroids. Although analgesic anti-inflammatory drugs are helpful, if there is a possibility that arterial involvement is present, it is probably better to use prednisone. The disease itself is usually self-limited, lasting from only a few months to as long as several years. The dosage can be titered, however, according to symptoms and the erythrocyte sedimentation rate. Frequently the patient can be controlled with doses of prednisone from 5 to 10 mg/day. Relief is often dramatic with a starting dosage of 20 mg/day and the patient will report almost complete cessation of all symptoms within a day or two. If arteritis is present then higher doses of prednisone should be used; as high as 60 mg/day. Doses at this level are indicated especially if the possibility of involvement of vessels to the eye is present. As the patient improves, the sedimentation rate will fall and the steroids can be titered by following the sedimentation rate. The patient's clinical symptoms are equally valuable in determining the dosage.

During the acute phase of the disease with involvement of the shoulder girdle this condition is sometimes mistakenly diagnosed as bursitis. The usual modalities for treating patients with bursitis, however, are found to be ineffective. Often the diagnosis of this condition is delayed until the correct diagnosis is made so they may have been incapacitated for some time.

Once the patient has been treated appropriately and is relieved of stiffness by appropriate therapy, then physical therapy to restore muscle function is of importance in returning patients to their usual state. Range of motion exercises for the shoulder and hip joints as well as muscle strengthening for the muscles in the shoulder and hip girdle are usually all that is necessary. Occasionally, in the patient who has some restriction of motion and muscle aching, the application of hot packs before therapy is advantageous.

SOFT TISSUE RHEUMATISM (FIBROSITIS)

By far the most frequent complaint of the elderly patient is soft tissue rheumatism. It has been pointed out by Swezey and Spiegel (31) that these soft tissue pain syndromes in elderly patients are a diagnostic problem because they are often incorrectly attributed to osteoarthritis. Osteoarthritis is frequently diagnosed in the patient who comes in complaining of pain around a joint and in whom this diagnosis is made when X-ray changes with osteophytes are found. As noted earlier the presence of osteophytes in the elderly patient does not necessarily correlate with the presence of disease and often the pain and disability are related to one of the soft tissue syndromes. These are fibrositis, bursitis, and tendonitis.

The usual laboratory tests for inflammatory disease are of little help, since the inflammation involved in these soft tissue conditions rarely produces any serological evidence of inflammation. The major disease from which these conditions must be differentiated, osteoarthritis, is noninflammatory so that here, particularly, there is no help in the differential diagnosis. Although these conditions cannot be distinguished by laboratory studies or by X-ray, they can be diagnosed by history and by a careful examination.

Substantial contributions have recently been made toward defining the "fibrositis syndrome" by Moldofsky et al. (21). The criteria in Table 1 are those that have been somewhat modified by Swezey and Spiegel (31).

Not all of these features are found in each patient. It is amazing, however, how many patients will be found who have a majority of the subjective and objective complaints in this list. Trigger points, or tender areas, which when pressed often reproduce the pain syndrome described by the patient, have been found in a number of the muscles of the back, shoulders, and hips. The etiology of these tender areas is as yet unknown. There have been a number of theories but very little clear-cut evidence has been found for an inflammatory lesion. The most interesting finding has been the relationship of patients who have fibrositis with abnormal sleep patterns. Smythe and Moldofsky (29) found interruptions of the nonrapid eye movement and normal delta wave sleep patterns in these patients. Clinically this is expressed by the patients as abnormalities in their normal sleep patterns, waking up frequently during the night, having difficulty getting to sleep, and having difficulty awakening in the morning. There often is depression, which is associated with the difficulty in sleeping and the pain.

Amitriptyline (Elavil®) given at bedtime has proved to be excellent therapy in these patients without the use of any other modalities. This seems to have

TABLE 1. *Criteria for fibrositis syndrome*

Subjective complaints
    Aching and stiffness for more than 3 months
    Chronic fatigue and poor work tolerance for more
      than 3 months
    Sleep disturbance for more than 3 months
    Morning aching and stiffness
    Reaction to weather
    Temporary relief with heat
    Poor appetite

Objective findings
    Palpable tender trigger points
    Unrestricted passive range of motion
    Dermatographia
    Normal complete blood count, erythrocyte sedi-
      mentation rate, antinuclear antibodies, rheuma-
      toid factor, creatine phosphokinase
    Nonspecific electromyographic findings
    Nonspecific muscle biopsy (no inflammatory cells)
    Abnormal nonrapid-eye-movement sleep

a beneficial effect on both the depression and the sleep pattern, with disappearance of the muscular complaints.

If the patient complains only of localized pain sensation without the other features of fibrositis syndrome, the trigger points can be treated by local therapy.

In my own practice I frequently find that once the trigger point is found, direct finger pressure over the area can sometimes be enough to break the pattern. The area can also be injected with anasthetic agents and/or steroids. They can also respond to ice massage and topical counter irritants.

BURSITIS

Bursitis is quite simply inflammation of a bursal sac and is a frequent problem in the aged. There are dozens of bursae in the body, some of which are prominent and, when involved in an inflammatory process, are amenable to local therapy. How many of those that lie deeper can be involved in a particular syndrome is unknown. Knowledge of the location of the bursa enables one to define a local syndrome more clearly. The bursae most frequently involved are over the shoulder, knee, hip, ischium, greater trochanter of the hip, and the anserina bursa below the medial aspect of the knee.

Bursitis is a mild inflammation causing the accumulation of fluid in the bursal sac but responsible for symptoms that include pain, tenderness, and restriction of motion. The cause of the bursitis is usually unknown, although in some such as ischial bursitis and prepatella bursitis, there is often good evidence that trauma was responsible.

The one most commonly involved is the subdeltoid bursa. Unfortunately in some cases it is difficult to tell tendonitis of the various portions of the rotator cuff from bursitis. The therapy, however, is much the same.

If inflammation persists then the decreased motion of the glenohumoral joint can lead to the development of frozen shoulder or adhesive capsulitis. This end stage usually is a result of the inflammation and decreased motion in the shoulder.

A number of therapies have been described for treatment of frozen shoulder including the use of injection of corticosteroids, or high dose steroids, by mouth with rapid tapering. However, there is no good evidence that these treatments are any better than conservative treatment with nonsteroidal analgesic anti-inflammatory agents. It has been pointed out that the natural history of this disease is that of a cycle of "freezing, frozen and thawing" (3), indicating that the disease is self-limited and the patient almost always returns to normal function after an average time of about one year. Active physical therapy can maintain some degree of motion until full motion returns. Weiser (32) suggested that manipulation under local anasthesia will return function in about two-thirds of the patients within two weeks.

One of the least known but often an important cause of knee pain and disability in the elderly patient is anserina bursitis. This has been recently emphasized by Brookler and Mongan (4). The anserina bursa is located over the medial surface of the tibia below the pes anserinus. It is located about 1 inch below the joint margin on the medial side. In my experience, about 10% of patients complaining of painful knees show some pain in this area as well as changes in the joint due to degenerative disease in the knee. Treatment by injection of lidocaine produces remarkable relief within minutes of the injection. Most of the time a single injection (with corticosteroids) suffices but in several patients up to three treatments were required over a period of a few months.

Just as the anserina bursa presents difficulties in diagnosis with pain due to a degenerative knee joint, the trochanteric bursa, when it is inflammed, can be mistaken for primary hip pain. This bursa, as its name implies, lies over the greater trochanter. The causes of inflammation of the trochanteric bursa are varied and, in general, as again with the anserina bursa, it may become involved due to imbalance and stress on the muscle groups contiguous to this bursa. The patients are seen complaining of pain around the hip. The pain can extend to the buttocks and down to the knee. The patients complain of pain when they lie on it or when they change positions and so cause stretching or movement of the muscles over the bursa.

Swezey (30) has pointed out that the differential diagnosis can be difficult when the X-ray films show degenerative changes in the hip or when there is lumbar discogenic disease so that the bilateral thigh pain radiating down the leg is confused with the bursal pain. The diagnosis is made by the physician's recognition that this bursa can be involved when the patient complains of hip pain. As with other bursae, pressure on the skin overlying the bursa elicits the pain. Injection of lidocaine into the bursa will frequently bring rapid relief. It is usually recommended that if relief is obtained in this way that it be followed by injection of a long-acting corticosteroid.

Treatment of "soft-tissue rheumatism" is not standardized. Some physicians feel that once the diagnosis is made, steroid injection of the area is the ideal therapy. However, the response to steroids cannot be predicted and only about 50% of the patients respond. Studies performed by Fearnley and Vadasz (11) showed that patients who had a higher erythrocyte sedimentation rate were those who were more likely to respond to steroid injection. This can be interpreted as meaning that if inflammation is present, the sedimentation rate is elevated and steroids are then effective. However, if the lesion is due to a mechanical process such as tear of fibers without inflammation, then it is less likely to respond to corticosteroids.

Other techniques such as ultrasound, hot and cold packs, rest with slings, analgesic anti-inflammatory drugs, and careful use of passive and active ranging can be effective. In the shoulder, for example, there should be rest in the initial stages with passive range of motion to prevent adhesive capsulitis (and subsequent limitation of shoulder motion).

It has occasionally been demonstrated that a calcific mass appearing on an X-ray film appears to be reduced in size at the same time that an acute bursitis develops. Since we know that these crystals may be the same type of crystals that are seen in pseudogout, then there seems to be some cause-and-effect relationship between not just the presence of the crystals but the fact that the crystals have probably been extruded or released into the bursal sac, setting up a crystal-induced inflammation. Because this is a type of inflammation, local steroid therapy might be the best way to treat since it would be expected to reduce the acute inflammation. However, it is rare that one can be this sure of the cause of the bursitis in a particular patient.

ARTHRITIS IN THE ELDERLY IN ASSOCIATION WITH OTHER SYSTEMIC DISEASES

There are a number of rheumatic disorders that have been found associated with diabetes mellitus in the elderly. For example, ankylosing hyperostosis appearing in the age range 60 to 69 was found in 21% of 122 diabetics compared to 4% of 148 nondiabetics (17). Ankylosing hyperostosis develops as bony outgrowth from the anterior lateral surfaces of the vetebral bodies almost exclusively on the right side. It is felt that the presence of the aorta and its movement on the left interfers with the development of the hyperostosis on that side. These growths can form bony bridges and lead to back pain, stiffness, and loss of motion (14). In addition, as one would expect, diabetic neuroarthropathy will present in the elderly patient. This is probably a feature of long-standing diabetes mellitus but most of the symptoms do occur from age 50 to 64. The foot is most often involved with unilateral painless swelling and the frequent appearance of ulcers under the metatarsophalangeal joints.

Pseudogout and gout, previously discussed, have been reported to have a higher incidence in persons with diabetes mellitus but this has not been proven. The same may be said for "frozen shoulder."

Dupuytren's contracture has been reported frequently in the elderly. These are fibrous nodules that appear in the palmar fascia on the ulnar side, causing contractures of the fourth and fifth fingers. There is a claimed association with diabetes, and it is said to appear in 1 to 3% of caucasians in middle and old age. Occasionally surgery will be of help but little else seems to do very much good.

Carpal tunnel syndrome is also said to have a high association with diabetes mellitus. However, as in some of the other conditions described, the association may be tenuous. It can appear as a primary manifestation but, in the elderly, the most important associated conditions in which it occurs are with the edema of hypothyroidism, tissue infiltration with amyloidosis, and in the presence of acromegaly.

Patients will complain of tingling and aching in the fingers in the distribution of the medial nerve, i.e., the thumb, index, middle, and occasionally the radial half of the ring finger. Patients often describe paresthesia at rest but the most common complaint is of waking during the night with the symptoms present and having to shake the hands vigorously to restore function. It is best diagnosed by Phalen's test of pressing the wrists together in marked flexion in a reversed prayer position and holding them in this position for about a minute to see if the symptoms can be induced.

Symptoms can be relieved frequently by the use of a wrist splint worn at night. Inexpensive splints can be obtained from most surgical supply houses. The best fit, however, will be with a splint made by an occupational therapist. Corticosteroid injections can occasionally help but if symptoms persist, definitive therapy will require surgery.

Another common rheumatologic problem claimed to be associated with diabetes mellitus is the occurrence of flexor tenosynovitis or trigger finger. Other inflammatory conditions such as rheumatoid arthritis may of course cause this. The condition also seems to have a high frequency in the elderly. It occurs more in women in the right hand and most often involves the thumb, middle, and ring fingers. The patients complain of locking or snapping of the finger with motion and occasionally it is so bad that the finger must be straightened manually with the other hand. This too can sometimes be helped by splinting or injection and again, as a last resort, by surgical release.

REFERENCES

1. Baker, S. B., Rovira, J. R., Campion, E. W., and Mills, J. A. (1979): Late onset systemic lupus erythematosus. *Am. J. Med.*, 66:727–732.
2. Basic data on arthritis knee, hip, and sacroiliac joints (1979): *Vital and Health Statistics* Series 11, No. 213. National Center for Health Statistics Public Health Service, Department of Health, Education and Welfare.
3. Bland, J. H., Merrit, J. A., and Boushey, D. R. (1977): Painful shoulder. *Semin. Arthritis Rheum.*, 7:21–47.
4. Brookler, M. I., and Mongan, E. S. (1973): Anserina bursitis: A treatable cause of knee pain in patients with degenerative arthritis. *Calif. Med.*, 119:9–10.
5. Brown, J. W., and Sones, D. A. (1967): The onset of rheumatoid arthritis in the aged. *J. Am. Geriatr. Soc.*, 15:873–881.
6. Byers, P. D., Pringle, J., Oztop, F., Fernley, H. N., Brown, M. A., and Davison, W. (1977): Observations on osteoarthrosis of the hip. *Semin. Arthritis Rheum.*, 6:277–303.
7. Currie, W. J. C. (1978): The gout patient in general practice. *Rheumatol. Rehabil.*, 17:205–218.
8. Eade, A. W. T., Morris, I. M., and Nicol, C. G. (1979): A health centre survey of rheumatism. *Rheumatol. Rehabil.*, 18:148–152.
9. Ehrlich, G. E., Katz, W. A., and Cohen, S. H. (1970): Rheumatoid arthritis in the aged. *Geriatrics*, 25:103–113.
10. Ellman, M. H., and Levin, B. (1975): Chondrocalcinosis in elderly persons. *Arthritis Rheum.*, 18:43–47.
11. Fearnley, M. E., and Vadasz, I. (1969): Factors influencing the response of lesions of the rotator cuff of the shoulder to local steroid injection. *Ann. Phys. Med.*, 10:53–63.
12. Gofton, J. P. (1971): Studies in osteoarthritis of the hip: Part IV. Biomechanics and clinical considerations. *Can. Med. Assoc. J.*, 104:1007–1011.
13. Grabias, S. L., and Mankin, H. J. (1979): Pain in the lower back. *Bull. Rheum. Dis.*, 30:1040–1045.
14. Gray, R. G., and Gottlieb, N. L. (1976): Rheumatic disorders associated with diabetes mellitus: Literature review. *Semin. Arthritis Rheum.*, 6:19–34.
15. Hernborg, J., and Nilsson, B. E. (1973): The relationship between osteophytes in the knee joint, osteoarthritis and aging. *Acta Orthop. Scand.*, 44:69–74.

16. Hunder, G. G., and Allen, G. L. (1978): Giant cell arteritis: A review. *Bull. Rheum. Dis.,* 29:980–986.
17. Julkunen, H., Karava, R., and Viljanen, V. (1966): Hyperostosis of the spine in diabetes and acromegaly. *Diabetologia,* 2:123–126.
18. Karten, I., Lee, M., and McEwen, C. (1973): Rheumatoid arthritis: Five-year study of rehabilitation. *Arch. Phys. Med. Rehabil.,* 54:120–128.
19. Kyle, R. A. (1975): Multiple myeloma. *Mayo Clin. Proc.,* 50:29–40.
20. McCarty, D. (1977): Calcium pyrophosphate dihydrate crystal deposition disease: Nomenclature in diagnostic criteria. *Ann. Intern. Med.,* 87:240–242.
21. Moldofsky, H., Scarisbrick, P., England, R., and Smythe, H. (1977): Musculoskeletal symptoms and non-REM sleep disturbance in patients with "fibrositis syndrome" and healthy subjects. *Psychosom. Med.,* 37:341–351.
22. Mosemann, G. (1968): Subacute rheumatoid arthritis in old age. *Acta Rheum. Scand.,* 14:14–23.
23. Mowat, A. G., and Camp, A. V. (1971): Polymyalgia rheumatica. *J. Bone Joint Surg.,* 53B:701–710.
24. Murray, R. O., and Duncan, C. (1971): Athletic activity in adolescence as an etiological factor in degenerative hip disease. *J. Bone Joint Surg.,* 53B:406–419.
25. O'Duffy, J. D. (1976): Clinical studies of acute pseudogout attacks. *Arthritis Rheum.,* 19:349–352.
26. Orozco-Alcala, J. J., and Baum, J. (1979): Regular and enteric coated aspirin: A re-evaluation. *Arthritis Rheum.,* 22:1034–1037.
27. Resnick, D., Niwayama, G., Goergen, T. G., Utsinger, D., Shapiro, R. F., Haselwood, D. H., and Wiesner, K. B. (1977): Clinical, radiographic and pathologic abnormalities in calcium pyrophosphate dihydrate deposition disease (CPPD): Pseudogout. *Radiology,* 122:1–15.
28. Silvoso, G. R., Ivey, K. J., Butt, J. H., Lockard, O. O., Holt, S. D., Sisk, C., Baskin, W. N., Mackercher, P. A., and Hewett, J. (1979): Incidence of gastric lesions in patients with rheumatic disease on chronic aspirin therapy. *Ann. Int. Med.,* 91:517–520.
29. Smythe, H. A., and Moldofsky, H. (1977): Two contributions to understanding of the "fibrositis" syndrome. *Bull. Rheum. Dis.,* 28:928–931.
30. Swezey, R. L. (1976): Pseudoradiculopathy in subacute trochanteric bursitis of subgluteus maximus bursa. *Arch. Phys. Med. Rehabil.,* 57:387–390.
31. Swezey, R. L., and Spiegel, T. M. (1979): Evaluation and treatment of local musculoskeletal disorders in elderly patients. *Geriatrics,* 34:56–70.
32. Weiser, H. I. (1977): Painful primary frozen shoulder mobilization under local anasthesia. *Arch. Phys. Med. Rehabil.,* 58:406–408.

Rehabilitation in the Aging edited by
T. F. Williams. Raven Press, New York © 1984.

Joint Replacement in the Elderly

Carl M. Harris

*Department of Orthopaedics, University of Rochester School of Medicine and Dentistry;
and The Genesee Hospital, Rochester, New York 14607*

"Total hip joint replacement (THR) is a relatively common procedure," according to a 1982 NIH report, "with an estimated 75,000 THRs performed in 65,000 patients annually in the United States. About 60% of these procedures are performed in patients older than 65 years with another 25% performed in patients between 55 and 64 years" (32). It is estimated that another 40,000 total knee arthroplasties are performed each year in the United States (22). Thus, joint arthroplasty may be considered a primary rehabilitative procedure for the elderly or near elderly.

The goal of joint arthroplasty is clearly stated in the opening paragraph of the introductory chapter of this volume: "To restore an individual to his/her former functional environmental status, or alternatively, to maintain or maximize remaining function."

In the vast majority of instances, when joint arthroplasty is done in a major weight-bearing joint, the intention is to relieve pain and its attendant disability. Restoration of movement is often a secondary gain. In non-weight-bearing joints, particularly the hands, restoration of function may be the most important goal, with pain relief secondary.

Surgery is generally reserved for patients who cannot achieve adequate pain relief or function by non-operative means. Joint arthroplasties are never carried out on a prophylactic basis.

In contemplating the merits of joint replacement arthroplasty, both patient and physician should have a clear indication of realistic goals. The spectrum of outcome varies from a rehabilitative triumph to dismal failure, and thought must be given to the resultant situation if failure occurs.

Joint replacement arthroplasties are almost always done as truly elective procedures. They should be done after (a) the patient (and family) is fully informed of the risks and potential benefits of the surgery, and (b) when the patient is in the best possible condition, both mentally and physically, to tolerate both the surgery and the physical requirements of the convalescence.

RISKS AND POTENTIAL BENEFITS OF JOINT REPLACEMENT ARTHROPLASTY

In simplest terms, the risks of joint arthroplasty fall into three broad categories:

1. The risks attendant with major surgery and the convalescence.

2. The risks attendant with the use of artificial materials.
3. The risks associated with failure.

As stated previously, the benefit from joint replacement in a major weight-bearing joint is usually pain relief. Pain is, of course, subjective; the person suffering pain is the only one in a position to evaluate its severity and consequent disability.

It is not uncommon for doctors who regularly see patients suffering from arthritis to see an anatomic abnormality that is not a disability. Many people, by various means of compensation, are able to accommodate to an anatomical deformity that could be potentially uncomfortable were it not for this compensation. It is also not uncommon to see people who tolerate considerable disability when in a position of enforced responsibility (a job, caring for a family member, or providing for a family). However, when these responsibilities are removed, the same anatomical situation may be the source of untenable disability. Another situation frequently encountered is one in which living circumstances change significantly, placing more demands on an individual who has some anatomical handicap. For example, a spouse who has been providing physical and emotional support may become disabled or die; the neighbor, who in the past provided a weekly shopping service, moves; children, who provided care for the household, grow up and move. In instances such as these, pain and disability may increase with no apparent increase or change in the anatomical situation.

A common observation from an individual with multiple joint abnormalities is that one joint is the source of most, if not all, complaints. It is frequently found that after successful arthroplasty of that joint, other joints then impose limitations in function that the patient clearly did not anticipate. It is an obligation in the preoperative discussion to try to anticipate these possibilities, if they exist, and to inform the patient of the possibility of multiple procedures being required to achieve the anticipated relief of pain and increase in function.

Once it is clear that non-operative treatment is not providing satisfactory relief of pain and disability, and it has been determined that joint replacement offers the best chance of correcting these problems, a thorough evaluation must be done.

In the majority of instances, the primary physician has good knowledge of the patient. However, there are some specific concerns, particularly in the older patient, that require special evaluation because they could influence the surgery or the convalescent course.

Special Concerns in the Evaluation of the Patient for Joint Arthroplasty

Patient Evaluation

The risks attendant with joint arthroplasty are not substantially different from those for any other major surgical procedure. In many senses, the actual risks of the operative procedure are fewer because it is usually possible to schedule it when the patient is in the best physical condition possible. Physicians, nurses, physical and occupational therapists, and social workers generally have the luxury of sufficient time to evaluate and appropriately inform and treat the preoperative patient. Preparation for surgery and in-depth discussion of risks and benefits should include an evaluation with particular emphasis on the following aspects:

Musculoskeletal

The status of the musculoskeletal system should be evaluated closely. The range of motion that can be achieved at all major joints, the strength of the various muscle groups, and some estimate of exercise tolerance ability need be documented. A standard method of reporting,e.g., that used for hip disabilities, is useful (21). Some thought must be given to planning the postoperative course. Such questions arise as: Will the patient be able to use a walkerette, crutches, or various forms of mechanical assists? Will platform walkerettes or crutches be appropriate? How much supervision is likely to be required? Is balance likely to be a problem, and will there be a need for additional help to provide standby assistance? Will special nursing be required?

An evaluation of the musculoskeletal system must include an adequate X-ray evaluation. This is discussed later in this chapter, but it is important to state that the musculoskeletal history and physical examination should complement the X-ray interpretation. Paget's disease can often be suspected on the basis of a physical examination and confirmed by X-ray; spinal stenosis with coincident lower extremity complaints may be suspected on the basis of history and a physical examination, and later confirmed by standard X-rays or computerized axial tomography.

A thorough evaluation of the neck should be done in anticipation of endotracheal intubation at the time of surgery. Any suspicion of abnormality should be confirmed by X-ray and, in certain instances, might be sufficient reason to recommend spinal or regional anesthesia. It is considered prudent to obtain cervical spine X-rays on all patients with rheumatoid arthritis in whom endotracheal intubation is anticipated (8).

Neurologic evaluation

A thorough neurologic evaluation should be carried out. Weaknesses that may be subtle in the sedentary individual can become profound when new motor skills are being learned in the convalescent phase or when the need to use some ambulatory assistance is required. Carpal tunnel syndromes, which may be mild in the sedentary individual, can easily be exacerbated in an individual who is attempting to use crutches or a walkerette.

Body stature and weight

This is an important aspect of evaluation and merits discussion from several points of view.

Vaughan (46) has stated that physiological risks of moderate degrees of over-weight (15 to 25%) are minimal. However, in an individual who is more than 30% overweight, there exists an increased morbidity and mortality. During the actual operative procedure, technical difficulties are encountered in securing intravenous lines, controlling the airway, placing percutaneous arterial lines, and achieving appropriate positions for surgical procedures. From a cardiovascu-lar standpoint, obesity is often associated with hypertension, altered serum lipids, and angina pectoris, as well as increased total central and pulmonary blood volumes. An increased cardiac output usually exists, and sometimes an elevated left ventricular and diastolic pressure (30). Pulmonary consequences of the obese include a reduction in the lung and chest wall compliance and an increase in the work and energy costs of breathing. Closure of peripheral lung units can occur, with consequence of low ventilation perfusion ratios, shunt, and systemic arterial hypoxemia (38).

Significant difficulties are frequently encountered in the postoperative period in initiating and establishing a partial or non-weight-bearing program in the overweight patient. Many obese people have poorly developed motor skills, and often have insufficient upper body strength to handle themselves easily in a partial or non-weight-bearing situation.

A not infrequent problem is the exasperation expressed by nursing personnel and therapists who meet with difficulty in handling an overweight patient. This can be a source of irritation to both the hospital personnel and the patient, with a resultant negative effect on patient rapport.

Another concern which will be dealt with in more detail later in this chapter is that there is a higher rate of late failure due to loosening, wear, and prosthetic breakage in the overweight individual.

If at all possible, it is recommended that the individual contemplating a joint arthroplasty try to get his or her weight near to an ideal level preoperatively. Coincident with this, there should be some regular preoperative program to develop motor skills and exercise tolerance.

Cardiopulmonary

Several cardiopulmonary concerns have been discussed as they relate to obe-sity; another major concern for which careful evaluation is required is coronary artery disease. In a 1972 study of approximately 35,000 patients, Tarhan et al. (45) reported that the risk of perioperative myocardial infarction was approxi-mately 6% if the patient had had a prior myocardial infarction, versus 0.13% if the patient had not. They reported that, if the prior myocardial infarction had occurred within three months, the risk was 37%; between three and six months, 16%. In addition, the mortality of such perioperative infarction was

50%. In 1978, Steen and co-workers (44) reported on a series of 73,000 patients, of whom 587 had suffered a documented prior myocardial infarction. Again, the overall risk of 6% was present and unchanged from the prior study, with a similarly high risk for patients within three months (27%), and within three to six months (11%) of an infarct (44).

It is useful to remember that a spinal anesthetic, or some type of regional anesthetic, can be utilized for many procedures. This becomes valuable where there are potential airway problems or risk with endotracheal intubation.

A potential source of cardiac irritability under anesthesia is related to potassium imbalance. It is known that acute hypokalemia does cause an increase in cardiac excitability with increased incidence of superventricular tachycardia and premature ventricular contraction. Chronic severe hypokalemia can lead to renal tubular dysfunction, and there may be sufficient impairment of muscle strength to necessitate mechanical ventilation.

In the presence of hyperkalemia, there may be considerable affect on skeletal and heart muscles. Muscle weakness may be sufficient to impair the patient's ventilatory capabilities. Muscle relaxants, inhalational anesthetics, and narcotics may potentiate dangerous hypoventilation (42). If the patient under consideration for arthroplasty has Parkinson's disease, recent stroke (up to six months), a major burn (up to three months), or some paralysis, succinylcholine may cause massive release of potassium. Within five days of many injuries, muscles become hypersensitive to succinylcholine. Additionally, hyperkalemic patients will be more susceptible to drugs that decrease cardiac contractility (e.g., local anesthetics) (18).

Any history of cardiac failure should be carefully evaluated keeping in mind that fluid balance during surgery and in the immediate postoperative period may be altered. It is well to remember that low molecular weight dextran (widely used for initial anticoagulation) is a volume expander, and can, under certain circumstances, cause cardiac failure.

Good pulmonary toilet in the immediate postoperative phase is imperative. In certain instances, it may be wise to have a pulmonary therapist evaluate the patient preoperatively, explaining some of the procedures that will be encountered in the immediate postoperative phase.

It should also be remembered that often the greatest cardiopulmonary stress may not come at the time of the actual surgery, but in the convalescent period when the patient may be inadvertently pushed to the limit of compromised exercise tolerance. It is necessary to be specific with physical therapists in outlining one's goals for the rehabilitative phase if there is concern regarding this type of stress.

Gastrointestinal

Most patients for whom joint replacement is being considered will have received various anti-inflammatory medications. The incidence of gastrointestinal distress and frank bleeding is high with many of these medications. Since almost all patients with lower extremity replacements, and many individuals with upper extremity arthroplasties, will be prophylactically anticoagulated, it is imperative that the physician be aware of any past or present problems.

Most patients will have prophylactic antibiotics during and immediately following joint arthroplasty, and any history of drug allergies or gastrointestinal sensitivities should be obtained. Ulcerative colitis or any history of pseudomembranous colitis will offer special problems.

Genitourinary

There is a high incidence of low-grade chronic infection in patients considering replacement arthroplasty; this represents a potential source of bacterial seeding of the joint arthroplasty. A second concern is that, in certain instances where there has been compromised function, there is exacerbation by postoperative electrolyte imbalance. Renal failure can be induced by low molecular weight dextran used for anticoagulation or from the various antibiotics that are used for prophylactic control of infection.

Hematologic

Iron deficiency anemia is frequently seen in older patients who have been on a long-time "tea and toast" diet, or who may have gastrointestinal blood loss. This should be recognized preoperatively and its cause(s) appropriately diagnosed and treated in the immediate preoperative and postoperative periods.

Peripheral vasculature

Mild peripheral arterial compromise may not be recognized easily in the sedentary individual, but can be a major problem in the postoperative phase if unusual demands are being placed on the patient. If history or physical examination suggests a problem of claudication, or if extensive arterial calcification is noted on the preoperative X-ray review, doppler studies or arteriography may clarify the problem.

In most instances where prosthetic replacement is carried out at the knee or distal extremities, a tourniquet will be used. This can be a concern in the presence of arteriosclerosis and may warrant a sophisticated preoperative vascular evaluation.

A history of phlebitis is extremely important to note. In lower extremity replacement, the instance of postoperative phlebitis is high. Studies have indicated that phlebitis may occur in over 50% of the patients undergoing total hip arthroplasty. Of these 50%, 1 in 10 may suffer a pulmonary embolus if prophylactic measures are not carried out (15,27,43).

These figures have justified the use of anticoagulation during the interoperative and/or the immediate postoperative phase. Any history of prior phlebitis increases these already high risks. Some surgeons feel that replacement should not be attempted within one year of a known phlebitis.

X-ray Evaluation

Complete x-ray studies are essential and should include:

1. The joint involved and its opposite member. As an example, if hip arthroplasty is being considered, X-rays should include the opposite hip, the pelvis, and the entire femur. If knee arthroplasty is being considered, the X-ray evaluation should include the entire femur and tibia.

2. Weight-bearing films are essential in considering total knee arthroplasty and can be of considerable help in all lower extremity replacements. For example, an apparent leg-length discrepancy assumed to be caused by an arthritic hip may be due in part to a fixed pelvic obliquity. This is frequently more apparent in a weight-bearing view of the pelvis and would be a reason to obtain views of the thoracolumbar spine. Weight-bearing AP or PA X-ray views of the knee are essential to the operative planning (Fig. 1). If a flexion contracture exists, it is desirable to take a weight-bearing PA view of the knee with the X-ray beam centered at the joint and at approximately 90° to the long axis of the tibia without superimposition of the femur, as would be seen in the weight-bearing AP view of the knee with a flexion contracture (Fig. 2). It is also recommended that infrapatellar views and intercondylar views be obtained.

3. Appropriate ancillary films are important. Cervical spine films should be obtained in patients with rheumatoid arthritis undergoing endotracheal anesthesia. Shoulder, elbow, hand, and wrist films would also be appropriate in rheumatoid arthritic patients if prolonged use of ambulatory assist is required.

4. Films of sufficient quality to estimate the size of the medullary canal, if intramedullary devices are to be used, as in the femoral component of a total hip replacement, are necessary. These should also be of sufficient quality to give an estimate of osteopenia that may be present either from disuse or disease.

Preoperative Physical Therapy and Occupational Therapy Evaluation

In our practice, it has been found to be of considerable benefit to have patients undergo preoperative evaluation by the physical therapist and occupational therapist. Included in this evaluation can be some instruction in preoperative muscle training and some instruction in the use of the ambulatory assistance that may be required postoperatively. The occupational therapist often has suggestions for the handicapped that are helpful both in the preoperative and postoperative phases.

As a considerable benefit, it has been found that an acquaintance made in the preoperative situation has been helpful in establishing good patient rapport with the therapists and has served to relieve some of the patient's anxieties that surround surgery.

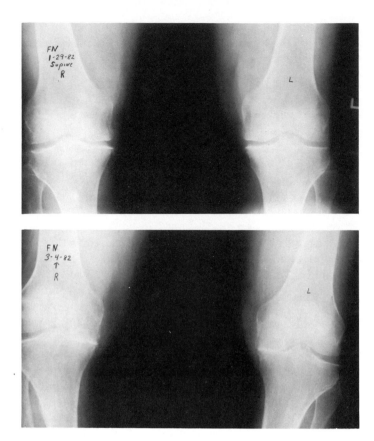

FIG. 1. Top: AP views of the knee showing an apparently normal medial joint space. X-rays taken supine. **Bottom:** The same patient with standing X-ray showing complete loss of medial joint space and a varus deformity.

Risks Associated with the Use of Biomaterials

At the present time it must be stated that there are no joint arthroplasty systems that have been demonstrated to last consistently without some degree of loosening, wear, or breakage. Occurrence of these complications is generally a function of patient activity and duration of use. Thus, they are less a problem in the elderly than in younger individuals. They can, however, occur at any age.

Because late failure can occur, many candidates for revision of a joint arthroplasty are elderly people who had their initial arthroplasty years before the failure. The metallic implants now in use have been developed so that corrosion found in earlier implants is no longer a problem. Most present implants consist of an articulation between one of our presently available metals and a plastic bearing.

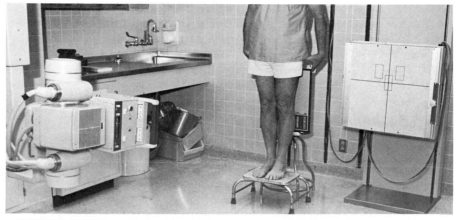

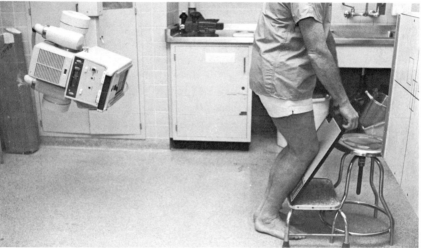

FIG. 2. Top: The technique of obtaining standing AP views of the knee. **Bottom:** The technique of obtaining standing PA views of the knee when a flexion contracture is present.

Charnley (10) should be credited for the development of total hip arthroplasty using ultra-high molecular weight polyethylene (UHMWP); it was developed for use as an acetabular cup in the total hip arthroplasty that he pioneered. Charnley first attempted using Teflon, which has a higher coefficient of friction than UHMWP, but he found it poorly tolerated. There was a rapid breakdown and development of large noncaseating granulomata around the joint (10).

Charnley, while not the first to use polymethyl methacrylate (PMM), should be credited also for early development of the technique of fixation of prosthetic components to bone using PMM. PMM, which is very similar to plexiglass, allows firm fixation of a prosthetic component to bone (47). After the operative site is prepared to accept the prosthesis, powdered polymer is mixed with a liquid monomer. Within minutes, a doughy plastic is formed. This is forced into the interstices of the cancellous bone of the joint. PMM is a grouting agent, and accomplishes the fixation by being spread over a large, irregular surface and not by adhesion.

While in the doughy stage, the prosthetic components are embedded in the PMM. Hardening of the plastic can be controlled by the ambient temperature, plus various additives that are placed in the monomer or powdered polymer. In the usual circumstance, hardening is designed to occur between 5 and 15 minutes.

The usual fixation is firm, and in great part accounts for the rapid pain relief and easy early motion.

When first developed, it was thought that wear of the UHMWP component would be the major problem necessitating a revision. This has turned out not to be so (40). However, several other problems have developed. Solutions to these problems have represented the major hurdles that have been—or are being—overcome with advances in our knowledge of biomaterials and biomechanics.

After the early glowing reports of total hip arthroplasty there were the scattered reports of femoral stem fractures. Ultimately, several causes were determined (3,9,35). One of the problems noted was poor positioning. It was found that a valgus position was necessary to eliminate stress risers on the metallic component. In simplest terms, this meant that the best position for the prosthesis was with the distal tip of the intramedullary portion of the prosthesis abutting the medial cortex when visualized in the AP X-rays. A second error was found in the use of small prostheses. Some early prostheses had small medullary stems which did not fill the canal and resulted in metal fatigue from toggling. A third error was due to inadequate cementing techniques. This was usually the result of failure to surround the prosthesis with PMM, which could cause one portion of the femoral stem to be fixed while another portion was free to move very slightly with stress. This resulted in metal fatigue.

Presently, most total hip femoral components are designed to completely fill the intramedullary canal or to permit some direct load-bearing on cortical bone at the calcar.

Initially, it was assumed that fixation between the bone and the PMM would be solid. However, it has been demonstrated that as a function of time and applied stress, loosening may develop (5). In most instances, loosening is not sufficiently severe to warrant revision. This is especially true in the older patient. The characteristic complaint with mild loosening of the femoral component is that of thigh pain on initiating weight bearing. In many instances, satisfactory relief can be obtained by the use of a cane or non-narcotic analgesic.

The apparent explanation for loosening is that shear zones develop between areas of different mechanical properties. Bone, PMM, metal, and UHMWP all have different elastic moduli. This means that under the same stress (or load) they will strain (or bend) to different degrees. Thus, at the interface between these materials, lines of potential shear develop as, under the same stress, they are straining or bending to different degrees. One attempt at solving this problem at the junction between bone and PMM has been to use pressure techniques to force cement further into the cancellous bone and thus increase the surface area and strength of the interface. By increasing the surface area there is less stress per unit area given the same load (47).

Another problem that has become apparent seems to result from firm fixation. In certain instances, best exemplified in a total hip, one may see osteolysis occur in the region of the remaining femoral calcar. This is an area where, in the natural state, one sees thick cortical bone and it is the area of maximum weight-bearing stress. As a function of time, it has been found that, in certain instances, this dense, heavy bone will become less visible. Two explanations have been advanced for this phenomenon. Some studies have suggested that the area may be devitalized by the surgical procedure, but another equally likely explanation is that the phenomenon is a result of "stress sparing." Stress sparing occurs when firm intramedullary fixation is obtained. Stress then applied to the femoral head is diverted through the prosthesis to a point more distal on the femur near the distal tip, and the area being spared undergoes atrophy (Wolff's law). As a result of this observation, one school of prosthetic design recommends that the femoral component should have a large flange that sits on the remaining calcar and thus prevents osteolysis by transmitting some load (13).

In earlier prosthetic designs, the ultra-high molecular weight portion of the prosthesis was small and unprotected. A classic example is the tibial component of the first Geomedic knees. Failures of prostheses with this design occurred because, with stress, deformities developed in the plastic. This problem seems to have been overcome by the use of a metal backing for small UHMWP components. In other designs, the thickness of the polyethylene has been increased to lessen the strain and deformation that occurs with physiologic stress (14).

At this writing, a major interest in prosthetic design is to obtain some type of "biologic bonding" of the prosthesis to bone. If this can be accomplished, it would eliminate the use of PMM, as bone would grow into the prosthesis. Current research indicates that to accomplish bony ingrowth into a prosthesis, one must apply a coating to the prosthesis that has a pore diameter of somewhere between 50 and 450 microns and a total porosity of at least 30%. Pore sizes less than or greater than these figures, or total porosity of less than 30%, appear to result in connective tissue ingrowth rather than bony ingrowth (6,7).

The porous materials under consideration for coating the prosthetic component include porous ceramics, scintered metals, and plastics. Porous ceramics are presently in use experimentally in some European centers. Scintered metal coatings on some prostheses are now available in the United States. With this design, small metallic beads are scintered on the metal component of the prosthesis. To bond the metal beads to the prosthesis requires a temperature approaching 1300°C. There was some concern that temperatures this high might weaken the grain structure of the casted prosthesis and lead to metal fatigue, but it is now thought by manufacturers that this potential problem has been overcome. A third method of obtaining a porous coat is with the use of scintered wire mesh. Currently this is promising, in the sense that it allows for reliable pore size and porosity.

If bony ingrowth is to occur, it will obviously be slow and not provide the instant fixation seen with PMM. At this time, it is presumed that early convalescence should be less vigorous and that there should be a longer period of protected weight-bearing than is now seen in cemented arthroplasties. Current thought is that this type of prosthesis will offer the greatest long-term advantage to the younger, more vigorous individual, and the advantages may not be as apparent to the older, more sedentary individual in whom rapid convalescence and early less restricted weight-bearing is desired.

Metal sensitivity has been reported, but in actual experience has not been a major problem. If there is concern about metal sensitivity in the patient undergoing total joint arthroplasty, testing should be carried out and a prosthesis selected that does not contain the offending metal (39).

The Risks of Failure

Fortunately, failures are not common. There is no question that total joint arthroplasties have added a new dimension to life for many and have allowed rehabilitation in every sense of the word. However, failures do occur, and the patient undergoing a joint arthroplasty must seriously consider the results.

Some failures should be classified as less-than-optimum results: The outcome may be considered a good result if viewed against the preoperative situation and not against a norm. For instance, it is unreasonable to expect that the individual who has been essentially chair-bound for an extended period of time will achieve the same range of motion and exercise tolerance after insertion of bilateral total hip arthroplasties and total knee arthroplasties as would an active person with osteoarthritis who had only a single painful joint. Nor is it reasonable to expect a patient who has a fused hip revised to a total hip arthroplasty because of back complaints to achieve the range of motion or gait that someone with a single joint osteoarthritis might expect. Both these cases could be considered successful if pain relief and improvement of function are viewed as goals and if the result is satisfactory to the patient.

Some patients' complaints would appear to be untreatable. For example, if, following total knee arthroplasty, the patient lacks sufficient flexion to climb stairs easily with a reciprocal gait but can walk without difficulty on a level surface, it must be accepted as a residual disability.

Mild patellar pain following a total knee arthroplasty, occurring only on changing from a sitting to an upright position, or in stair-climbing, is difficult to treat and must be accommodated by the patient.

Most of the immediate problems faced by the patient and the physician in the surgical and post-surgical period that could result in failure are of a general nature and could be considered complications of almost any major operative procedure.

There have been several special problems seen with joint arthroplasties that can result in failure.

Infection: Infection in the immediate postoperative period is not commonly seen. There are several reasons for this. In most instances surgery has been scheduled with the patient in optimum health. Any occult infection, such as a dental abscess, a urinary tract infection, or a stasis ulcer should have been adequately treated.

Replacement arthroplasties in most instances are carried out by individuals well-schooled in various techniques and frequently are done in special environments that include special rooms utilizing various combinations of limited access, laminar flow, high efficiency air filters, ultra violet lights, special gowning techniques, or special exhaust systems for the operating room personnel (34).

The concern has been to limit introduction of bacteria into the wound at surgery. It has been demonstrated that, to be transmitted as aerosols, bacteria must be on particles greater than 0.5 microns in diameter, and efforts have been made to limit the number of these particles in the ambient air, or to sterilize them by use of air filtration, ultra violet lights, topical antibiotic irrigation, or other germicidal irrigation.

In most instances, prophylactic antibiotics are given for varying lengths of time in the operative and postoperative phase. PMM, when introduced in the dough phase, undergoes an intense exothermic reaction. Surface temperatures can exceed 100°C. It is postulated that this devitalizes tissue at the bone cement interface and that an undetermined amount of tissue is damaged. It is assumed that this tissue has a poor host resistance and could serve as a medium for infection if a bacteremia subsequently developed. This reasoning is used to justify the use of a prophylactic antibiotic; clinical experience has shown that there is significantly less infection with antibiotic prophylaxis (2,16,34,41).

It has also been demonstrated that there are higher instances of infection in certain patient groups. Persons with rheumatoid arthritis, especially those on steroids, have been shown to be at considerably more risk for postoperative infection than the general population (11,36).

Tissue reaction: Slow healing in patients with rheumatoid arthritis with vasculitis, or on steroids, has been observed to the point of wound dehiscence during the early phase of convalescence. This has led some physicians to restrict activities more in these patients than in others. Difficulty in wound closure, particularly around the knees, with resultant closures under tension, has resulted in instances of wound breakdown.

Myositis ossificans or heterotopic bone formation is a special problem, occurring most frequently about the hip. While it may occur in as many as 50% of all cases of hip surgery, it is sufficiently extensive to become a disability in less than 2% (37). Those most likely to develop myositis ossificans are individuals who have undergone previous hip surgery, have ankylosing spondylitis, or have hypertrophic osteoarthritis.

In high risk individuals various medications (29) and postoperative radiation have been used with some success (12).

Patient–physician over-optimism This can be a problem if the preoperative assessment has suggested a higher level of activity than develops, or if the patient sets an unrealistic goal.

Salvage of the Unsatisfactory Result

If a biomaterial failure occurs, in most instances it is possible to carry out revision surgery. It must be remembered that the risks faced at the original surgery are not only still present, but the risk of failure has increased. Some of the reasons are as follows:

1. The patient is usually considerably older.
2. Revision surgery is technically more difficult than the original surgery.
3. Bone stock is usually lost as a result of the original surgical procedure and has often been compromised by the failure.
4. Special prostheses are frequently required.
5. The risks of infection and myositis ossificans increase.

In the instance where infection occurs, one of three things can occur. In those situations recognized early, where good prosthetic fixation remains, a certain number can be salvaged by various types of drainage procedures, debridement, and antibiotics (25). In some instances, this may include the removal of the prostheses and reinsertion. A second situation is sometimes found in which it is not possible to cure the infection, but it may be possible to control it by use of long-term antibiotics (19). In these instances, the prostheses invariably loosen. To accept this situation, the patient must be prepared to accept the disability associated with loosening. Usually this can only be accomplished in a low-demand situation. The alternatives of a resectional arthroplasty or fusion should be less attractive than the disability associated with the need for life-long antibiotics and a loose prosthesis. A third situation can occur, in which the infection cannot be cured or controlled with the prosthesis intact. In this case, the salvage procedure usually consists of a fusion or a resectional arthroplasty. Which method is used will depend on the decisions made by both the physician and the patient.

In the vast majority of cases in which failure occurs at the hip or shoulder, a resectional arthroplasty will be carried out. In the hip, subsequent ambulation is usually carried out with the aid of an ischial weight bearing brace and some additional type of ambulatory aid (cane, crutch or walkerette). For most elderly people, particularly those with other joint disabilities, the brace represents a considerable handicap, and the energy expenditure for ambulation is quite high.

In the shoulder, the advantage of having some remaining glenohumeral motion frequently outweighs the pain relief by fusion. There is also considerable difficulty in obtaining a fusion.

In the knee, the procedure of choice is generally knee fusion. While there have been several reports of difficulty in obtaining fusion after removal of total knee components, we have obtained rapid fusion in a small series by using intramedullary nails and compression techniques (20).

STAGING OF PROSTHETIC INSERTIONS

Replacement arthroplasty, with very rare exceptions, is elective surgery. If it is known that multiple arthroplasties are to be carried out, there are a few general principles that are to be followed:

1. If it is anticipated that a hip and knee arthroplasty are to be done, one generally does the hip as the first joint. There are two reasons: (a) If the hip has a flexion contracture, there will either be compensatory lordosis or compensatory knee flexion to allow an upright weight-bearing stance. Correction of the hip flexion contracture will obviate the need for compensatory knee flexion on weight bearing and thus make it more likely that a successful knee arthroplasty with full extension will be obtained. (b) During hip arthroplasty without trochanteric osteotomy, the knee must frequently be flexed to near 90° with some varus and external rotation stresses applied. Theoretically, this could damage a knee arthroplasty. During knee arthroplasty, no extremes of position are required of the hip and no unusual stresses are applied. Therefore, it is safer to do knee arthroplasties following hip arthroplasties rather than vice versa.

2. Most surgeons doing upper extremity replacement arthroplasties would prefer their patients not use crutches, walkerettes, or canes. Therefore, if it is anticipated that both upper and lower extremity arthroplasties are to be done, it is preferable to do lower extremity surgery first and complete this prior to upper extremity arthroplasty.

3. As will be discussed later (in *Discharge Planning*), many surgeons find that staging arthroplasties at roughly three-month intervals allows close to full convalescence from one procedure before the second is attempted. In most instances, this seems to result in better overall satisfaction with the individual prosthesis. Staging of the prostheses at this interval, rather than doing multiple arthroplasties simultaneously, allows for better treatment if complications develop. For example, if a patient is to develop heterotropic new bone formation about the hip, it is well to know this prior to the second arthroplasty so that preventive measures can be taken, because it is known that those who have previously suffered myositis ossificans are more likely to have it on this occasion. If total hip arthroplasties are carried out at the same sitting, and bilateral heterobone develops, a severe disability can result.

SPECIFIC ARTHROPLASTIES

The Hip

The total hip arthroplasty is by far the commonest arthroplasty done and the arthroplasty about which most is known at this time.

As it is commonly performed, total hip arthroplasty involves replacing the proximal femur with a metallic ball and replacement of the acetabulum with a socket made of UHMWP (Fig. 3).

In most instances, the components are cemented with PMM, although, as noted earlier, there is an effort being made to develop a porous, coated prosthesis that will utilize a biologic bond to bone without the use of cement. There is increasing tendency to develop UHMWP components that have a metal backing, minimizing stress across the plastic.

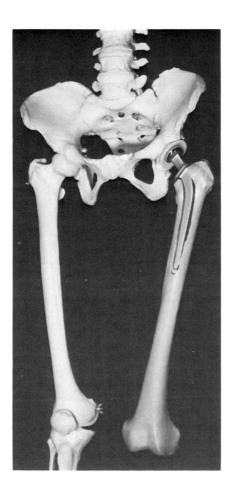

FIG. 3. Positioning of components of a total hip arthroplasty as seen in a skeleton. The acetabular component is ultra-high molecular weight polyethylene, and the femoral component metal. The femoral component is in the intramedullary canal.

The indication for total hip replacement is most often pain not satisfactorily relieved by nonoperative measures. Elderly persons, or more specifically, those who by reason of age or associated problems or illness are not likely to require revision, and are the best candidates (Fig. 4).

The actual life expectancy of the hip prosthesis is uncertain. Materials hold up well and abrasive wear, per se, does not appear to be a major factor. The problems for which revision is required are generally prosthetic breakage, loosening of the components, or infection.

Prosthetic loosening remains a problem, related to several factors. Clearly, the size of the individual and the use to which the prosthesis is being subjected are strong influences. The heavy patient who is very active tends to loosen his or her prosthesis more frequently than the lighter, less active patient (9,35). Improvements in prosthetic design, including porous coating, give promise to reduce this rate of loosening.

Knowledge of biomaterials and biomechanics has reduced the incidence of loosening. Prostheses with larger intramedullary stems that directly abut cortical bone are now being widely used. This allows stresses to be placed through femoral cortical bone as well as cancellous bone. Placement of a prosthesis in a valgus position to eliminate stress risers on the proximal femoral shaft has previously been discussed.

The use of a flanged prosthesis, which allows some weight-bearing load on

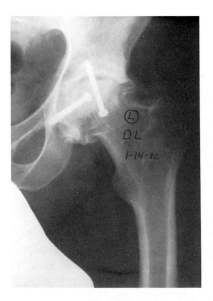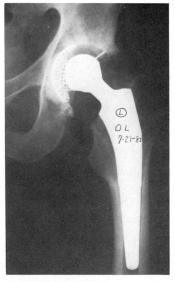

FIG. 4. Left: Preoperative X-ray of a man with degenerative arthritis and avascular necrosis of the left hip secondary to a fracture/dislocation of the hip. **Right:** The postoperative X-ray on the right demonstrates an uncemented porous coated Dual Lock® femoral component with a cemented acetabular component.

the proximal femur at the point where the femoral head was resected from the neck of the femur, has been advocated as a means of distributing weight-bearing stresses in a more normal fashion and thus minimize loosening. The use of cement introduced under pressure to allow greater penetration of the cancellous intramedullary bone, as many now advocate, may reduce the incidence of loosening of the bone cement junction.

The surgical approach used for insertion of total hip arthroplasty is generally a lateral or anterolateral approach to the proximal femur; a minority of surgeons prefer a posterior approach. However, the posterior approach may be used if previous surgery has been carried out through this approach (for instance, an Austin-Moore hemiarthroplasty or a previous fixation of an acetabular fracture).

In most instances, it is possible to insert the components without the removal of the greater trochanter. This is currently the most popular means of approach, and it eliminates the risk of one complication, i.e., of the trochanteric non-union.

While removal of the trochanter for better visualization of the acetabulum and the femoral shaft is not now done routinely by most surgeons on the initial operative procedure, it is widely employed when technically difficult procedures are done, such as revision of a failed total hip replacement, acetabular reconstruction for congenitally dysplastic hips, or when there is a total knee arthroplasty in the same limb. When a total knee arthroplasty is present, one aims to minimize the stresses at the knee that are required to expose the shaft for inserting the femoral component.

When the trochanter is removed, it must be reattached by various means: Wire fixation techniques and cancellous screws are commonly used. Protective weight-bearing is usually carried out until early union is noted. This is often a period of 8 to 12 weeks, but can be of longer duration. In spite of all precautions, there remain instances of non-union of the trochanter that approach 10%. In most instances, when bony union fails to develop, a fibrous union does occur and allows for adequate gluteal function. In a relatively small percentage of cases there is gluteal weakness and a partial disability.

Prophylactic antibiotics and prophylactic anticoagulants are widely used. Depending upon the preference of the surgeon and other physicians, these are started before, during, or immediately after the operative procedure. Numerous protocols are used governing both the type and duration of anticoagulation. It is generally accepted that any anticoagulation be continued until the patient is fully ambulatory and any suggestive signs of dependent swelling have disappeared. The use of elastic stockings on both extremities during the postoperative phase is widely accepted. Some surgeons advocate a mechanical-pulsed extremity compression as an adjunct to anticoagulation.

In the postoperative phase, the initial physical therapy typically consists of muscle setting and gentle active ranges of motion of the hip, knee, and ankle. In the first 24 hours, there is usually a drainage tube in the wound, and all medications are given intravenously, so that vigorous mobilization is difficult.

The leg is held in some type of immobilization in the immediate postoperative period. This can be balanced suspension and skin traction, or can consist of a sling at the knee and skin traction to prevent external rotation and extension. Immobilization is carried out until active control of the extremity is achieved and the patient is past the risk of dislocation on simple transfers. It should be realized that in all procedures, the tensor fascia lata is incised and small amounts of the gluteal muscles are detached. This results in some weakness of the extremity, and until this weakness disappears, the limb must be protected in transfers.

The position to be avoided varies with the surgical approach. When an anterior approach has been used, the patient is at most risk for dislocation if the extremity is extended and externally rotated. Therefore, the best position is one of slight flexion at the hip with the leg in neutral or internal rotation. This can be accomplished with a sling or balanced suspension and rotation straps if necessary.

If a posterior approach has been used, the patient is most at risk for dislocation when the hip is flexed or internally rotated (the opposite of the anterior approach). The risk of dislocation following posterior approach can be minimized by keeping the limb in extension at the hip, maintaining some slight abduction, and by immobilizing the knee in a proprietary splint. By eliminating the ability to actively flex the knee, flexion at the hip becomes more difficult.

After motor control is achieved (when the patient can extend the knee against gravity and set the quadriceps and gluteal muscles), assisted movement out of bed can be achieved safely. If a bed-to-chair regimen or extreme changes of position are attempted before good voluntary motor control is achieved (e.g., transfer from bed to an X-ray table), proper positioning of the extremity must be maintained.

As soon as good voluntary motor control is noted, the immobilization can be removed. A flexion sling attached to an overhead bar on the bed is a valuable self-help device that can be used as a flexion assist for both the hip and the knee. It will allow active quadriceps exercise against gravity and assist in hip flexion and adduction.

Sitting upright in a chair can be started early in the postoperative course. It is generally not wise to have the patient sit more than 30 minutes at any one time. Venous compression can occur and dependent swelling develop; this will predispose to phlebitis or a stasis problem.

Walking can usually be instituted within a day or two of the time the patient can be out of bed safely. Initially, this is best accomplished with a walkerette with transition to other types of aids, such as a cane or crutch, as rapidly as the patient's stamina and balance will allow.

In the majority of cases, partial weight-bearing is allowed. It should be remembered that non-weight-bearing will be unrealistic for many of the elderly, especially those with musculoskeletal disabilities or balance problems.

The amount of weight-bearing allowed will vary with several factors. Some surgeons are reluctant to allow full weight-bearing for a period of at least six weeks under any circumstances; others allow weight bearing as tolerated from the onset.

When trochanteric osteotomy has been performed, restriction to partial weight bearing is usually carried out until early union of the trochanter can be noted.

In most instances, it is advisable that the patient use a cane until full recovery (a period of six to twelve weeks).

The Knee

The normal knee is not a hinge, but a finely articulated joint which, in normal bending, is undergoing a complex sequence of motions. In the first 70° of flexion from full extension, there is a rolling and gliding motion occurring at the femorotibial junction with a constantly changing axis of rotation in the distal femur that describes an ellipse. Coupled with this, there is some rotation of the tibia on an axial line in relation to the femur (28). To date, no prosthetic knee has successfully duplicated all these motions. This results in some forces on the prosthetic knee that predispose to wear of the component or, in cases of a fixed hinge prosthesis, has transmitted rotational stresses to the bones at an interface. Loosening of the fixed hinge prosthesis at the bone cement interface is so common that this design has been virtually eliminated and most prosthetic knees now have some degree of variable rotation built within the design (Fig. 5) (17,26,31).

In all knee arthroplasties, long-term success of the arthroplasty depends to a considerable degree on proper alignment. In order to carry out the procedure properly, a knowledge of the alignment and the kinetics is important. (See *X-Ray Evaluation.*)

The various knee arthroplasty prosthetic devices available can generally be divided into two types: an unconstrained prosthesis and a constrained prosthesis.

An unconstrained prosthesis is a surface replacement of the articular surfaces of the distal femur and the proximal tibia; and occasionally the articular surface of the patella. Stability in the joint will be due, in large part, to the retained collateral, cruciate and capsular ligaments.

A constrained total knee arthroplasty prosthesis has inherent stability to allow it to be used in a situation where there are inadequate ligaments or extreme capsular laxity.

There are numerous devices commercially available; most consist of a metal femoral component and an ultra-high molecular weight polyethylene tibial component (frequently with metal backing) (Fig. 6). If used, a patellar replacement is of high molecular weight polyethylene. As with the hip, these components are cemented to the bone with polymethyl methacrylate.

When the primary problem is the loss of articular cartilage and small amounts of subchondral bone, as in the majority of cases, it is possible to use one of many available unconstrained knees; with these, the major ligaments and capsu-

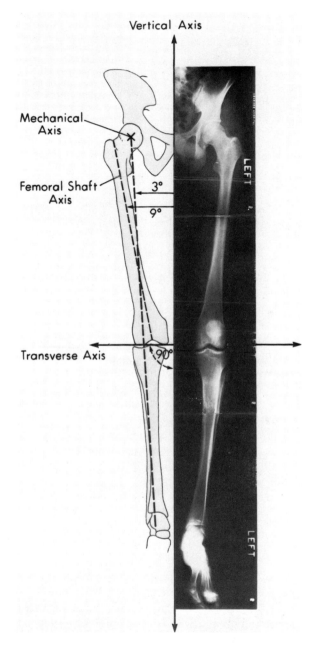

FIG. 5. Composite of anatomical relationships in the lower extremity. Several factors are important: (a) In a normal standing configuration, a plumb line dropped from the hip will pass through the knee and bisect the talus. (b) Axial lines drawn down the shaft of the femur and tibia subtend an angle of approximately 6°. The degree of varus (bowing) or valgus (knock-knee) is measured from this point. (c) The weight-bearing surface of the knee should be at right angles to the plumb line.

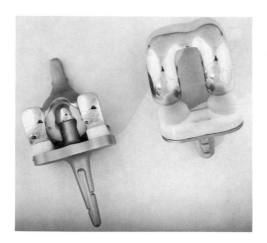

FIG. 6. **Left:** A constrained Spherocentric® total knee as seen from a posterior view. Note the ball and socket arrangement that allows rotation, gives lateral stability, but allows an arc of flexion well past 90°. Plastic runners on the tibial component stabilize the varus/valgus moment (rocking) and partially limit rotation. This would be used primarily in situations where inherent stability of the knee was lacking. **Right:** An unconstrained Multiradius® knee, used where there is remaining bony ligamentous and capsular stability. The femoral component is metal and the tibial component UHMWP supported by metal.

lar structures will be intact. In certain instances, however, where extreme angular deformities have developed, there may be sufficient ligamentous laxities due to stretching so that it would be difficult to obtain stability without some secondary procedures that tighten ligaments.

As a general rule, it has been found that, when combined angular deformities as viewed in a weight-bearing knee approach 40°, there will be difficulty in achieving postoperative stability with an unconstrained knee. An example is a 20° fixed knee flexion contracture with a 20° valgus deformity. In these situations one must be prepared at the time of surgery to carry out ligamentous or capsule repair or to use a constrained knee prosthesis.

In the preoperative assessment of the ligamentous integrity of the knee, the collateral and capsular ligaments are most important. During insertion of most unconstrained and all constrained prosthetic devices, the anterior cruciate is usually sacrificed and, with certain prostheses, the posterior cruciate is sacrificed as well.

Postoperative Regimen for the Knee

Considerable variation will be found in the postoperative regimens (Figs. 7, 8, and 9). Some of the variations are generated by philosophical considerations that differ with surgeons, but some are imposed by anatomic considerations. The anatomic considerations are especially critical when soft tissue reconstructions have been carried out coincident with the knee arthroplasty. However, certain generalizations can be made.

1. In most postoperative regimens, some type of compression dressing or pulsed boot is used in conjunction with limb elevation in the immediate postoperative period in an attempt to minimize phlebitis. It is of paramount importance to remember that, if true elevation is to be carried out, the ankle should be

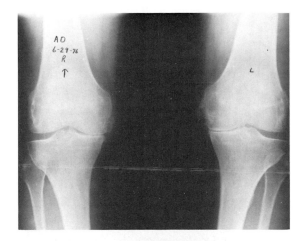

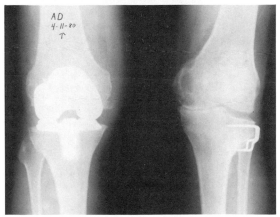

FIG. 7. Top: Degenerative arthritis in the knees of a 72-year-old farmer. Note the valgus posture with complete loss of medial joint space. **Bottom:** The same patient after bilateral operative procedures. A tibial osteotomy was performed on the left knee and an unconstrained total knee arthroplasty placed in the right. Both procedures are working well.

above the knee and the knee above heart level. A "jack-knife" position should be avoided; it can account for some venous constriction of the pelvis or proximal femoral vessels.

2. In the majority of cases, prophylactic antibiotics will be used. Most surgeons employ the same regimen as in total hip arthroplasty.

3. Following an arthroplasty of the knee, there is a period of time when quadriceps weakness is present. This will vary considerably from patient to patient. It will generally be shorter if quadriceps exercises were used as part of the preoperative situation. During the period of weakness, many surgeons prefer to protect the knee by some type of immobilization. This may include a bulky dressing with a light plaster shell or, possibly, the use of a proprietary

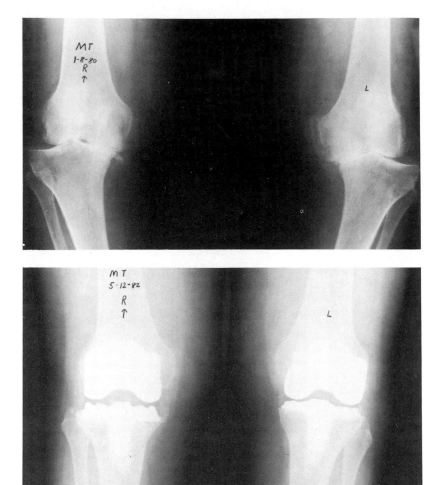

FIG. 8. Top: Severe degenerative arthritis of both knees with a marked varus deformity and subluxation in a 75-year-old woman. **Bottom:** Successful treatment using bilateral unconstrained prostheses.

splint. (It is the author's practice to maintain the limb in a bulky dressing that extends from the toes to the groin.) This is continued until there is sufficient quadriceps function to allow the patient to protect the limb in transfers. The actual time of immobilization rarely exceeds four to five days.

4. Suction drainage is usually placed in the knee joint and is continued until the drainage is less than 30 ml. per eight-hour shift, but should not exceed 72 hr. If bleeding in excess of this amount is still occurring after 72 hours, serious consideration should be given to reexploring the wound.

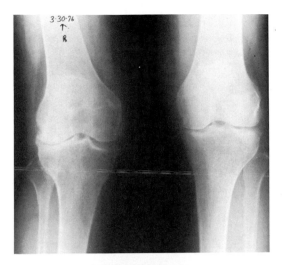

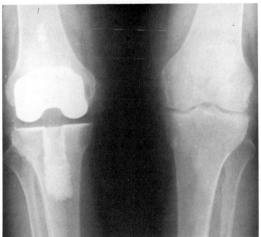

FIG. 9. Top: A marked valgus deformity in the right knee of a 68-year-old woman. **Bottom:** Successful treatment using an unconstrained total knee arthroplasty.

5. After removal of the bulky dressing, active flexion and extension exercises are begun. Various flexion assist slings are used as well as supervised physical therapy. In certain instances, passive continuous flexion is being used through a motorized exercise device attached to the bed. In routine cases, the author seeks to have the patients actively flexing through an arc of 90° from a position of active full extension in two weeks. If it appears that this goal cannot be reached during this period of time, consideration for manipulation under anesthesia is given. At approximately two weeks, it is frequently found that gravity alone will provide sufficient force to disrupt any intraarticular adhesions that

are occurring and that appear to be limiting activity. Manipulation is not carried out beyond a point of five weeks following surgery because of a view that the excessive stress required at that time may cause prosthetic loosening or damage.

6. *Weight-bearing:* As with total hip replacement, the recommendation for the amount of weight-bearing to be allowed will vary among surgeons. Although no extensive studies have been reported, most published regimens advocate weight-bearing as tolerated with the use of a walkerette, crutches, or a cane. Most surgeons recommend the use of at least a cane until maximum recovery of strength and motion has occurred. If stability is a problem, some type of walking aid is recommended indefinitely.

7. Support stockings should be used for at least six weeks or longer if there is any suggestion of dependent edema.

8. A regimen of daily unsupervised exercises is set up for the patient to assure that range of motion and muscle strength are maintained.

Other Arthroplasties

Hip and knee arthroplasties are the most frequently performed. Although clear statistics are not available, probably the next most commonly performed arthroplasties are the metacarpophalangeal (MCP) joints in the severely handicapped patient with rheumatoid arthritis. As stated earlier, many surgeons prefer to have all anticipated lower extremity surgery completed before considering upper extremity surgery, because they do not want their patients to use a cane or crutches after arthroplasty of the hand, wrist, elbow, or shoulder.

MCP joint arthroplasty is frequently a part of a staged procedure to restore grip strength and dexterity to the hand and wrist as well as to improve the cosmetic appearance. Preoperative assessment of the patient requires a thorough knowledge of upper extremity functional anatomy because the hand cannot be considered independent from the shoulder, elbow, or wrist. It is not uncommon to have to carry out fusion or replacement arthroplasty of the wrist, or perhaps even shoulder arthroplasty in anticipation of MCP joint surgery in order to achieve a desired result.

The preoperative assessment of the patient differs little from that required for lower extremity arthroplasty. However, it should be remembered that, with the exception of the shoulder, most upper extremity surgery can be carried out under regional anesthesia and the concerns that accompany a general anesthetic are not necessarily present.

The postoperative regimen following MCP joint arthroplasty is frequently a tedious one requiring regular and frequent periods of exercise. In many instances, the exercise program must be tailored to the individual and is difficult to generalize. For example, special concerns may be directed toward stabilizing a painful wrist while exercising the MCPs, or in other instances, special resting splints may have to be fashioned. Customized splints with exercisers made from rubber bands are commonly used (4).

In recent years, shoulder arthroplasty has been receiving increased favor.

Several problems that resulted in a high incidence of failure early in the development of shoulder arthroplasty seem to be responding to modifications of the prosthetic devices.

It has become apparent that an intact rotator cuff is the key to a successful arthroplasty. The bony portion of the gleno-humeral—or shoulder—joint is mechanically unstable in the sense that the humeral head is spherical and much larger than the relatively small and flat socket of the glenoid. Stability at the shoulder joint is gained by the four muscles that comprise the rotator cuff. These muscles, acting in concert, keep the humeral head well centered on the glenoid, and permit the more powerful muscles such as the deltoid, pectoral, and biceps muscle to work around a stable fulcrum. If the rotator cuff, particularly the supraspinatus, is torn or otherwise inadequate, proximal subluxation of the humeral head may occur with resultant pain and inefficiency.

The most reliable and successful shoulder arthroplasties are possible for patients who have intact rotator cuffs and in whom the arthroplasty essentially consists of resurfacing the glenoid with a polyethylene implant and replacing the humeral head articular surface with a metallic ball (33).

In instances where the rotator cuff is not intact, prostheses have been designed to provide partial correction. One type of prosthesis attempts to prevent proximal subluxation of the humeral head against the undersurface of the acromion by a proximal lip on the glenoid component that contains the humeral head. The second method is by use of a constrained ball and socket type joint.

A concern with the constrained joint is that the glenoid fixation is difficult to obtain, because of the size of the socket and the relatively thin bone of the glenoid and scapula that are not amenable to bulky fixation. Thus, constrained prostheses have a fairly high rate of loosening of the scapular component.

Elbow prostheses are still in a state of development, although there have been several recent publications that would indicate that success with these prostheses is improving (23).

As with total shoulder arthroplasty, total elbow arthroplasty replacements meet with difficulty with fixation of the components, especially when there has been inadequate soft tissue stability. Both the elbow and shoulder are subjected to extremely high compressive forces because they act as fulcrums. The load they must bear is usually held in the hand, and the muscles that stabilize the joint act over short distances.

Replacement arthroplasties of the ankle and the metatarsophalangeal joints are done less frequently in the elderly individual than those mentioned earlier. Ankle arthroplasty continues to be in a developmental stage. Replacement arthroplasty of the metatarsophalangeal joints seems best indicated in those individuals who have primarily hallux valgus and who will be sufficiently active so that they would be unhappy with the disability imposed by the more commonly done resectional arthroplastics.

In order to accomplish satisfactory exercise programs, it is invaluable for the surgeon to work closely with specially trained physical therapists or occupational therapists who are knowledgeable not only in the functional anatomy of the disease process, the type of surgery carried out, but who are also capable of fabricating special splints and exercise devices. It has become apparent that the greatest number of satisfactory results in upper extremity arthroplasties come from those centers that are capable of providing sophisticated postoperative exercise regimens.

DISCHARGE PLANNING

Discharge from closely supervised convalescent care is related more to performance than time. Prior to discharge, it is preferable to have the patient independent. By independence, it is meant that the patient should be able to transfer, unassisted, from either a bed or chair to an upright position, be able to perform an exercise regimen without supervision, and be able to use a commode and climb stairs without assistance.

Realistically, most patients without other significant handicaps will be able to be independent, by this definition, within 10 to 21 days following surgery. However, most individuals, following this or any other major surgery, find that their exercise tolerance is markedly diminished. They find that most of these things can be accomplished, but not as frequently or with the vigor that is desired. Depending on the patient, it may take 6 to 12 weeks for sufficient stamina to return so that activities of daily living are performed easily in a repetitive manner. As previously noted, this observation has led many orthopaedic surgeons to recommend a three-month interval between consecutive joint arthroplasties. While this generalization is not followed by all, it seems to have considerable merit for many patients.

As soon as early wound healing appears assured, it is possible to shower. This is often preferable to a bath because of the extreme hip and knee flexion required to get into a bathtub. When balance or weakness is a problem, it is recommended that a walkerette be carried into a shower.

In the early convalescence, dressing is frequently a problem. Assistance with various self-help devices can aid in accomplishing these tasks. In most instances, elastic stockings cannot be applied independently—some help is required. The use of elastic hose to minimize peripheral edema and the occurrence of phlebitis is widely recommended. This is generally continued until there is no evidence of dependent edema, or for at least six weeks.

Driving is usually not allowed until the sixth postoperative week. In addition, while traveling as a passenger, scrupulous use of a seatbelt is important. Irreparable damage has been done to hip and knee arthroplasties when the recovering patient has been thrown against a dashboard in a collision or sudden stop.

Because the risk of phlebitis remains for some period of time in the postoperative phase, it is not wise for the patient to remain in a sitting position for a long period of time. Our present recommendation is not to drive or remain in a sitting position in excess of 90 minutes without a brief period of walking or some change of position.

There is a slight risk of late infection following joint arthroplasty. Figures are not available as to the incidence, but it cannot be doubted that deep infections around the prosthetic device have occurred when there has been bacteremia or septicemia with the source of infection elsewhere.

Because bacteremia may follow a dental procedure, many physicians and dentists follow the recommendations of the American Heart Association for prevention of cardiac infection and use penicillin (1). However, Jacobsen and Murray have presented data suggesting that erythromycin, clindamycin, or a penicillinase-resistant penicillin (methicillin or nafcillin) would be better to protect against seeding of a joint arthroplasty (24).

REFERENCES

1. American Heart Association, A Committee Report (1977): Prevention of bacterial endocarditis. *J. Am. Dent. Assoc.,* 95:600.
2. Andrews, H. J., Arden, G. P., Hart, G. M., and Owen, J. W. (1981): Deep infection after total hip replacement. *J. Bone and Joint Surg.,* 63B:53.
3. Andriacchi, T. P., Galante, J. O., Belytschko, T. B., and Hampton, S. (1976): A stress analysis of the femoral stem in total hip prostheses. *J. Bone and Joint Surg.,* 58A:618.
4. Beckenbaugh, Robert D., Dobyns, James H., Linscheid, Ronald L., and Bryan, Richard S. (1976): Review and analysis of silicone-rubber metacarpophalangeal implants. *J. Bone and Joint Surg.,* 58A:483.
5. Beckenbaugh, Robert D., Ilstrup, Duane M. (1978): Total hip arthroplasty: A review of three-hundred and thirty-three cases with long follow-up. *J. Bone and Joint Surg.,* 60A:306.
6. Bobyn, J. D., Pilliar, R. M., Cameron, H. U., and Weatherly, G. C. (1980): The optimum pore size for the fixation of porous-surfaced metal implants by the ingrowth of bone. *Clin. Orthop.,* 150:263.
7. Bobyn, J. D., Pilliar, R. M., Cameron, M. B., Weatherly, G. C., and Kent, G. M. (1980): The effect of porous surface configuration on the tensile strength of fixation of implants by bone ingrowth. *Clin. Orthop.,* 149:291.
8. Cabot, Anthony, and Becker, Alfred (1978): The cervical spine in rheumatoid arthritis. *Clin. Orthop.,* 131:130.
9. Chao, Edmund Y. S., and Coventry, Mark B. (1981): Fracture of the femoral component after total hip replacement: An analysis of fifty-eight cases. *J. Bone and Joint Surg.,* 63A:1078.
10. Charnley, J., Follacci, F. M., and Hammond, B. T. (1968): The long-term reaction of bone to self-curing acrylic cement. *J. Bone and Joint Surg.,* 50B:822.
11. Colville, James and Raunio, Pauli (1978): Charnley low-friction arthroplasties of the hip in rheumatoid arthritis: A study of the complications and results of 378 arthroplasties. *J. Bone and Joint Surg.,* 60B:498.
12. Coventry, Mark B., and Scanlon, Paul W. (1981): The use of radiation to discourage ectopic bone: A nine year study in surgery about the hip. *J. Bone and Joint Surg.,* 63A:201.
13. Crowninshield, R. D., Brand, R. A., Johnston, R. C., and Pedersen, D. R. (1981): An analysis of collar function and the use of titanium in femoral prostheses. *Clin. Orthop.,* 158:270.
14. Ducheyne, Paul, Kagan, Abbott, II, and Allen, Lacey J. (1978): Failure of total knee arthroplasty due to loosening and deformation of the tibial component. *J. Bone and Joint Surg.,* 60A:384.
15. Evarts, C. M., and Alfidi, R. J. (1973): Thromboembolism after total hip reconstruction. *JAMA,* 225:515.
16. Fitzgerald, Robert H., Declan, R. Nolan, Ilstrup, Duane M., VanScoy, Robert E., Washington, John A., III, and Coventry, Mark B. (1977): Deep wound sepsis following total hip arthroplasty. *J. Bone and Joint Surg.,* 59A:847.
17. Goodfellow, John, and O'Connor, John (1978): The mechanics of the knee and prosthesis design. *J. Bone and Joint Surg.,* 60B:358.
18. Gravlee, G. P. (1980): Succinylcholine-induced hyperkalemia in a patient with Parkinson's disease. *Anesthesia and Analgesia,* 59:444.
19. Harris, C. M. (1982): Infection following total joint arthroplasties. *(Submitted for publication.)*
20. Harris, C. M. (1982): Knee fusions for failed total arthroplasties. *(Submitted for publication.)*
21. Harris, William H. (1969): Traumatic arthritis of the hip after dislocation and acetabular fractures: treatment by mold arthroplasty: an end-result study using a new method of result evaluation. *J. Bone and Joint Surg.,* 51A:737.

22. Hori, Roy H., Lewis, Jack L., Zimmerman, Jerald R., and Compere, Clinton L. (1978): The number of total joint replacements in the United States. *Clin. Orthop.,* 132:46.
23. Inglis, Allan E., and Pellicci, Paul M. (1980): Total hip replacement. *J. Bone and Joint Surg.,* 62A:1252.
24. Jacobsen, P. L., and Murray, W. (1980): Prophylactic coverage of dental patients with artificial joints: a retrospective analysis of thirty-three infections in hip joints. *Oral Surg.,* 50:130.
25. Jupiter, Jesse B., Karchmer, Adolf W., Lowell, J. Drennan, and Harris, William H. (1981): Total hip arthroplasty in the treatment of adult hips with current or quiescent sepsis. *J. Bone and Joint Surg.,* 63A:194.
26. Kaufer, Herbert, and Matthews, Larry S. (1981): Spherocentric arthroplasty of the knee: clinical experience with an average four-year follow-up. *J. Bone and Joint Surg.,* 63A:545.
27. Kelsey, Jennifer L., Wood, Philip H. N., and Charnley, John (1976): Prediction of thromboembolism following total hip replacement. *Clin. Orthop.,* 114:247.
28. Kettelcamp, Donald B., and Nasca, Richard (1973): Biomechanics and knee replacement arthroplasty. *Clin. Orthop.,* 94:8.
29. Lowell, J. Drennan (1982): Heterotopic ossification in revision arthroplasty. In: *Revision Total Hip Arthroplasty,* 2nd ed., edited by R. H. Turner and A. D. Scheller. Grune and Stratton, New York.
30. Mann, George V. (1974): The influence of obesity on health (first of two parts). *N. Engl. J. Med.,* 291:178.
31. Murray, David G., and Webster, Dwight A. (1981): The variable-axis knee prosthesis: two-year follow-up study. *J. Bone and Joint Surg.,* 63A:687.
32. National Institute of Health Consensus Conference (1982): Total hip joint replacement in the United States. *JAMA,* 248:1817.
33. Neer, Charles S., Watson, Keith C., and Stanton, F. Joann (1982): Recent experience in total shoulder replacement. *J. Bone and Joint Surg.,* 64A:319.
34. Nelson, J. Phillip, Glassburn, Alba R., Jr., Talbott, Richard D., and McElhinney, James P. (1980): The effect of previous surgery, operating room environment, and preventive antibiotics on postoperative infection following total hip arthroplasty. *Clin. Orthop.,* 147:167.
35. Pellicci, Paul M., Salvati, Eduardo A., and Robinson, Harry J. (1979): Mechanical failures in total hip replacement requiring reoperation. *J. Bone and Joint Surg.,* 61A:28.
36. Poss, Robert, Ewald, Frederick C., Thomas, William, and Sledge, Clement B. (1976): Complications of total hip-replacement arthroplasty in patients with rheumatoid arthritis. *J. Bone and Joint Surg.,* 58A:1130.
37. Riegler, Hubert F., and Harris, Carl M. (1976): Heterotopic bone formation after total hip arthroplasty. *Clin. Orthop.,* 117:209.
38. Rochester, Dudley F., and Enson, Yale (1974): Current concepts in the pathogenesis of the obesity-hypoventilation syndrome: mechanical and circulatory factors. *Am. J. of Med.,* 57:402.
39. Rooker, G. D., and Wilkinson, J. D. (1980): Metal sensitivity in patients undergoing hip replacements: a prospective study. *J. Bone and Joint Surg.,* 62B:502.
40. Rose, Robert M., and Radin, Eric L. (1982): Wear of polyethylene in the total hip prosthesis. *Clin. Orthop.,* 170:107.
41. Salvati, Eduardo A., Wilson, Philip D., Jolley, Michael N., Vakili, Fayegh, Aglietti, Paolo, and Brown, George C. (1981): A ten-year follow-up study of our first one hundred consecutive Charnley total hip replacements. *J. Bone and Joint Surg.,* 63A:753.
42. Schwartz, Allan B. (1978): Potassium-related cardiac arrhythmias and their treatment. *Angiology,* 29(3):194.
43. Sikorski, J. M., Hampson, W. G., and Staddon, G. E. (1981): The natural history and aetiology of deep vein thrombosis after total hip replacement. *J. Bone and Joint Surg.,* 63B:171.
44. Steen, Petter A., Tinker, John H., and Tarhan, Sait (1978): Myocardial reinfarction after anesthesia and surgery. *JAMA,* 239:2566.
45. Tarhan, Sait, Morfitt, Emerson A., Taylor, William F., and Giuliani, Emilio, R. (1972): Myocardial infarction after general anesthesia. *JAMA,* 220:1451.
46. Vaughan, Robert W. (1980): Obesity: implication in anesthetic management and toxicity. 1980 Annual Refresher Course Lectures, Number 240. American Society of Anesthesiologists, Inc., Las Vegas.
47. Weinstein, Allan M., Bingham, Dennis N., Sauer, Barry W., and Lunceford, E. M. (1976): The effect of high pressure insertion and antibiotic inclusions upon the mechanical properties of polymethylmethacrylate. *Clin. Orthop.,* 121:67.

Rehabilitation in the Aging edited by
T. F. Williams. Raven Press, New York © 1984.

Rehabilitation in Ophthalmology for the Aged

Abraham L. Kornzweig
(1900–1982)

*Department of Eye Research, Jewish Home and Hospital for the Aged; Mount Sinai
School of Medicine of City University of New York; and Mount Sinai Hospital,
New York, New York 10025*

Any procedure, device, activity, drug, or method which will help visually handicapped aged individuals improve their visual capacity can be considered rehabilitation.

In this chapter the most common serious problem affecting vision, the development of cataracts, is addressed first. Even though its primary treatment (and thus rehabilitation of vision) is a surgical procedure performed by an ophthalmologist, awareness of the new developments in cataract extraction and lens replacement is important for any physician dealing with rehabilitative aspects of aging. Vitrectomy, another new development, is also discussed. The remainder of the chapter is devoted to low vision aids for persons for whom surgical or medical correction of the visual disability is impossible. Throughout it is assumed that properly fitted corrective lenses will be provided and rechecked periodically.

CATARACT

The most important cause of loss of vision in aged persons is cataract formation. The need for surgery to remove the cataractous lens depends on the degree of visual loss and the visual requirements of the patient. Many an older person with a cataract in one eye but fairly good vision in the other is able to carry on the daily activities quite well. But when the good eye loses vision by a developing cataract and the person is thereby visually handicapped, removal of the cataract becomes necessary. A person whose occupation requires good visual acuity may decide on cataract removal sooner than another person without such need. These facts have to be taken into consideration by the ophthalmologist. There must also be assurance that the retina behind the cataract is healthy and the prospect of good vision following surgery is expected. There should be good light perception and projection in all quadrants of gaze. Macular function has to be tested to make sure that there is no significant degeneration. In those rare cases where retinal detachment or vitreous hemorrhage is suspected, an ultrasonic scanning is indicated. These tests are all done preparatory for surgery in those cases where visual loss from other causes besides cataract formation is suspected.

The most important procedure is the removal of the cataractous lens and its replacement by spectacles, contact lenses, or an intraocular lens implant. The success rate for this operation varies, depending upon the type of procedure. The customary operation of intracapsular cataract extraction in capable hands is successful in 90 to 95% of cases. Phacoemulsification, another method, is also successful in a large percentage of cases and is preferred by some surgeons because of the small incision that is made and the quick return to relatively normal activity. This operation is limited to those surgeons who have spent the time to learn the technique and acquired the necessary equipment. The principle behind the procedure is the use of an ultrasonic probe that emulsifies the lens, which is then aspirated by the same probe. The patient's stay in the hospital is shortened to about 24 hr. In some favorable cases the patient may be allowed to go home several hours after surgery. He is then followed postoperatively on a daily basis until the wound is healed, and spectacles or contact lenses are prescribed. Within two weeks the patient returns to his regular activities. The operation is preferred by persons who are not too old and in whom the lens is not so sclerosed or hardened as to make emulsification more difficult.

For persons who may have difficulty postoperatively wearing the usual cataract spectacles or contact lenses, the latest operation of the intraocular lens implant has been particularly helpful. In this procedure, a clear sterile plastic lens is placed inside the eye to replace the cataractous lens. Once the lens is in place and the incision closed, the patient is able to see almost as well as before the cataract formation and doesn't require any additional glasses except for reading and other close work. The operation is relatively new and the overall success rate has been reported to be around 80% (3,4,6). In one series of cases in which the patients for this operation were carefully selected—with exclusion of patients who were diabetic, had a history of glaucoma or an eye infection such as uveitis or iritis, or were found to be highly myopic—the success rate improved to 93 to 97%. A control series of cases who had the usual type of cataract surgery had the same improved success rate (6).

The lens implant operation, however, is still considered experimental by some ophthalmologists, and in fact twice the number of complications have been reported as were found in a control series of customary cataract operations. Thus further evaluation is necessary before this procedure can be recommended for more general use (3).

VITRECTOMY

There are several other eye conditions in older persons that were formerly considered untreatable that can now be helped to some degree by a surgical procedure. The most important condition in this group is the vitreous hemorrhage that occurs occasionally in patients with diabetic retinopathy. Vitreous hemorrhages tend to recur in this disease and eventually vision may be completely lost. The new procedure is called vitrectomy (1). A special probe is introduced into the vitreous body with which the hemorrhage is aspirated and vitreous strands and adhesions to the retina are cut. The removed vitreous tissue is replaced by clear sterile solutions. Vision has been restored in cases in which the retina is still in fairly good condition. Even a slight or moderate improvement in vision is considered a successful result in what would otherwise be a blind eye. Pre-retinal membranes that occasionally form as a result of retinitis can also be removed with the same vitrectomy technique. Illumination inside the eyeball is now available by a fiber optic probe which produces a cold sterile light.

Vitrectomy is now being used for vitreous hemorrhage due to other causes, such as injury or central retinal vein occlusion. The same operative procedure is also being used for removal of intraocular foreign bodies and parasites, although these conditions are not frequent in the aged.

Older individuals with retinal detachments are now operated on with good expectations of improvement in vision in the affected eye. The introduction of the binocular operating microscope has been a major advance in ophthalmic surgery. It enables the surgeon to use finer instruments and sutures, which can be more accurately placed. It has been especially helpful in corneal transplants, and cataract and glaucoma operations. New sutures of hairlike thinness and great tensile strength made of silk or synthetic material are now available. They result in more accurate and firmer closing of incisions, lesser postoperative hemorrhages and infections, and early ambulation of patients with fewer postoperative vascular complications, especially important in aged patients.

LOW VISION AIDS

There are eye conditions in the elderly which cause loss of vision, and which cannot be helped by surgery or medical therapy. Chief among these is macular degeneration. Other conditions are corneal opacities, vitreous hemorrhages, injuries to the eyes, and occlusive vascular diseases of the retinal and choroidal vessels. When the vision in the better eye is reduced to 20/70 or less, help is needed to read ordinary newspaper print, to telephone, to type, to sew on black material and to do work requiring good central vision. Vision reduced to 20/200 or less incapacitates the individual for performing any activity for ordinary work. Such persons are considered severely visually handicapped—industrially blind. In such persons rehabilitation is most important if possible. Ophthalmologists and optometrists are aware of these needs which are included in the term *low vision aids*—usually provided in low vision clinics,[1] but also in private offices of ophthalmologists and optometrists.

The types of low vision aids are many depending upon the degree of visual impairment. For those only mildly or moderately impaired, hand-held magnify-

---

[1] Up-to-date lists of low vision clinics in the United States are available from the American Foundation for the Blind, 15 West 16 Street, New York, N.Y. 10011.

ing glasses are used. The magnifying lens must be held at its focal point. A fixed focus magnifying glass can be used with the reading material placed on a desk or table. The reader moves the lens along the line and reads matter magnified from 2 to 10 times. Such reading is slow, but with patience and persistence greater speed can be acquired. Some of these lenses have direct illumination by flashlight attachments. Good illumination is necessary for improved results.

Spectacles for individuals with poor reading vision are available that may give a magnification from 2 to 10 times. These glasses require the individual to hold reading matter much closer to the eyes than most people are accustomed to doing. Many resent the necessity to do this and give up the effort. They must be reassured that the eyes are meant to be used for seeing, just as other organs have special capabilities. Continuing use of the eyes is desirable and necessary to prevent further deterioration from disuse (2,5).

Older individuals who are still capable of traveling and going outdoors by themselves but who have poor distant vision can occasionally be helped by telescopic lenses. This type of lens can be used temporarily when needed to see an approaching bus number or street address, or to identify a person at a distance. It can be used in theaters and movies to see the person on a stage. It can be placed permanently on a pair of spectacles for use in driving a motor vehicle in order to read directional signs from a greater distance. The telescopic lens is placed on the upper edge of the glass so as not to interfere with the view in driving. When a sign has to be read, the head is dropped for a few seconds and vision is directed through the telescopic lens. Usually the lens is placed in front of the better eye, and only one telescopic lens is necessary. Telescopic lenses for both eyes, binoculars, are occasionally used for viewing the television screen from a greater distance or for the larger screen at the movies. It has been my experience that aged visually impaired persons seldom use telescopic lenses. They find them too cumbersome and difficult to focus. The single hand-held telescopic lens that is used to see a specific object is preferred.

Large Print Newspapers and Books

An important adjunct for the visually impaired is the use of large print newspapers, books, and some magazines. The *New York Times* has a weekly edition in large print, and *Reader's Digest* has a large print monthly. In this field the National Association for the Visually Handicapped has been a pioneer. This endeavor, begun by the executive director, Lorraine Marchi, 25 years ago, has resulted in a large collection of books in many fields of interest that are available for purchase and even for distribution to institutions as additions to their libraries. A newsy publication in large print called *Seeing Clearly*[2] comes out occasionally

---

[2] Available from the National Association for the Visually Handicapped, 305 East 24 Street, New York, N.Y. 10010.

and is distributed without charge to low vision clinics and individuals who are on the mailing list.

Closed Circuit Television

During the past decade closed circuit television equipment has been used as an aid to the visually handicapped.[3] Each set contains a television screen of variable size, a camera to pick up the reading material, and a powerful lens to enlarge the image seen by the camera anywhere from 4 to 60 times. The reading matter on the screen may appear dark on a light background or the reverse, whichever is more comfortable to the user. These instruments are expensive when used on an individual basis, but could be used by senior centers or homes for the aged, where many individuals can have access to it. They come in various sizes, some of which are portable. Most of the manufacturers will allow for trial periods to determine if the person or the group at an institution can learn how to use the instrument—or if they are capable of manipulating the controls effectively.

These instruments are used most efficiently by people in the younger age group who are more flexible. Older people who are visually handicapped may have additional disabilities that add to the difficulty of making the necessary adjustments. This was the experience at a home for the aged with which I am acquainted. After a trial period of a month, using two supervisors to assist and explain the workings of the instrument, the conclusion was that the complexities of the instrument were beyond the capabilities of the home's residents, whose average age was above 80 years.

Radio Reading Services

The Radio Reading Service is a relatively recent addition to the rehabilitation of the visually handicapped aged person confined to his room who is unable to read a newspaper.

A single channel broadcast by a special radio center provides service at particular hours of the day, in some areas up to 20 hr, and in other areas at specified times. Daily news, sporting events, and weather reports are covered, and books are read. The special receiver is not too expensive and in some places is provided free of charge to the residents of homes for the aged. The patient does not feel isolated because of his visual or physical handicap.[4]

---

[3] Among the manufacturers of these electronic visual aids are: (a) Visualtek, 1610 26 Street, Santa Monica, Calif. 90404; (b) Pelco Industries Inc., 351 East Alondra Boulevard, Gardena, Calif. 90248; and (c) Apollo Electronic Visual Aids, 6357 Arizona Circle, Los Angeles, Calif. 90045.

[4] More information about these radios may be obtained from the Radio Reading Service, 15 West 16 Street, New York, N.Y. 10011; and the organization In Touch, 322 West 48 Street, New York, N.Y. 10038. There are many other centers across the United States combined in the

Follow-up Care

Follow-up care in the use of low vision aids is important for many elderly patients. Some are easily discouraged and need continuing support and repeated instructions. Others complain of the difficulty in holding reading matter too close to the eyes for any extended period because of weakness or instability of the arms and hands. Where this is true, spectacle aids or fixed focus magnifiers may be used.

Older people often lose interest in reading, preferring radios or television viewing—where they can sit closer to the instrument for better viewing or hearing. For a low vision aid to be successful it must be accepted by the patient, encourage him to use his available vision, stimulate his interest, and be comfortable in its use. Motivation to improve the visual status is an important asset for success (2,5).

REFERENCES

1. Blankenship, G. W., and Machemer, R. (1978): Pars plana vitrectomy for management of severe diabetic retinopathy. An analysis of results five years following surgery. *Ophthalmology,* 85:553–559.
2. Faye, E. E. (1970): An analysis of success or failure of visual aids. In: *The Low Vision Patient, Clinical Experience with Adults and Children,* p. 114. Grune and Stratton, New York, London.
3. Food and Drug Administration (1979): Intraocular lens complications. Reprinted from the Academy Argus of the American Academy of Ophthalmology, Vol 2, p. 1.
4. Hoffner, K. J. (1978): Survey on the use of intraocular lenses. *Ophthalmology,* 85:400–407.
5. Kornzweig, A. L. (1976): A low vision clinic in a home for aged. *J. Am. Geriatric Soc.,* 24:538–541.
6. Stark, S. J., Hirst, L. W., Ship, R. C., and Maumanee, A. E. (1977): A two year trial of intraocular lenses at the Wilmer Institute. *Am. J. Ophthalmol.,* 84:769–774.

Association of Radio Reading Services whose publication is called HEAR$_R$Say–ARRS; the address is Box 1988, Cleveland, Ohio 44106.

The two main sources of supplies for low vision aids in the New York area are The American Foundation for the Blind, 15 West 16 Street, New York, N.Y. 10011, and the "Lighthouse," also called the New York Association for the Blind, at 111 East 59 Street, New York, N.Y. 10022. These institutions are national in scope and their facilities are open to everyone.

Rehabilitation in the Aging edited by
T. F. Williams. Raven Press, New York © 1984.

Dental Care for Rehabilitation of the Aging

Sidney I. Silverman

New York University, College of Dentistry, New York, New York 10010

Dental disease is generally a chronic disorder with occasional acute episodes. Like most chronic pathology, dental disease has biologic stigmata that can be observed at the biochemical, cellular, tissue, and organ systems levels. The signs of dental disease readily observed in acute problems are inflammation, infection, and necrosis in the soft tissue of the tongue, lips, oral mucosa, and the dentoalveolar supporting bone of the teeth. These signs are usually associated with pain, limited or altered motion of the jaws and difficulty or distortions in mastication, deglutition, and, occasionally, in speaking.

The more chronic signs of dental disease leading to the acute problems are numerous. These include: abrasion, erosion, loss of tooth structure; displacement and malalignment of the teeth and dental arch form by trauma, caries, and habit formation; gingivitis and advanced periodontal disease of the investing ligaments and alveolar bone of the teeth; inflammatory, hemorrhagic, and keratinizing defects in the oral mucosa; infection, tumor and osteoclasia of the residual maxillary bones; degeneration and arthritic changes in the position and motion patterns of the temporomandibular joint; and disorganization in the neuromuscular mechanisms regulating mandibular motion and dental occlusion. Acute episodes that bring dental problems to the attention of patients and providers of health care with an urgency have a very low incidence and are of short duration when measured against the time of pain-free periods during a life span.

Dental disease not only destroys the teeth and the dentoalveolar bone; it significantly alters the tissues of the adnexae and impairs the several functions of the oropharyngeal structures. Litvak et al. (17) describe a number of sequelae of the loss of form, bulk, strength, speed, and specificity of motion of the muscles of the face; diminution of sensory nerve endings in the mucosa; alteration in tactile, stereognostic, and position sense of jaw posture; and alterations in esthetics of face form, masticatory, deglutive, and speaking skills. In additional recent investigations by Silverman and Block (35), there are suggestions that dental disease alters visual and acoustic processes associated with posture, gait, and vocational skills. These studies also include psychological and emotional aspects of adjusive behavior and self-concept in socialization experiences. Medical disorders and their treatments are also contributory to the etiology and exacerbation of dental disease; these are discussed further on in this chapter.

Dental care for the aging has a history of neglect based in part on myth,

biomedical misinformation, and serious social, economic, and political deprivation. As significant as this neglect is, it is no worse than the history of unfulfilled
dental health needs of other segments of our population. For example, there
has been until recent decades serious neglect of children in general and more
specifically almost total neglect of handicapped, physically disabled, and chronically ill children. In addition, young and older adults confined to long-term
health facilities such as psychiatric hospitals, nursing homes, and other extended
care services, receive relatively minimal care; usually only limited acute care
is available. Also included in this group of underserved populations are the
ethnic minorities—the blacks, Indians, and Hispanics, and other economically
deprived and low income families such as migrant workers, alcoholics, drug
addicts, and persons confined to penal institutions. Finally, according to Weinberger and Milham (39), there is the unfortunate attitude prevailing in all segments
of the population of no perceived need for dental care for the aging (5,15,21).
Unfortunately, old people themselves have a very low perception of their own
dental needs (10).

The significance of identifying these people who have little or no care is
that each of these subgroups has its share of aging persons (6). In effect, we
have a higher proportion of the aging population in these disadvantaged groups
with acute dental disease than in the general population. In absolute numbers,
there are over 22 million people 65 years old and over (10% of the population)
(8), more than half of whom are widowed or single women living on substandard
incomes. There are at least another 10 million prematurely aging persons between
50 and 65 years of age who, because of biomedical problems or severe economic
dysfunction, may be considered as aging. This group is included in aging because
they experience some adjusted levels of function and they need significant medical
and/or social agency support services.

The extensive dental need is presently worldwide, as recent studies in other
English-speaking countries indicate. Studies by Burgess and Beck (7) indicate
that 92.6% of the population 60 and over wear removable denture prostheses
in New Zealand; in Britain, according to Hobdell et al. (12), 37% of all adults
wear removable prostheses. Thus one notes that even in countries where health
system plans make dental service more accessible than in countries without
such insurance, the dental health is less than desirable. To improve the quality
of dental health, the answer lies not only in funding but in overcoming the
many social, psychological, and cultural processes inhibiting access to dental
health services.

MYTHS ABOUT DENTAL CARE

The myths that perpetuate this deplorable dental health situation are numerous. It is not uncommon for older persons to say, "Why should I spend money
and time to restore my teeth. I don't have long to live!" or, "I don't have the
money and I won't burden my children." "My wrinkles are caused by age, so

what can you do about it?" or, "I don't go anywhere so what difference does it make how I look?" These are self-imposed judgments about the inevitability that one looks old at some scheduled calendar age, as reported by Silverman (31).

The myth about looking "old" and "wrinkled," as synonomous related effects, is reinforced by cartoon caricatures of old crones who are toothless, by mass media appealing to older women and men, and by use of youthful models made to look older. In truth, collapse of the oral-facial tissues because of loss of teeth and dentoalveolar bone in young people makes them look old. As stated by Moore (23), Rembrandt, in many of his paintings of old persons (Figs. 1 and 2), makes them look youthful and vigorous because he painted the differential topography of the face such as the philtrum of the upper lip, the proper contours, and the demarcation separating the vermilion from the skin portion of the lips (Fig. 3). He included the wrinkling of the face, which is related to the loss of elastic properties and collagen changes in the skin. Rembrandt understood, as do morticians, that topography of the face can look youthful and vigorous when support is provided by the teeth of the dentoalveolar bone or the replacement prosthesis. It is not true that loss of teeth and the "old" look is natural. Conversely, it is true that retaining and caring for teeth will sustain the "vigor of life look" through the eighties and nineties of any given person.

The worst myth perpetuated on older persons is that expressions of sexuality and physical attractiveness are not appropriate attitudes for aging persons. Men who smile and greet women with cordiality and descriptive language indicating beauty and attractiveness of women are "dirty old men." Women who dress smartly in vogue and use facial cosmetics and hair couture are acting "cute" or "silly" or inappropriately "kittenish." In truth, older men and women have interest in sexual encounters, and enjoy banter and many of the social amenities and physical contact with sexual partners. Since humans are face oriented and have all their special senses organized in a cephalic position, and since all verbal and nonverbal communication is face-to-face, it is cruel to deny and even deplore

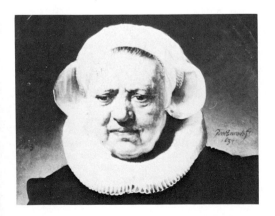

FIG. 1. Rembrandt (1606–1669), in his portrait of an elderly woman, demonstrates his awareness of the differentiated facial topography when the teeth and alveolar bone are intact. Note the tubercle and the fullness of the vermilion aspects of the lips, the clear lateral oblique shadow of the nasolabial sulcus, and the appropriate depression of the geniolabial sulcus.

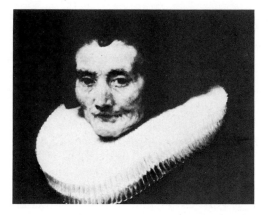

FIG. 2. Rembrandt knew how to paint the portrait of an edentulous person. Note the disorganization of the facial topography around the depressed lips. This portrait reveals the corrugation of the skin as the unsupported buccinator muscle fails to fill out the facial contours.

the consciousness of sex. Sexuality in all its forms is a human right of all people and especially the aging for whom it is one of the vital urgent needs for expression of the human condition. Providing dental health care can help dispel this cruel myth that sexuality is not for the aging. (See also G. P. Bray, *this volume.*)

The myth that older people can survive without teeth because there are ade-

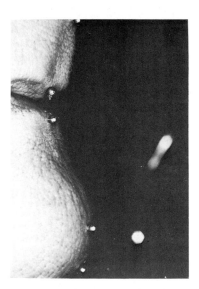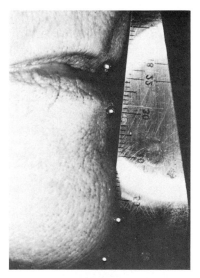

FIG. 3. The most significant profile landmarks are revealed in these illustrations. A recent study indicates the major displacement in the upper lip after the loss of teeth causes a dorsal anteroposterior collapse of the tubercle. When teeth are restored, the displacement forward may be from 2 to 10 mm. The study also indicates the major direction of displacement of the junction of vermilion and skin portion of the lower lip is a collapse and recovery of 0 to 12 mm. **Left:** Note the position of the lips marked with steel balls attached to tissue. This patient is edentulous and not wearing dentures. **Right:** Note the forward movement of the lips when dentures are in the mouth.

quate soft diets and food supplements to sustain life without teeth is a hoax qualified by partial truth. It is true that acute disease and death are not immediate consequences of the loss of teeth. It is, however, equally true that people without adequate teeth to masticate food develop nutritional patterns containing high water, high carbohydrate foods that may contribute to water and electrolyte imbalance, obesity, and generalized protein depletion. This often complicates dietary regimens for patients with endocrine dysfunction, cardiovascular problems, and other special dietary requirements. In addition to these nutrient problems, the patients do not enjoy the psychological and socialization benefits of their eating experiences. Institutionalized patients may spend 50% of their working day preparing for mealtime, waiting for meals in dining rooms, and talking about food (29). In one study, Silverman (30) reported a hostile reaction to the medical staff and administration because of the prevalence of soft high caloric diets. There is also increased likelihood of aspirating foods because of the inability to slow the deglutive process when eating soft diets. Chewing food with teeth slows ingesting; people eat less and enjoy their food more. Contrary to the myth that people like and prefer soft mushy food, older people like to chew food and enjoy the gustatory flavor of most vegetables, fruits, and nuts as they experience the masticatory resistance to fibrous and chewy foods. They select soft diets because they have no teeth, not because they like them.

Another myth is that old people are antisocial, preferring to be alone during meals. It is observed in clinical practice that people who drool and dribble saliva because they are edentulous or people who are nonverbal because they are unintelligible when speaking with teeth cannot enunciate bilabial, lingual, and labiodental consonants. They, therefore, tend to eat with people who are similarly afflicted or they choose to eat alone. Given teeth with which they can eat, their self-concept often improves, their communication skills improve, and they enjoy the socialization experience.

THE PREVALENCE OF DENTAL NEED

The need for comprehensive dental care for the aging is extensive (18), and the availability, accessibility, and utilization for such skilled care has been reported to be relatively diminishing (3,11). Successive studies in the United States, from 1962 to the present, suggest a discouraging future for the dental health of the aging. The earliest studies by the National Center for Health Statistics indicated that in a national sample of persons age 55 to 74 years, 44.4% required dental care as soon as possible; among those age 75 to 79 years, 53.9% needed immediate attention by a dentist (2,25). Succeeding surveys have pointed out the same patterns of dental need among the aged (22). In another survey in 1965, the number of older persons who were edentulous was found to be 38.1% in the age group 55 to 65 years, 55.4% among those 65 to 74, and 67.3% among those 75 years and older (13). A follow-up study for the period 1971 to 1974 found 45.5% of the population 65 to 75 years of age to be edentulous in both upper and lower jaws, only a 10% reduction from the state of edentulousness in the 1965 survey (14). In addition, 55% of the same group age 65 to 74 had periodontal disease on their remaining teeth. This fact, when considered as a function of 100% of the total population between 65 to 74 years of age, indicates that 45% were edentulous and 30% had serious periodontal disease affecting those with teeth. Thus 75% of the age group required ongoing dental health care for edentulousness or periodontal disease. When frequency of dental visits is assessed for these older persons, approximately 45% had not been to a dentist within one year, 17% had not been within two to four years, and 24.1% had not seen a dentist within five years.

Dental needs are even greater within nursing home populations than the general populations of the same age range (40). In a study of the Washington Dental Service from 1963 to 1965, approximately two-thirds of examined nursing home residents were determined to be in need of dental treatment (S. Lotzkar, *unpublished report*). In Michigan, 54% of nursing home patients were found to need dental treatment (S. Lotzkar, *unpublished report*). Despite this large proportion of nursing home residents in need of immediate dental care, few receive it. A 1973 nursing home sample disclosed only 18.9% of nursing homes provided dental services.

A significant study in 1972 (10) indicates the low level of perceived need among older people compared to the high level of objective need for dental care. The same study suggests a very vigorous dental health program for older people is desperately required to increase utilization of accessible treatment resources. The serious neglect and undertreatment in providing dental care for the aging is without doubt related to economic factors inhibiting provision of care. Public assistance, private insurance, and Medicare programs generally exclude any significant reimbursement for dental care (1,28). In 1971, New York City health data (1) indicates only 10.5% of total costs for dental care was public supported; patients paying 89.5% from private funds. By contrast, 71.5% of physicians' fees were paid by public and third party funds.

SIGNS AND SYMPTOMS OF DENTAL DISEASE

Caries in the older patient is a different clinical process and is more often found in root surfaces; it has a different morphogenesis than tooth caries in children and adults. Periodontal disease states, often chronic and long-standing as marginal gingivitis or tooth mobility, have different clinical implications in regard to treatment. Disease processes move more slowly, particularly caries, and the factor of diminished longevity compared to youth may modify technique. Endodontics required for pathological conditions of the pulp is a useful technique to keep teeth for overdentures. The processes of loss of face height, jaw stability, and occlusion associated with edentulousness and changes in tonicity of the tongue and facial muscles affecting speech, head posture, and deglutition are all functions of aging.

Caries

Caries, a universal pathologic process, is essentially an infectious disease that alters and/or destroys the hard tissues of teeth. Studies in animals demonstrate that carious lesions can be induced in germ-free animals by inoculation with cariogenic masses from decaying teeth. The microorganism from these transferred masses generate acids to demineralize the enamel, dentine, and cementum, leaving vulnerable the residual organic matrix to digestion and tooth substance loss.

Caries is produced throughout life and although the acid formation, demineralization, and organic matrix are similar at all ages, the organisms differ by age in the location on the tooth, and the speed and character of the caries process (20). In children, a lactobacillus attacks the pits, fissures, and crevices on the coronal surface of the teeth. This organism invades the fusion areas of the tooth cusps (fissures) where readily biogradable glycoproteins are in relatively higher concentration. The pit and fissure chemistry is altered with age, acquiring sulfhydryl groups from saliva, and becomes harder, leathery, and dark brown. Thus in the elderly they are less vulnerable to decay.

In the young adult, the principal microorganism is the *Streptococcus mutans,* which although present from infancy through old age is especially virulent during adolescence and young adulthood. It attacks the smooth enamel and penetrates quickly to the pulp with the inflammatory and infectious process often causing pain, periapical, and periodontal infection. Beyond age 35 the organism is also less destructive, partly due to uptake and increased density of fluoride content in the enamel.

In the mature and aging adult, the dominant microorganism associated with caries is the *Odontomyces viscosus.* The tongue is the normal habitat of this microorganism, proliferating among the filiform papillae as a normal component of the flora in the oral cavity. As salivary secretion diminishes with age, the ondontomyces become pathogens, proliferating as white or brown masses on the tongue and spreading along root surfaces into the gingival crevices. Root surface plaque shelters the organism and slow, literally expanding erosive rather than the quickly penetrating *Streptococcus mutans* caries are generated. The cementum and dentine, slowly demineralized and discolored, are especially vulnerable in marginal crevices and periodontal pockets. In persons who have been irradiated for tumor lesions of the head and neck, the dehydration and resultant xerostoma accelerate and potentiate the destructiveness and rate of penetration of the caries through the root structure. Xerostoma is also a concomitant of the high frequency of utilization of drugs in older people, which diminishes salivary flow.

In light of the etiology and microbiologic agents causing tooth decay in the aging, the following fluoridation and oral hygiene practices are considered to be effective in preventing decay and tooth loss.

Fluorine, an essential trace element in nutrient requirements for health, is found in practically all soils, plant, and animal life. However, its distribution is variable in many regions of the earth. Accordingly there are many areas where fluorine is deficient in both diet and water intake. For example, in the southwest there are many parts per million in water, and in the northeast there are only minimal, inadequate trace amounts required for healthy teeth and bone mineralization.

Fluoridation provides protection to the teeth through one or more mechanisms (9). Fluoride ions in low concentration can form acid-resistant hydroxyapatite crystals within the dental enamel; fluoride ions in high concentration can be incorporated into tooth structure during and after eruption. The free fluorides can also inhibit caries although the mechanism is not clearly understood. Fluorides can concentrate in plaque, preventing the firm attachment of the plaque to tooth surfaces and thus diminishing the acid action of hard structure dissolution.

These actions of fluorides are effective inhibitors of caries in the aging. Toothbrushing with a fluoride-containing toothpaste inhibits plaque formation and resultant caries. Patients who have diminished saliva associated with pharmacotherapy or with radiation therapy can be helped with a fluoride gel placed within a night guard appliance over the teeth during sleep. An effective artificial saliva for reducing the trauma and decay-producing effect of xerostoma has been developed (24).

Fluoride treatment of water and in dentifrices has already proven an effective public health measure, even if one considers only the number of edentulous persons in America. In the 30 years that fluorides have been used, the number of Americans over 30 who wear one or more complete artificial dentures has dropped from 35.2% in 1960 to 24.7% in 1975. Admittedly there are other causes for tooth retention such as more access to dental care and higher utilization of services, but this is offset in part by a rapid increase in longevity.

Fluoridated water is medically safe. In repeated sample studies of the 105 million people drinking fluoridated water by 1970, the World Health Organization (WHO), the U.S. Public Health Service, and numerous state and other official agency research organizations have demonstrated repeatedly the effectiveness and safety of fluoridation. In studies repeated again by the WHO in 1975, by the National Cancer Institute in 1976, and the U.S. Center for Disease Control and Blood Institute in 1977, no evidence was found linking fluorides with cancer rates.

Fluoridation has also been found to be associated with improved salivary flow, which provides not only a mechanical coating for the enamel, dentine, and exposed cementum, but also protection from the external environment that threatens the health of teeth. This protection includes bacterial agglutination and the removal by lavage of pathogens inhibiting bacterial growth. It has a favorable metabolic effect on normal resident flora, providing specific immunity. In addition, the saliva, of course, provides digestive enzymes.

Modification of the Tooth Structures and Investing Tissues, Periodontal Membrane and Alveolar Bone

Conditions prevalent in older persons include: occlusal attrition, marked formations of secondary dentin, apical migration of the periodontal attachment, increased cementum deposition, deepening of gingival pockets, and increased mobility and migration of teeth (Figs. 4 and 5).

Degenerative Changes in Oral Mucosae

These may take the form of hyperkeratosis, loss of elastic properties, or tissue fragility. Clinically observed ischemia and an associated increased predisposition to traumatic ulcerations during therapy or with prosthesis may also be encountered. Extensive ulceration may be present without pain or hypersensitivity, or minimal trauma may be present without overt signs of tissue damage (Figs. 6 and 7).

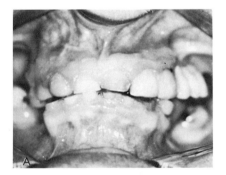 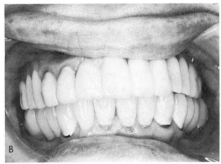

FIG. 4. The abraded teeth in **(left)** were caused by prolonged loss of the patient's posterior teeth, resulting in a loss of 8 mm of face height measured in vertical plane. The lost dimension was recovered **(right).** This photograph was taken 12 years after restoration. Note the minimal recession on the lower anterior teeth after many years of regular prophylaxis every 3 months.

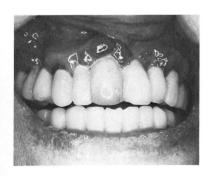

FIG. 5. Advanced inflammatory proliferative periodontal disease associated with poor oral hygiene practices and inadequate restorative and prosthetic care. This disorder responded favorably to treatment.

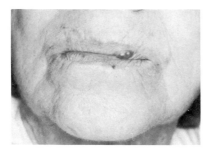

FIG. 6. Benign hemorrhagic lesion of the lip. Patient bites lip repeatedly because the anterior teeth are in an edge-to-edge position in free closure. The teeth should be reset to avoid further injury.

Degenerative Changes of the Maxilla, Mandible, and Temporomandibular Joint

The bodies of the jaws often present signs of the osteoporosis that is common with aging. The temporomandibular joint may develop varying degrees of subluxation, and the latter may be associated with poor muscular tone, maladaptive positions related to malocclusion, or arthritis. Disturbances in the facial components of the skeletal system may also be due to arthritic changes, such as rheumatoid arthritis, and other endocrine and metabolic disorders in addition to osteoporosis, such as acromegaly, Paget's disease, and osteomalacia. Infections, tumors, and congenital deformities of bones and joints may cause myofascial pain, limitation of jaw motion, disturbances in occlusion, and impaired hand-mouth skills for feeding or self-care and oral hygiene.

Distortion of Neuromuscular Stimulation

Loss of teeth and their periodontal membranes, whose proprioceptive end organs aid in regulating jaw posture, results in lack of maintenance of normal posture. The loss of teeth also causes a reduced tonus of the facial musculature. Thus the facial landmarks become distorted, displaced, or missing in both the relatively static state of respiratory rest or the dynamic states of swallowing, speaking, and chewing. The landmarks that may be affected are the philtrum, the tubercle and vermilion border of the lip, the nasolabial sulcus, and the commissure of the mouth. The skin may also be observed to be markedly corru-

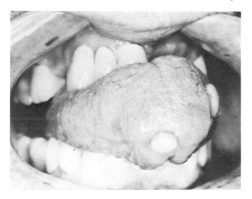

FIG. 7. A benign fibrotic lesion of the tongue that the patient had for 20 years. However, recurrent laceration required the tissue to be removed. Healing was uneventful.

gated as its elasticity is diminished because of changes in the elastic fibers and the ground substance of the connective tissues.

There is so much sensory distortion of oral perception in the aging that it has produced a language of pain, which patients communicate with both verbal and nonverbal behavior. Three categories or groups of pain expression have been identified: (a) sensory (organic), described as temporal, spatial, punctate, incisive, and thermal; (b) effective (psychologic), described as fear, punishment, and anxiety; and (c) evaluative (mixed), described as bad, violent pounding, throbbing, burning, nagging, and tiring.

The descriptive language and observed nonverbal behavior must be related to morphologic and physiologic response mechanisms. The facies and body habitus reflect attitudes about self-worth. These are coupled with the physiologic responses including the circulatory changes and sweating, and somatic motor activity including masseter jaw muscle clenching, postural body tension, and rapid eye movement.

MEDICAL-DENTAL CONSIDERATIONS

Systemic disorders of the aging and their respective therapeutics not only present oral stigmata but may also potentiate the signs of dental disease. The following are among those frequently observed in dental practice.

Tardive Dyskinesia

Use of phenothiazine drugs as psychotropic agents may lead to this condition, characterized by excessive perioral contraction, facial grimaces, and grossly protruded tongue movement when initiating speech (Figs. 8 and 9). Affected persons may also exhibit uncontrolled acceleration and deceleration patterns of movement when opening and closing the jaws during speech. This causes trauma

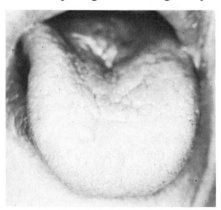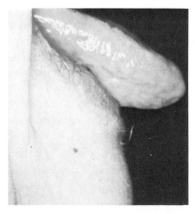

FIG. 8. Left: Frontal view of patient experiencing tardive dyskinesia. When initiating a speech sequence, her tongue was uncontrollable and she protruded it. **Right:** Profile view of protruded tongue when initiating speech.

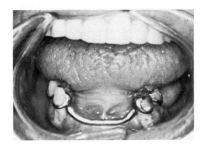

FIG. 9. A training aid attached to the teeth in a patient was used to discharge initial proprioceptor stretch stimulus and response. Patient placed tongue tip against the bar held in position by vitalium clasps. After pressure of the tongue was achieved, patient was able to talk without protruding tongue.

to the teeth and periodontal tissues by excessive impact forces when teeth occlude. An additional serious sequela of tardive dyskinesia is aspiration of food particles during deglutition.

Reduced Salivary Secretion

Many drugs that aging patients ingest have an inhibitory effect on salivary secretion. This action exacerbates the problem of diminished secretion, which normally accompanies the aging process. The marked diminution of saliva removes the usual lavage and lubricant effect of saliva cleansing the teeth, the mucosa, the gingiva, and the tissue crevices in the pharyngeal, buccal, and sublingual spaces of the mouth and throat. The clinical syndrome of the "dry mouth" associated with diminished secretion is the burning mouth syndrome. Sometimes described as a "killing, blinding, or burning pain," it is usually a low grade chronic pain, occasionally accompanied by minor mucosal ulceration or keratotic reactions. The patient sometimes complains of postural disorientation of the head, neck, and jaws as a consequence of dental treatment. When the postural complaint is so acute and persistent, akin to visual or acoustic hallucination, it suggests a schizoid behavioral pattern. The symptom is characterized as the Verkrümmt Kupf syndrome (32).

The dryness is also associated with aspiration of food. It is suggested that older patients always have some fluid available when eating to assist in swallowing. In addition to the knowledge of diminished secretion, it is suggested all dentists and auxiliary support personnel should be trained in cardiopulmonary resuscitation techniques, with special training in recognition of foreign object obstruction of the airway in both conscious and unconscious patients.

The second major problem resulting from diminished salivary secretion is the rapid onset of caries with special vulnerability on the root surfaces of the teeth where dental plaque accumulates (Fig. 10). Plaque, inducing root caries and periodontal disease, requires daily cleansing and is present almost universally in the remaining teeth of older persons. Institutionalized patients should have daily surveillance of oral health care. Older people living at home or in institutions should be seen by dentists for caries, periodontal disease, and cancer detection every three to six months. This examination is suggested even for patients who have no natural teeth, whether or not they have artificial dentures, because inflammation and tumor may exist without pain.

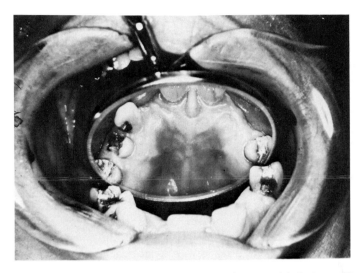

FIG. 10. Characteristic inflammation of palate seen under a partial denture without clasps and rests. The sustained unsupported pressure of the denture on the palatal mucosa coupled with poor oral hygiene reveals an inflamed area.

Oral Mucosal and Gingival Inflammation

Prolonged antibiotic therapy may cause monilia infections anywhere in the oral mucosa and especially on the palate and tissue folds in the buccal mucosa. The monilia often incubates in artificial dentures, especially those with soft resins that are porous and have high water sorption properties. The infection is often associated in denture wearers with a papillomatous hyperplasia of the mucosa on the hard palate, providing excellent crevices for propagating the monilia. Changing the antibiotic agent, cleansing the dentures or even constructing new ones, and a strict regimen of oral hygiene is required to eliminate the monilial infection.

Corticosteroid drugs, used for their anti-inflammatory effect in various systemic diseases may indirectly exacerbate periodontal disease through diminishing the normal protective response. It may be necessary to decrease steroid therapy until oral tissues are treated and then provide a strict home treatment program for self-care of the teeth before again initiating therapy.

Anticoagulants

Anticoagulants may require modification in dosage when periodontal treatment or other oral surgery treatment is required. Prolonged bleeding time of simple wounds in these procedures may cause extreme anxiety for patients or may result in clots within a necrotic wound on exposed bone. This "dry socket" is extremely painful during the healing period and although it rarely causes secondary infection it can be most uncomfortable.

However, if properly managed, anticoagulants need pose little risk to patients undergoing surgery (4,27). When the prothrombin time is maintained at 1½ to 2 times the control time, and when careful surgical technique is used, dental surgery for these patients leads to no significant bleeding problem.

Mucosal Ulceration

Elderly persons with dementia or depression, or who are receiving analgesic medications for any cause, may have high thresholds of pain perception in the oral cavity. They may wear an ill-fitting prosthesis or bite their lips or tongue, causing infected and bleeding ulcerations and not be aware of the injury. Sometimes a malignancy as large as a walnut is present without a patient's awareness. Other causes of ulcerations include blood dyscrasias and long reactions. It is strongly recommended that all institutionalized patients not only be examined by a dentist on admission but that daily inspection be done by ward attendants, nurses, and other professional persons observing lips and face, eating habits, and oral hygiene.

Motor Disorders

Disorders such as parkinsonism, cerebral palsy, Bell's palsy, neurogenic tumors, and cerebrovascular accidents are often associated with disorders of mastication, deglutition, speech, and respiration (Fig. 11). The pain and aberrant motion are associated with trauma to tooth substance and the investing periodontal tissue.

Sensory Disorders

Sensory changes affecting the mouth and face in older people may be associated with cerebrovascular accidents, trauma, tumor, and the effects of drugs.

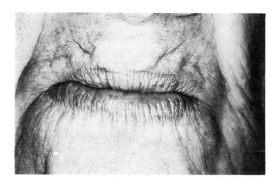

FIG. 11. Degenerative neuropathies cause asynchronous lip movements affecting speech, esthetics, chewing, and swallowing. Food and saliva dribble at the corners of the mouth and lateral lisping during speech is often present. The tooth alignment in dentures must attempt to cope with this asynchrony.

Sensory distortion may manifest itself in the burning mouth syndrome, a facial pain syndrome associated with inappropriate management of pain in oral function. A new clinical syndrome of head posture hallucination, the Verkrümmt Kupf syndrome (32), is related to severe psychopathological personality disorders. Loss of tactile discrimination is present in older persons who lose their teeth. Denture replacement usually improves tactile and stereognostic sense (17) (Fig. 12).

TUMOR DETECTION AND DENTAL CARE

Current data indicate that 26,000 persons annually in the United States are diagnosed to have oral cancer, causing 9,000 deaths each year. These oral cancers can be detected in early stages by dentists, with a higher incidence of cure than when detection is late. The lips account for 18%; the tongue, 17% (Fig. 13); and the salivary glands, 8%. Approximately 28% is located in the pharynx between the mouth and the esophagus. Although the direct causative agents and processes have not been known, many factors contributing to oral and pharyngeal cancers have been identified. These include care for oral hygiene, chronic irritation caused by jagged teeth, and projecting ill-fitting dental filling materials and artificial dentures. When these problems of dental care are accompanied by excessive smoking of cigarettes, cigars, and pipes as well as chronic heavy alcohol drinking, the patient is a high risk candidate for oral cancer.

Tumors of the larynx should be suspected and searched for when patients have a change in voice quality and pitch such as hoarseness, nasality, denasality, excessive and spontaneous coughing unrelated to colds, or prolonged aphonia. Spontaneous bleeding and proliferation of fragile oral mucosa and gingival papilla may indicate the presence of blood dyscrasias including leukemia.

Squamous cell neoplasms of the oral cavity account for approximately 5% of all cancer in men and 2% in women (19). It has been stated that "although the oral cavity is easily accessible and is examined frequently by physicians and dentists, 60% of all oral cancers are well advanced by the time they are detected" (19). The five-year survival rate of all oral cancers is only 30%; by comparison, skin and lip cancers have a 90% survival rate.

The major traditional lesion of concern has been the white lesion, especially leukoplakia, traditionally labeled (perhaps unjustly) as the most common precancerous lesion in the oral cavity. Another type of lesion has recently been recognized as suggestive of cancer, namely, erythroplasia. This is essentially a red minimally keratinized smooth nongranular lesion. Unlike a nonspecific inflammatory lesion, the mucosal surface of the carcinoma appears atrophic and slightly eroded. The boundaries of the erythroplastic lesions may be poorly defined and are irregular, sometimes revealing speckled-like blending of inflamed and normal mucosa.

A further recent detection procedure for oral cancer is examination by an intraoral smear from saliva or the surface of a lesion to determine the presence

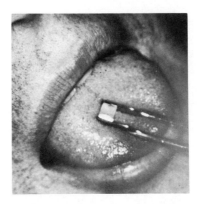

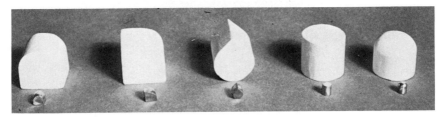

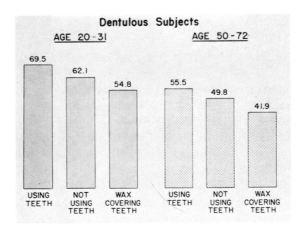

FIG. 12. Oral stereognostic discrimination skills of older patients diminish with passing decades. **Top:** Varied small steel configurations were placed in a blindfolded patient's mouth. **Middle:** The large chalk models that the patient had to identify when blindfold is removed. **Bottom:** The mean stereognostic scores under different conditions reveal younger patients with teeth scored higher in identification of forms, 69.5% compared to 55.5% in older patients with teeth. When teeth are covered with wax to eliminate periodontal nerve endings in the skill test, the difference in age performance persisted.

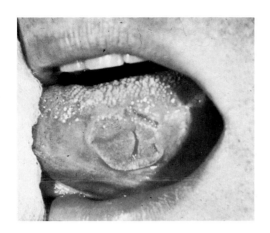

FIG. 13. A typical carcinoma of the ventral surface of the tongue, which requires biopsy for confirmation.

of carcinoembryonic antigens. These antigens may indicate cancer in a suspicious lesion (38).

COMMUNICATION SKILLS AND DENTAL CARE

Dental care requires a high degree of participation by the aging person as a cotherapist. Not only must the person be responsible for self-care in oral hygiene, but the neuromuscular skills for speaking and chewing must be learned and relearned. This implies the person must first have adequate levels of hearing to have aural feedback to learn new tongue-tooth position and jaw movement patterns used in speech production. To produce appropriate vowel production with new dentures requires positioning the jaw, tongue, and lip and pharyngeal structures in new positions to relearn just the production of vowels. Figure 14 indicates the position of the tissues for vowels and Fig. 15 demonstrates tongue and tooth relationships in producing consonants. Older patients who are hearing-impaired require longer periods of time and persistent supervision to learn to wear artificial dentures effectively.

ORAL FUNCTIONAL DISORDERS

Many systemic disorders have oral sequelae affecting dental treatment. These systemic disorders may be biochemical, subcellular processes that affect electrolyte-water balance; metabolic processes, such as infection, injury, inflammation, and wound repair; cellular processes, including cellular regrowth and energy utilization and circulation; or organ system processes affecting speech, swallowing, and mastication. These disorders may be manifested as dysfunction of jaw motion, occlusion instability, poor prognosis for dental arch realignment, and alterations in face height and profile. The neuromuscular asynchrony may affect

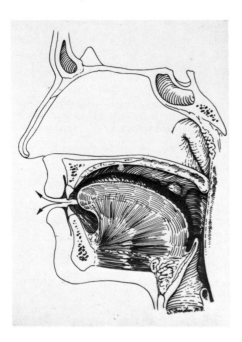

FIG. 14. A schematic drawing showing open tube-like channel for uninterrupted air to produce a vowel sound.

FIG. 15. Typical configuration of speech channel through oral cavity to produce a consonant. Note air flow is interrupted as it passed from lungs and larynx by placing posterior and dorsum of tongue against soft palate and pharynx to produce *k* or *ng*.

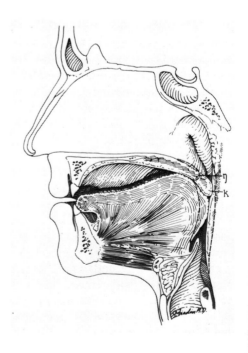

speech and hearing communication; it also may affect the general sensations of pain and touch including two-point and stereoagnostic discrimination.

The following review of the morphogenesis and the physiological and clinical characteristics of the oral functions will help clarify the relationship between systemic and dental problems.

Morphogenesis

The morphogenesis of the orofacial complex of skeletal, muscular, and epithelial structures sustains the original design of the conducting digestive and respiratory tubes (Fig. 16). The oropharyngeal tissues form a split tube in which valving mechanisms expedite the sequential or simultaneous activities of breathing and speaking, and chewing and swallowing. The skeleton expedites the activity of the muscles by a system of supportive and lever mechanisms for fixation. These mechanisms facilitate speed and specificity of motion necessary to perform a highly selective, low-energy movement for speech or a high-energy movement for mastication.

The muscle groups, through their radial distribution and fiber arrangement, the number and location of muscle attachments, and their contiguous facial and connective tissue attachments, create the movement and the contour of the spaces for vowel production, trituration of foods, or ingestion of nutritional substances.

The valving mechanisms, in consequence of high innervation, present a remarkable synthesis of the activity of the orofacial structures. The cranial nerves that serve the orofacial structures are the apotheosis of the whole evolutionary history of the branchial arch derivatives. The cranial nerve complex has a high autonomic nervous system component that mediates the visceral function of the jaws, lips, tongue, and soft palate. The hierarchy of evolutionary development allows the earliest function of swallowing to persist even when speech and chewing, later skills, are impaired or lost.

Mastication

This learned function is usually associated with unilateral jaw motion within a volume of motion of the mandible, characterized by wide, excursive, lateral displacement (Fig. 17). Chewing is also a voluntary sensory-motor function depending in large measure on the available opposing occlusal contact surfaces, which neurologically condition the static and dynamic position of the mandible during mastication.

Mastication is not only learned, but becomes resistant to change once motion patterns are habituated for an extended period of time (years). Many dentists attempting to restore the lost position, contour, and movement of the face and mandible encounter prolonged, discouraging treatment experiences. Often patients will complain to their physicians that dentists cannot provide comfortable dentures. The dentist should first construct treatment or "learning" dentures to decondition the old habituated proprioceptive jaw position experience, and by incremental changes in jaw position and tooth arrangement create new tactile and proprioceptive stimuli to stimulate recovery of facial masticatory muscle form, strength, and specificity of response. This treatment is more costly than the simple replacement of teeth when no biologic changes are induced. Physicians understanding the esthetic and functional requirements of new dentures should reinforce patients to cope with the stress of the conditioning or learning therapy.

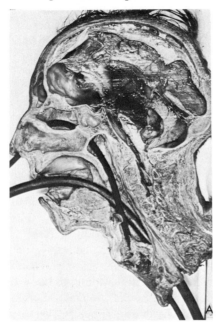
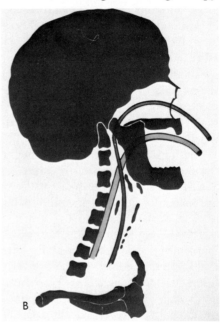

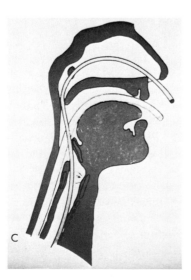

FIG. 16. A: Sagital view of mouth, nose, and pharynx with tubes placed in airway and food passage. Note how they cross in the oropharynx. Loss of neurologic integrative function in keeping valve action synchronized causes aspiration of food. **B:** Schematic drawing demonstrating airway and food tubes in relation to skeletal elements of head, neck, and inframandibular elements. Note that a high degree of flexibility is possible to support and maintain muscles that must keep airway patent. **C:** Schematic drawing demonstrating soft tissues of tongue, lips, and pharynx in relation to airway and food passage. Even when skeletal elements are diseased or missing by trauma, disease, or congenital defect, the soft tissues can swallow and breathe effectively. The skeleton only expedites skill learning, speed of motion, and strength of movement.

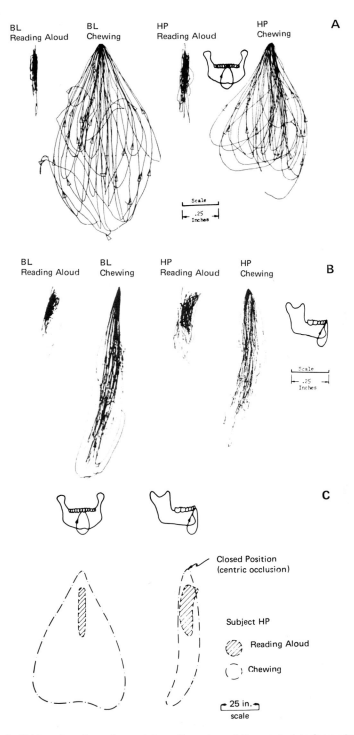

FIG. 17. A: Orbits of motion of a point on the edge of the central incisor, viewed in the frontal plane for speech and chewing. **B:** Orbits of motion of a point on the incisal edge of a lower incisor, as viewed in the sagittal plane for speech and chewing. **C:** Typical composite areas of speech and chewing for patient with normal and so-called ideal occlusion.

It is akin to physical therapy for patients who must learn to walk again after an orthopedic and neurologic accident. Similarly, skill learning for denture use is the function of time and cooperation.

Patients also need instruction on how to select and prepare food that they can effectively masticate. Some patients who have low or no manual dexterity must also receive instructions in improving hand-mouth skills during feeding. An additional consideration in mastication is the knowledge that head posture is very variable during the day and, since gravity as well as the muscles of mastication dominate the position and motion of the mandible, it is recommended that a consistent head and neck posture be maintained during meal time. When a patient is bedridden or slouches in a wheelchair, the body posture and associated jaw movement is usually more difficult than when the patient sits erect at a table while eating. Lying supine when eating not only does not allow teeth to occlude effectively, but makes patients vulnerable for aspiration of food particles.

Deglutition

Deglutition, more visceral than mastication, is present at birth as an innate biologic function. It is a symmetrical, modified peristaltic action initiated at the lips moving a masticated and triturated food bolus rapidly through the fauces, the linguo-, and laryngopharynx to the esophagus. To achieve the rapid movement, the mandible must be fixed in position allowing the larynx to be elevated in a forward thrust by the contraction of the suprahyoid muscle. The action shields the larynx under the base of the tongue, permitting the esophageal valve to open to receive the bolus. When teeth are absent the tongue is used to fix the mandible. This tongue action offers less stable resistance, and the swallow is reinforced by head "bobbing." This results in less control over the bolus and contributes to aspirating food. Dentures and/or stable healthy natural teeth, even a few that offer predictable reliable tooth contact positions, provide better swallowing skills and a more secure patient during eating.

The sequence of illustrations (Fig. 18) selected from a cineradiographic sequence of swallowing a radioopaque bolus, demonstrates the action of lips, tongue, pharynx, the skeletal elements, and the involved processes. A synchronized swallow sequence is predicated on an intact highly integrated nervous system. Aging persons may demonstrate problems in memory sequencing, acceleration-deceleration pattern of alternating body part movements and response time and patterning in both visceral and somatic functions. Observation of mastication and swallowing helps to identify abnormalities affecting both autonomic and voluntary neuromuscular functions.

FIG. 18. A cineradiographic sequence demonstrating selected successive stages in movement of a radiopaque bolus during swallowing. **Top:** The bolus is confined to the oral cavity. **Middle:** The fine radiopaque line over the back and dorsum of the tongue indicates the elevation of the soft palate prior to the passage of the bolus into the oropharynx. **Bottom:** This indicates the forceful movement of the bolus toward the esophagus. Note the sharp angulation on the soft palate above the midportion of the bolus. This is caused by the action of the tensor palati with its downward movement and the elevation action of the levator palati pulling the palate upward.

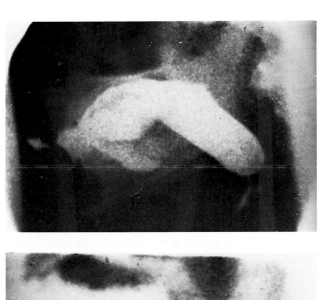

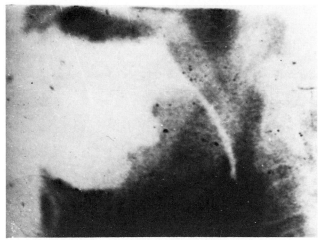

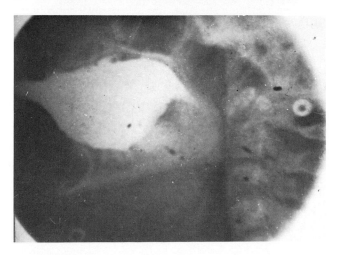

Speech

Speech may provide diagnostic signs of both dental-oral disorders and systemic disease. Short inhalation-exhalation sequences are present in persons with emphysema, lung cancer, and cardiovascular or neurologic disorders. The person's inability to prolong inhalation for speech sequencing should suggest that all intraoral procedures be of very short duration. When foreign objects, like impression trays and materials, are placed, the head should be flexed about 30° forward after initial placement of the foreign body to allow gravity to move fluids and debris ventrally out of the mouth. Suction apparatus should be used to remove saliva and thus avoid the need to swallow and breathe forcefully. The slight flexion allows easily controlled breathing associated with clinical procedures and should not be confused with the extension of the head and protrusion (elevation) of mandible during cardiac and pulmonary resuscitation in emergency situations where forced breathing is required.

The second component of speech performance is the voice quality and resonance characteristics of speech. Any aberration in loudness, harshness, or nasality should be noted. The vowel sounds, which may be voiced or unvoiced, are partly produced by the larynx and modified by the configuration of the pharynx. Basically, however, they are completed into their unique acoustic effects by the configuration of oral space from the fauces to the lips. The separation of the jaws, the opening of lips, and the space between the dorsum of the tongue and hard palate provide the area for vowel production. Dentoalveolar disease or inappropriate ill fitting prostheses interfering with the vowel space can impair intelligibility. More seriously, they mute the unique quality of a person, diminishing not only loudness but also the stress on words that gives affective meaning to speech, expressing feeling, intent, and mood in excess of the semantic-linguistic component of sounds and words.

Finally, the teeth alone or in combination with the tongue and the lips produce, respectively, the interdental, the linguodental, and the labiodental consonant sounds. The teeth are thus critical to the proliferation of the high frequency speech sounds. When teeth are missing, the loss or distortion of dental sounds like *t,d,p,v,s,* and *f* can make speech unintelligible, especially when speaking or conversing with a hearing-impaired person, as is a common situation when one elderly person is attempting to converse with another.

Visual Sense

Various studies (16,35) suggest that when teeth are decayed or missing, or when undue pain and pressures exist, with changes in occlusion of the jaws, the central focus of the visual field as well as head and neck posture may change; and hand-mouth, eye-hand, and location skills may be altered if not impaired by dental problems.

Hearing

Persons with hearing disability tend to hold their heads rotated to hear speakers best. Thus when the right ear is impaired the person rotates the head and neck slightly to the right in a rather steady postural state so the left ear is turned closer to a speaker. The head rotation may be in conflict with the person's head position dominated by eye coordinates when chewing and swallowing. The conflict of posture may cause premature closing contact of teeth and dentures during daily repeated swallows causing irritation and loose dentures. It may be necessary for a dentist to refine the shape of the teeth and dentures to accommodate the visual and hearing positions when they relate to speaking or chewing.

Esthetics Problems

Oral functions are also related to the self-concept of the older person, who perceives and evaluates a static and dynamic facial topography that relies on normal tooth position for esthetically pleasing contours. The normal tonicity of the musculature of the face and the normal histochemical composition of the skin, with its collagen and elastic fiber content, reflect the facial configurations that remain throughout life in a healthy person. When teeth are lost or diseases alter the skin, then the tubercle, the junction between skin and the vermilion aspects of the lips, and the position and planes of the nasolabial and geniolabial sulci may be altered, missing, or distorted (Fig. 19).

In summary, the major function of the oral tissues—mastication, deglutition, respiration, speech, and appearance—maintain a mutual interdependence, diminishing or reinforcing one another in health and disease.

DENTAL THERAPY

The techniques of dental care for older patients are similar in instrumentation and materials to those for other patients. Pathological conditions differ in rate of development, location in the dental arch, state of muscle tonicity, and degeneration of mucosa. Repair and wound healing are similar in detail but differ in time of response. Older people require more time to learn to wear dentures and to learn skills for home care and speech and esthetic improvement. Principles and methodology of an incremental therapy program follow.

Comprehensive Care Procedures

The recommended treatment program provides acute care, prophylaxis, diagnosis, and definitive treatment. The acute care and examination procedures are usually a reliable predictor of patient capacity to benefit from treatment. Patients who cope well with preliminary treatment can benefit from periodontal, endodontic, and even minor orthodontic care. Provisional prostheses may also be supplied by modifying old prostheses or constructing new, short-term prostheses (Fig. 20). When good function, healthy periodontal tissue, and caries reduction have been achieved, long-term fixed or removable prostheses may be constructed. The sequence of limited goal stages of care is termed an *incremental care program*.

An incremental care program should be planned so treatment can be interrupted or terminated without difficulty. Economic hardship, illness, retirement, and migration to other parts of the country are common in the lives of older patients.

Surgical Management

Soft tissue management includes provision of all surgical, periodontal, and endodontic treatment available to younger patients. These include vestibular reduction or augmentation, bony defect filling, rotational flaps of mucosa, autoge-

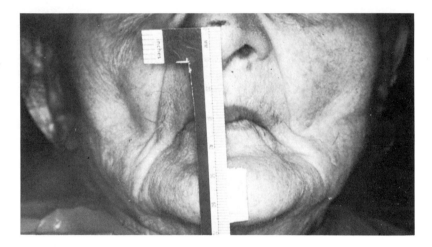

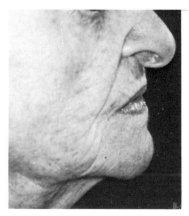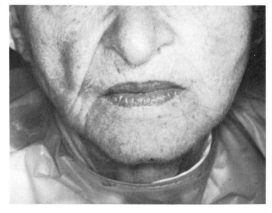

FIG. 19. Top: Severely disorganized facial topography with a loss of 12 mm in face height and 7 mm in anteroposterior dorsal collapse of the lips. **Bottom:** The recovered profile (19 mm) and full face (12 mm) views, respectively, after dentures restored the facial contours.

nous transplants of mucosa, extensive gingivectomy, and hemisection and molar root therapy. It is very important to keep cuspid teeth for overdentures by using advanced periodontal and endodontic techniques.

The surgical procedures for ridge reduction or augmentation are appropriate for older patients. Consultation with the patient's physician is recommended to ascertain dosages for medications the patient may be requiring such as anticoagulant drugs and insulin. It is generally unnecessary to reduce palatal or mandibular tori; it is recommended that sharp bony spicules that are painful on digital pressure be reduced. Alveoloplasties are also recommended to assist in prosthodontic treatment. There is undue concern about the effect of the loss of alveolar bone on the retention of a denture prosthesis. This is not a concern, since dentures are retained essentially by areas of hard and soft tissue coverage and the soft palate seal at the denture periphery.

Prosthodontic Management

New practices in dental prosthetics include interim or transitional prostheses, recovery of lost vertical height and profile, retention of maxillary teeth when a full mandibular denture is constructed, and recall and maintenance programs that provide prosthesis care and supportive psychological counseling, self-care training, and frequent adjustment (36). A recall program requires at least an examination every three months.

Care of older patients with sequelae of congenital defects or acquired defects from trauma, tumor, or degenerative neuropathy requires special techniques. The principal problems in patients with congenital defects are arch form disorganization and speech rehabilitation; patients with acquired defects may have domestic and vocational problems and face the constant threat of reactivation of the tumor process. Degenerative neuropathies and arthritides cause severe problems in jaw motion caused by asynchrony or temporomandibular joint problems.

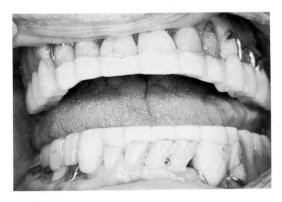

FIG. 20. The provisional short-term prosthesis provided to restore lost tooth structure and to correct lateral displacement of jaws.

Maintenance and Follow-Up Care

Contrary to prevailing custom, older people require more frequent adjustment and correction of occlusion, denture base fitting, and esthetic corrections than younger people. Dentures are more unstable in older persons than in younger denture wearers. Older persons also require more frequent periodontal treatment and prophylactic care. They should be selectively recalled at least every three months, and sooner in many instances. The hygienist is an essential professional in health care for the elderly, not only in the provision of primary care, but in the administration of services and in the preventive care associated with follow-up services.

In conclusion, one of the major problems in providing dental care is the lack of a reliable method for evaluating the quality of care and a more cost-effective utilization of funds, resources, and trained personnel. Peer review of quality of dental care is difficult at best even for younger adults (26,37).

SUMMARY

The options in the selection of dental care for the aging include the full spectrum of treatment procedures generally available to all age groups. They include endodontic, periodontic, orthodontic, surgical, restorative, and prosthodontic procedures for treatment of root and coronal caries, acute and chronic periodontal and surgical disorders. One of the most prevalent disorders is complete or partial edentulousness, which seriously alters mastication, deglutition, and the speech and language skills of the aging. These dental problems furthermore affect the self-concept and self-esteem of older persons who often perceive their facial esthetics as faulty and unsightly. The selection, sequence, and extent of dental procedures are patient-specific and should not be generalized solely by dental disorders but rather treated in concert with attention to those medical and psychosocial problems that are typically also present (33,34).

REFERENCES

1. Avnet, H. H., and Nikias, M. (1967): *Insured Dental Care.* Group Health Dental Insurance, Inc., New York.
2. Baird, J. T., Jr., and Kelly, J. E. (1962): *Need for Dental Care Among Adults.* Series 11, No. 36. Division of Health Examination Statistics, Department of Health, Education and Welfare.
3. Banting, D. W. (1972): A study of dental care cost, time and treatment requirements of older persons in the community. *Can. J. Public Health,* 63:508–514.
4. Behrman, S. J., and Wright, I. S. (1961): Dental surgery during continuous anticoagulant therapy. *JAMA,* 175:483–488.
5. Bell, B. D., and Stanfield, G. F. (1973): Chronological age in relation to attitudinal judgments: An experimental analysis. *J. Gerontol.,* 28:491–496.
6. Brotman, H. B. (1974): The fastest growing minority: The aging. *Am. J. Public Health,* 64:249–252.
7. Burgess, W. C., and Beck, D. J. (1969): Survey of denture wearers in New Zealand. *N.Z. Dent. J.,* 65:223–232.

8. Burnham, C. E. (1971): *Edentulous Persons.* Series 10, No. 89. National Center for Health Statistics, Department of Health, Education and Welfare.
9. Collier, D. R. (1980): Fluorine: An essential element for good dental health. *N.Y. State J. Med.,* 6:1338–1339.
10. Giddon, D. B., Mosier, M., Colton, T., and Bulman, J. R. (1976): Quantitative relationships between perceived and objective need for health care—dentistry as a model. *Public Health Rep.* 91:507–514.
11. Henderson, R. M. (1971): Shortage of dental care for the chronically ill and aged. *J. Mich. Dent. Assoc.,* 53:306.
12. Hobdell, M. H., Sheinhan, A., and Cowell, C. R. (1970): The prevalence of full and partial dentures in British populations. *Br. Dent. J.,* 128:437–442.
13. Johnson, E. S., Kelly, J. E., and Van Kirk, L. E. (1965): *Selected Dental Findings in Adults by Age, Race and Sex.* Series 11, No. 7. Division of Health Examination and Statistics, Department of Health, Education and Welfare.
14. Kelly, J. (1974): *Basic Data on Dental Examination Findings of Persons 1–74 Yrs.* Series 11, No. 214. National Health Survey, Department of Health, Education and Welfare.
15. Kogan, N. (1961): Attitudes toward old people: The development of a scale and an examination of correlation. *J. Abnorm. Soc. Psychol.,* 62:44–55.
16. Landa, L., and Silverman, S. I. (1966): *Cephalometric Study of Head Posture and Vertical Dimension of Rest by Radiography.* Presented to Greater N.Y. Academy of Prosthodontics. (Abstract)
17. Litvak, H., Silverman, S. I., and Garfinkel, L. (1971): Oral stereoagnosis in dentulous and edentulous subjects. *J. Prosthet. Dent.,* 25:139–151.
18. Marshall, J. Y. (1975): Policies on community dental health; Council on Dental Health. *Am. Dent. Assoc.,* 1:26–27.
19. Mashberg, A., and Garfinkel, L. (1978): *Early Diagnosis or Oral Cancer: The Erythroplastic Lesion in High Risk Sites.* American Cancer Society, Professional Education Publication, New York.
20. Massler, M. (1980): Geriatric dentistry root caries in the elderly. *J. Prosthet. Dent.,* 44:147–149.
21. Miller, S., and Heil, J. (1976): Effect of an extramural program of dental care for the special patient on attitudes of students. *J. Dent. Educ.,* 40:740–744.
22. Moen, B. D. (1962): Statistics relating to dental care for the aged. *J. Am. Coll. Dent.,* 29:94–97.
23. Moore, H. (1980): Television Broadcast: WNET, June, New York.
24. Nakamoto, R. Y. (1979): Use of a saliva substitute in postradiation xerostomia. *J. Prosthet. Dent.,* 42:539–542.
25. Putnam, W. J. (1962): Programming dental care for the chronically ill and aged. *J. N.J. Dent. Soc.,* 33:327–332.
26. Schonfeld, H. K. (1969): Peer review of quality of dental care. *Am. J. Dent. Assoc.,* 79:1376–1382.
27. Scopp, I. W., and Frederics, H. (1958): Dental extractions in patients undergoing anticoagulant therapy. *Oral Surg.,* 11:470–474.
28. Sereno, E. (1966): *Current Availability of Dental Care Under Welfare Provisions: Provision of Dental Care in the Community,* University of Michigan, Ann Arbor, Michigan.
29. Silverman, S. I. (1958): Nutrition and dental care in a physical medicine and rehabilitation program. *Arch. Phys. Med. Rehabil.,* 39:555–559.
30. Silverman, S. I. (1959): *Dental Care and Nutrition in the Aging.* Conference on Aging. New York Medical College, Department of Physical Medicine and Rehabilitation, New York.
31. Silverman, S. I. (1973): *Psychology of Esthetics.* Esthetic Medcom Learning Systems. New York.
32. Silverman, S. I. (1975): The burning mouth syndrome. *J. Dent. Assoc. S. Afr.,* 30:163–166.
33. Silverman, S. I. (1979): Correlation of biologic, psychologic and clinical aspects of dental care for the aging. In: *Geriatric Dentistry: Clinical Application of Selected Biomedical and Psychosocial Topics,* edited by C. J. Toga, K. Nandy, and H. N. Chauncey, pp. 195–214. Lexington Books, Heath, Lexington, Mass.
34. Silverman, S. I. (1979): Geriatric dentistry. In: *Current Concepts in Dental Hygiene,* edited by W. Reynolds and S. Boundy, pp. 47–67. Mosby, St. Louis.
35. Silverman, S. I., and Block, M. (1970): Visual motor function, dental occlusion, proprioception and intersensory function. *I.A.D.R.* (Abstract). International Association Dental Research, p. 218.

36. Silverman, S., Silverman, S. I., Silverman, B., and Garfinkel, L. (1976): Self image and its relation to denture acceptance. *J. Prosthet. Dent.,* 35:131–142.
37. Soricelli, D. A. (1968): Methods of administrative control for the promotion of quality in dental programs. *Am. J. Public Health,* 58:1123–1139.
38. Toto, P. D. (1979): Fluorescent antibody detection of CEA in oral squamous cell carcinoma. *J. Oral Med.,* 34:45–46.
39. Weinberger, L. E., and Milham, J. (1975): A multi-dimensional, multiple method analysis of attitudes toward the elderly. *J. Gerontol.,* 30:343–348.
40. Wilder, M. H. (1973): *Current Estimates from the Health Interview Survey.* Series 10, No. 95. National Center for Health Statistics, Department of Health, Education and Welfare.

Rehabilitation in the Aging edited by
T. F. Williams. Raven Press, New York © 1984.

Specific Cardiac Disorders

Nanette Kass Wenger

Department of Medicine (Cardiology), Emory University School of Medicine; and Cardiac Clinics, Grady Memorial Hospital, Atlanta, Georgia 30303

Approximately 25 million people in the United States are aged 65 and older, and half of them have some cardiac disorder. Indeed, cardiovascular disease is the major cause of death after age 65, accounting for more than 40% of deaths in this age group (15). Coronary atherosclerotic heart disease remains the most frequent clinical problem, hence its emphasis in this chapter. The combination of coronary atherosclerotic heart disease and hypertension is also common. Congestive heart failure, from a variety of causes, increases with increasing age. Arrhythmias and electrocardiographic abnormalities have an increased incidence with aging (4).

Cardiac disease in the elderly is complicated by the fact that it rarely occurs in isolation; there is typically other major systemic illness. Protein-calorie malnutrition is frequent. Additionally, changes of aging are seen in other organ systems; because of these varied limitations of function with aging, an increased incidence of drug sensitivity is encountered.

GENERAL CONCERNS OF REHABILITATION RELATED TO CARDIAC DISORDERS

Inactivity and deconditioning, because of a variety of medical problems in the elderly, may cause cardiovascular disability or may exacerbate underlying cardiac disease.

Prolonged inactivity and bedrest quickly and markedly impair cardiovascular functional capacity (22). Other associated problems include a negative nitrogen and protein balance, thrombophlebitis and pulmonary embolism, and the fear of becoming a cardiac cripple.

More often than the younger counterpart, the elderly cardiac patient fears major deterioration of function, recurrent myocardial infarction, and major infirmity, and may be excessively concerned about failure of life-sustaining equipment, e.g., a cardiac pacemaker.

All too often, the physician potentiates the problem by prescribing excessive bedrest for the elderly cardiac patient and by overmedication to relieve discomfort and assure rest. In general, physicians know little about the activity habits of their elderly patients; and limited data about physical activity, both in health and with cardiovascular disease, are available for individuals over age 65. Even prior to illness, many elderly patients decrease their level of physical activity due to a varied combination of musculoskeletal instability, depression, and inappropriate admonitions from the physician or from family members (2). Additionally, because of the decreased aerobic capacity with aging, any submaximal task is perceived as requiring increased work because of its increased relative energy cost. Relative inactivity thus potentiates the decreased physical work capacity in the elderly, often threatening their independent lifestyle. This can be averted, and indeed functional capacity improved, with the institution or reinstitution of physical activity (11).

The changes in cardiac function with aging (N. K. Wenger, *this volume*) often potentiate the cardiovascular functional impairment due to disease. Emphasis in the rehabilitative approach to the elderly patient with cardiac disease must have the dual aim of preserving physical function, including mobility and self-sufficiency; and of preserving mental function—self-respect, alertness, minimizing anxiety and depression, and encouraging readjustment to society.

CORONARY ATHEROSCLEROTIC HEART DISEASE

Coronary atherosclerotic heart disease accounts for over two-thirds of cardiac deaths in the elderly population. Additionally, the clinical manifestations of coronary disease differ significantly from the classic presentations encountered in younger individuals.

Angina pectoris in the aged may not be described as typical effort angina, predominantly because of the sedentary lifestyle of many older patients. It is often arthritis, other musculoskeletal problems, or claudication that causes the limitation of activity before anginal pain is initiated. Elderly patients with previously asymptomatic coronary atherosclerosis may have angina precipitated by hypertension, anemia, or arrhythmia. Correction of these features may improve the cardiac status and rehabilitation prognosis.

Myocardial infarction, too, has a different and more subtle presentation (18,19). Pain is limited or atypical with advancing age, and painless myocardial infarction is not unusual. The more frequent presentations include sudden unexplained dyspnea or even pulmonary edema, an exacerbation of preexisting congestive heart failure, profound weakness, nausea or vomiting, agitation, restlessness or acute confusion, syncope, cerebrovascular accident, and peripheral arterial embolism. Less commonly, evidence of progressive renal failure may herald myocardial infarction. Often the painless myocardial infarction is precipitated by another problem with associated hypotension, hypoxemia, or anemia. The male preponderance of myocardial infarction decreases with age, with an essentially equal sex incidence over age 70. Attention to teaching energy-conserving techniques in household work thus constitutes an important feature of rehabilitation of the elderly woman with myocardial infarction.

Myocardial infarction in the elderly tends to be more severe. In general, the infarctions are larger and are characterized by more and typically severe complications, by increased morbidity and mortality, and by a protracted hospital stay for the survivors. Indeed, the hospital mortality for patients over age 70 is 30 to 40%, approximately twice that of younger patients. Probably because of the increased severity of infarction, the elderly patients tend to have more residual invalidism and increased late deaths.

As regards the clinical course, cardiogenic shock, pulmonary edema, and congestive heart failure, major determinants of severity and mortality, are far more common in the elderly. Conduction defects and heart block occur with increased frequency, as do atrial fibrillation and atrial flutter (23,31). Cardiac rupture during the first week or so is particularly frequent in the elderly and is heralded by hypotension, recurrence of chest pain, and, preterminally, by electromechanical dissociation, transient persistence of cardiac electrical activity as evident on the electrocardiogram in the absence of ventricular pumping function.

Nevertheless, the elderly patient benefits from the skills and services available in a coronary care unit, and intensive coronary care has decreased the mortality for the elderly as well as for the younger patients. Older patients respond as well to defribillation as younger ones. It deserves emphasis that a substantial number of elderly patients have an essentially uncomplicated clinical course, and these individuals have an excellent prognosis for recovery and rehabilitation despite their age; however, the prognosis worsens with recurrent myocardial infarction.

Therefore, age should not be a bar to admission to a coronary care unit (6,31). With the institution of this concept, the clinical picture of myocardial infarction in the elderly has been reported as changed. More elderly patients admitted to coronary care units present a more classic pain syndrome, but that may be the reason for their coronary care unit admission. This explanation is reinforced by the fact that there are fewer self-referrals to the hospital among the elderly, so that coronary care unit admission may reflect physician selection. However, even those elderly patients with typical pain commonly have associated dyspnea. The elderly patient is more frequently at rest at the onset of myocardial infarction, possibly a reflection of the more sedentary lifestyle. Nevertheless, the prior medical history of patients admitted to the coronary care unit is similar in older and younger individuals in regard to antecedent angina pectoris and prior myocardial infarction, treated hypertension, and diabetes mellitus (23,31).

In the coronary care unit, the elderly patient tends to have more disorientation and cerebral dysfunction, possibly related to the increased occurrence of hypotension, dysrhythmia, and sensitivity to medications, particularly narcotics, analgesics, and sedatives. They may be increasedly anxious, fearing death, and may have problems understanding the monitoring devices, the multiplicity of personnel and procedures, and so on. Careful and repeated explanations must be part of the early rehabilitation. When age is no barrier, about one-fifth of all coronary care unit admissions are over age 70. Other problems encountered with increased frequency in the elderly patient with myocardial infarction include difficulty with urination, particularly in the male with prostatic enlargement receiving diuretic therapy; a stool softener and a soft diet will often avert common gastrointestinal complications. The use of atropine to reverse sinus bradycardia may precipitate glaucoma, urinary retention, or confusion; alternate therapy such as temporary pacing may be preferable.

However, for the elderly patient with an uncomplicated clinical course, early ambulation helps prevent cardiovascular deconditioning. Even several hours of sitting in a chair each day may obviate the orthostatic intolerance generated by protracted bedrest. The demonstration that physical activity will not produce cardiac symptoms provides immeasurable reassurance. Gradually progressive physical activity during the hospitalization is comparable to that for younger patients. This will enable the physical performance of personal care and daily living activities on return home and may avert or delay the need for institutional care. The subsequent maintenance of an appropriate physical activity level often requires reinforcement and encouragement, both from the physician and other health professionals and from family and friends. In the rehabilitative approach, risk factor modification is far less relevant than in the younger patient, except for advice to discontinue cigarette smoking because of its association with increased sudden cardiac death and fatal reinfarction. Blood pressure control is indicated to prevent cerebrovascular complications and improve the management of angina pectoris and heart failure. Emphasis should be on return to preinfarction lifestyle, while defining the importance of regular physical activity with intervening rest. Because of the decreased aerobic capacity with aging, the energy expenditure of walking constitutes a significant percentage of total aerobic capacity. Thus walking is an effective physical conditioning stimulus in the elderly, even walking as slowly as 3 or 3½ mph (11). An ideal posthospitalization physical activity regimen is therefore a walking program, gradually increasing the pace of walking and the distance walked. Continued social and recreational activities should be encouraged, as should return to a light job when appropriate, and return to prior patterns of sexual activity.

Clear and specific instructions are requisite regarding diet, activity, and medications. Difficulties to be anticipated include visual and memory impairments that may complicate medication-taking; and the combined medical, psychological, and social problems often encountered in the patient with multisystem degenerative disease.

Restoration of normal physical activity and prior lifestyle are major deterrents of anxiety and depression, both of which pose therapeutic problems in the elderly cardiac patient. Most psychotropic drugs are contraindicated after infarction because of their adverse effects on heart rate, blood pressure, and cardiac rhythm. Benzodiazepine drugs appear safest. In encouraging participation of older patients in physical activity programs after myocardial infarction (or other illness), several distinctive features must be appreciated. Warm-up or limbering-up exercises appear particularly important in permitting effective training to occur.

After exercise, an increased amount of time is required for the heart rate to return to resting levels. This necessitates design of the training program to incorporate longer intervals of rest or of low-level activity between the exercise training periods. Because the training intensity is low-level, and perhaps related to a slower initial adaptation to and acceptance of a training regimen, older individuals require a longer time to attain a training effect. Only after more prolonged training is there a decrease in heart rate and blood pressure response to any level of submaximal work.

Additional benefits of physical activity include the maintenance of joint mobility and neuromuscular coordination; general coordination and flexibility also improve. Exercise increases muscle and tendon strength, which enhances joint stability, helping prevent damage with sudden, unexpected activity demands.

Nevertheless, running and jumping exercises should be limited for elderly individuals, as they produce excessive orthopedic problems. Additionally, inasmuch as older patients have a decreased ability to sweat efficiently and to tolerate heart stress, high-level physical activity should be avoided and even moderate exercise limited in hot and humid environments.

Exercise-increased energy expenditure is an adjunct to dietary therapy in weight control.

AORTIC VALVE DISEASE

Aortic Stenosis

A short, early-peaking basal systolic murmur is the most common cardiac murmur in the elderly, occurring in one-third to one-half of patients. It is typically encountered in an asymptomatic individual, is associated with a normal carotid pulse, has no hemodynamic consequences, and is termed the murmur of aortic sclerosis. Another proposed mechanism is turbulent aortic blood flow in a dilated aorta (3,20).

To be differentiated from this benign problem is hemodynamically significant aortic stenosis, occurring in the minority of patients with a basal systolic murmur. The typical clinical history in elderly individuals hospitalized for significant aortic stenosis includes symptoms of congestive heart failure in over one-half of patients. The incidence of angina varies, possibly related to the variable coexistence of coronary atherosclerotic heart disease. About one-third of these patients have syncope, often exertional in character. Indeed, hemodynamically significant aortic stenosis is the most common anatomic cause of syncope in the elderly.

Physical examination defines a slowly rising carotid pulse, at times with a thrill, although on occasion the rigid blood vessel wall may permit a relatively brisk carotid upstroke and mask the diagnostic carotid pulse abnormality. The left ventricular impulse is sustained; the aortic component of the second heart sound is diminished or, at times, absent; and reversed splitting of the second heart sound (S_2) is occasionally described. A fourth heart sound may be audible. The basal systolic crescendo-decrescendo murmur is long, loud, harsh, and late-peaking, at times associated with a thrill and often radiating into the neck. The transmitted, often holosystolic, high-frequency components heard at the lower left sternal border and toward the apex must be differentiated from the murmur of mitral regurgitation. On occasion, an aortic regurgitant murmur may be present. The electrocardiogram typically shows left ventricular hypertrophy, and dense aortic valvular calcification is seen on the chest roentgenogram.

Cardiac catheterization is warranted in the symptomatic patient to determine the severity of the aortic stenosis, as the clinical examination may be misleading and echocardiography and other noninvasive tests cannot reliably assess severity (7). Aggressive surgical management is indicated (7,28), as patients with hemodynamically significant aortic stenosis have a high mortality after the onset of congestive heart failure, angina, or syncope. Even in old age, aortic valve replacement significantly increases survival and improves the quality of life; it is the indicated rehabilitative procedure.

Aortic stenosis is common in old age, and is seen more frequently in men under age 80 and in women over age 80. The 20% of patients with associated mitral valve disease are presumed to have a rheumatic etiology. Far more common, however, is calcific change either in a congenitally bicuspid aortic valve (among the younger of the elderly patients) or calcific degeneration of a tricuspid aortic valve, more frequently encountered in patients over age 75 to 80 (21) (Fig. 1). Bacteremia may result in aortic endocarditis with any underlying valve abnormality; education regarding endocarditis prophylaxis is an important component of care.

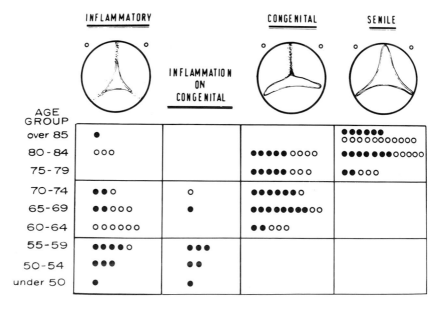

FIG. 1. Age and sex distribution of the different pathological types of isolated aortic stenosis. *Closed circles,* men; *open circles,* women. (Reproduced from ref. 21, with permission.)

Aortic Regurgitation

The murmur of aortic regurgitation is the most common diastolic murmur in old age. When there is associated mitral valve disease, a rheumatic etiology should be suspected; rheumatic aortic valve disease is more common in men than in women.

As previously mentioned, calcific aortic valve disease is often associated with a soft regurgitant murmur. The prognosis is far less satisfactory in luetic aortic regurgitation, which is often hemodynamically severe and frequently associated with aortic aneurysm.

By contrast, isolated aortic regurgitation, probably due to dilatation of the aortic root, rarely has hemodynamic consequences, and the prognosis is excellent. For patients with any of these lesions, prophylaxis against infective endocarditis must be emphasized.

HYPERTROPHIC OBSTRUCTIVE CARDIOMYOPATHY

Hypertrophic obstructive cardiomyopathy (idiopathic hypertrophic subaortic stenosis) is often not suspected in the elderly, despite the relative frequency of

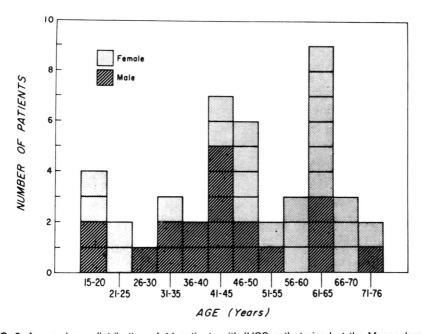

FIG. 2. Age and sex distribution of 44 patients with IHSS catheterized at the Massachusetts General Hospital from January 1, 1964 to June 1, 1970. Note that under the age of 60 years, there were equal numbers of male and female patients, whereas among the older patients women predominated ($p < 0.025$). IHSS, idiopathic hypertrophic subaortic stenosis. (Reproduced from ref. 30, with permission.)

elderly patients in the population of individuals with this disorder (Fig. 2). In the elderly patient, confusion with valvular aortic stenosis or coronary disease with papillary muscle dysfunction is common (30).

The older patient with hypertrophic obstructive cardiomyopathy has been described in some reports as more disabled by chest pain or dyspnea and more frequently reporting dizziness, palpitations, and syncope. Other studies define symptoms as comparable to those of younger patients. Women predominate among the older patients with hypertrophic obstructive cardiomyopathy.

The diagnosis can be suspected by the response of the murmur to provocative maneuvers and can be made definitively by echocardiography.

Differentiation from valvular aortic stenosis is important in that remission of symptoms often occurs with discontinuation of nitroglycerin, diuretic drugs, and cardiac glycosides, which may exacerbate the outflow obstruction, and with the institution of beta adrenergic blocking agents (9). These patients, too, require education about prophylaxis against infective endocarditis.

RHEUMATIC MITRAL VALVULAR DISEASE

Rheumatic heart disease is the most common cause of mitral valvular disease in the elderly individual, although this pattern may change in subsequent years with the marked diminution in childhood rheumatic fever. Two-thirds of patients have predominant mitral regurgitation, and one-third predominant mitral stenosis; one-half have associated aortic valve disease.

The prognosis is generally good, with three-quarters of middle-aged patients with asymptomatic mitral valve disease, most typically mitral stenosis with regular sinus rhythm, alive and well 20 years later. The onset of atrial fibrillation appears to be the main feature determining deterioration.

Among elderly patients hospitalized with mitral valve disease of greater hemodynamic severity, 40% have congestive heart failure as the major complication; the 10% with angina usually have associated coronary atherosclerotic heart disease. Pulmonary embolism may further complicate congestive heart failure. Systemic embolism is not unusual, particularly when atrial fibrillation is present. Careful education of patients requiring ambulatory anticoagulant therapy is important in minimizing bleeding complications.

NONRHEUMATIC MITRAL VALVE DISEASE—MITRAL REGURGITATION

The two most common causes of nonrheumatic mitral regurgitation in the elderly are papillary muscle dysfunction, typically following myocardial infarction, and calcification of the mitral annulus. The latter can be relatively definitively diagnosed by the characteristic X-ray picture and at echocardiography. Calcification of the mitral annulus is more frequent in women than in men and is typically clinically unimportant.

Myxomatous degeneration of the mitral valve may cause mitral valve prolapse with a mitral regurgitant murmur. Arrhythmias and atypical chest pain are encountered. Hemodynamic severity varies (10) but, with progression to chordal rupture, severe and often life-threatening cardiac decompensation can be expected.

Less common causes of nonrheumatic mitral regurgitation include a left atrial myxoma (which more often mimics mitral valvular obstruction) and the mitral regurgitation associated with hypertrophic obstructive cardiomyopathy.

CARDIAC SURGERY IN THE ELDERLY

In general, cardiac surgery in the elderly is complicated by cardiovascular, cerebrovascular, and peripheral vascular insufficiency; atherosclerotic changes in the aorta and large vessels; impaired renal function; prostatic obstruction; pulmonary problems; and the often debilitated and malnourished state of elderly individuals (28).

The most frequent valvular surgery, as previously discussed, is aortic valve replacement for hemodynamically significant calcific aortic stenosis. The prognosis of the medically treated patients is extremely poor, with few patients surviving three years after the onset of heart failure, angina, or syncope; sudden death is common. Because left ventricular function is typically well preserved, even after the onset of heart failure, valve replacement in these Class III and IV patients carries only a 10 to 20% mortality even in the elderly patient. The

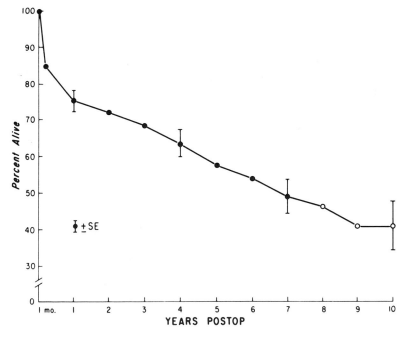

FIG. 3. Survival curve for 221 isolated aortic valve replacements in patients over 60 years of age at the University of Oregon Medical School. *Open circles* indicate fewer than 20 patients at risk. (Reproduced from ref. 27, with permission.)

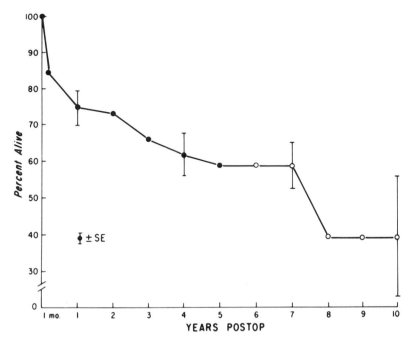

FIG. 4. Survival curve for 89 isolated mitral valve replacements in patients over 60 years of age at the University of Oregon Medical School. *Open circles* indicate fewer than 20 patients at risk. (Reproduced from ref. 27, with permission.)

relief of symptoms is often spectacular, warranting an aggressive approach to aortic valve replacement if the patient is alert and has no complicating medical illness (1) (Fig. 3). Concomitant coronary bypass surgery may be indicated (25). Gradually progressive early ambulation is appropriate after successful surgery and decreases postoperative complications.

The results of mitral valve replacement are far less dramatic and satisfactory (28) (Fig. 4). The increased mortality is probably related in part to the underlying left ventricular dysfunction; and the often needed long-term anticoagulant therapy poses added risk in the older individual.

Coronary artery bypass surgery affords the same symptomatic relief in older as in younger subjects, but carries an increased morbidity and mortality. The effect on longevity is doubtful, and careful patient selection is warranted. As previously indicated, early ambulation and gradually progressive physical activity are part of the postoperative management.

HYPERTENSION AND HYPERTENSIVE CARDIOVASCULAR DISEASE

Much of the cardiovascular morbidity and mortality in the elderly is related to hypertension. This is true for both isolated systolic hypertension and systolic-diastolic blood pressure elevations (17). Over age 65, about 40% of white and over 50% of black individuals have either isolated systolic hypertension or systolic-diastolic hypertension. Severely elevated diastolic blood pressure (110 mm Hg or above) is three times as common in elderly blacks as in elderly whites (16). Hypertension increases the risk of myocardial infarction, congestive heart failure, and stroke, much as it does in the younger individual. Control of hypertension has the potential to decrease cardiovascular morbidity and mortality.

Blood pressure increases with age in most population samples; systolic blood pressure continues to increase into the seventh and eighth decades, whereas diastolic blood pressure levels off in the fifties and sixties (Fig. 5). Nevertheless, at any age, elevation of the blood pressure is associated with an increased risk of cardiovascular events in both men and women (16).

In addition to accelerated atherogenesis (myocardial infarction and congestive heart failure), hypertension adversely affects cardiac performance, renal function, and cerebral blood flow; increases aortic aneurysm rupture and dissection; and increases the incidence of cerebrovascular bleeding (Table 1).

In the elderly patient, most recommendations are for drug treatment for a blood pressure in excess of 160/95. There is little evidence whether antihypertensive therapy alters the course of asymptomatic elderly individuals without evidence of end-organ damage from isolated systolic hypertension. Nevertheless,

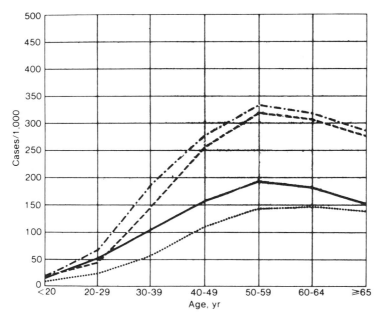

FIG. 5. Prevalence of elevated blood pressure at screening (diastolic ≥ 95 mmHg). *Solid line,* White Male; *dotted line,* White Female; *dotted and dashed line,* Black Male; *dashed line,* Black Female. (Reproduced from ref. 26, with permission.)

TABLE 1. *Incidence of cardiovascular disease according to hypertensive status in men and women age 65–74*[a]

	Coronary heart disease		Brain infarction		Congestive heart failure		Intermittent claudication	
	Men	Women	Men	Women	Men	Women	Men	Women
Blood pressure status								
Normotensive	5.35	2.20	0.70	—	1.05	1.25	3.60	1.70
Borderline	11.55	6.55	2.15	2.15	2.85	2.65	1.85	1.45
Hypertensive	14.85	11.30	3.50	3.95	8.90	5.15	3.80	2.85
Regression coefficient	0.508	0.728	0.751	1.044	1.113	0.708	−0.034	0.341
t Value	2.98	3.92	2.10	2.98	3.84	2.69	−0.12	1.13
Hypertensive vs. normotensive								
Difference in risk	9.50	9.10	2.80	3.95	7.85	3.90	0.20	1.15
Attributable risk (%)	64	81	80	100	88	76	5	40
Risk ratio	2.8	5.1	5.0	—	8.5	4.1	1.1	1.7

[a] Framingham study: 18-Year Follow-up. Five-year incidence per 100 at risk.
From Kannell (12), with permission.

isolated systolic hypertension doubles the risk of cardiovascular complications, so that the risk, expense, and inconvenience of therapy must be compared with the benefits of systolic blood pressure lowering (16).

With any antihypertensive drug regimen, dosage should be very gradually increased; the hypovolemia and decreased baroreceptor activity common in the elderly may accentuate responsiveness to antihypertensive agents. The therapeutic goal is a reduction of diastolic blood pressure below 90 mm Hg. If isolated systolic hypertension is treated, the target blood pressure is 140 to 160 mm Hg (17). General recommendations for antihypertensive therapy in elderly individuals include the use of a thiazide diuretic with supplementary potassium. Dietary inadequacies in the elderly render them increasedly susceptible to hypokalemia. Reserpine may be effective, but should be avoided in the individual with associated depression. Beta adrenergic blocking agents seem advantageous in patients with predominant systolic hypertension; however, these agents appear less effective in elderly than in younger patients (16). They have the advantage of effectively lowering blood pressure without producing orthostatic hypotension. Associated aortic regurgitation constitutes a moderate contraindication to beta blockade because of the longer diastolic interval available for regurgitant flow as the heart rate slows. Dietary sodium and calorie restriction may be helpful. In following the response to therapy, blood pressure should be measured in both the sitting and standing positions because of the common orthostatic decrease in blood pressure in elderly individuals.

Complications of antihypertensive therapy are more frequent in the elderly individual, both because the diminution of renal function increases the incidence of drug toxicity and because the aged patient with less sensitive baroreceptor responses is more susceptible to the orthostatic complications of volume depletion. Gradually assuming the upright posture may avert dizziness and syncope.

LESS COMMON FORMS OF HEART DISEASE

Pulmonary Heart Disease

Pulmonary heart disease frequently coexists with coronary atherosclerotic heart disease and hypertensive cardiovascular disease, but in its severe form is uncommon in old age. It may be that severe pulmonary heart disease, especially that associated with heart failure, shortens life expectancy.

There is an age-dependent loss of lung function, with the elderly individual having a decreased maximum breathing capacity, decreased vital capacity, decreased forced expiratory volume (FEV), and increased residual volume. Although these changes present little problem with usual activity, they may limit the maximum capacity for physical activity.

The important components of care include control of infection, relief of bronchospasm, and liquefaction of sputum. The management of the associated congestive heart failure includes the standard control of sodium and water retention and the relief of respiratory failure.

Although kyphoscoliosis is common in old age, the severe kyphoscoliotic heart disease characterized by congestive heart failure is unusual.

Pulmonary embolism (see H. Keltz, *this volume*) is common in older individuals, especially in the setting of prolonged immobilization. Anticoagulant therapy is associated with an increased risk of bleeding in the elderly.

Thyroid Heart Disease

Thyrotoxic heart disease (13) is a not uncommon cause of high-output failure in the elderly. It is characterized by atrial fibrillation, cardiac enlargement, and congestive heart failure. It may exacerbate the clinical manifestations of coronary atherosclerotic heart disease, hypertensive cardiovascular disease, or other causes of congestive heart failure. In the elderly patient, the hypermetabolic aspects may be masked, and the cardiovascular symptoms may dominate the presentation. Control of the dysrhythmia and failure depends on control of the hypermetabolic state.

Myxedema heart disease is less frequent, presenting as sinus bradycardia, cardiac enlargement, and pericardial effusion. Administration of thyroid hormone reverses the problem. This, however, must be done cautiously in the elderly patient with symptomatic coronary atherosclerotic heart disease.

Congenital Heart Disease

Atrial septal defect is the most common congenital lesion encountered in the elderly. In the absence of pulmonary hypertension and atrial fibrillation, patients are often asymptomatic.

INFECTIVE ENDOCARDITIS

The clinical diagnosis of endocarditis is less commonly made in older than in young patients (29), despite the fact that one-third of cases of infective endocarditis occur in elderly individuals. There is often no known antecedent valvular disease; when present, common underlying valvular lesions in the aged include calcified or deformed aortic valves (13) and rheumatic mitral valvular fibrosis. At times elderly patients are afebrile and/or without cardiac murmurs, and present with anemia, renal failure, coma, or hemiplegia. The prognosis is far more serious in the elderly, where infective endocarditis is associated with a high mortality.

ARRHYTHMIAS

Any severe tachy- or bradyarrhythmia that decreases the cardiac output is of concern in the elderly because it may compromise vital organs impaired by aging and disease.

Aged patients often have significant dysrhythmia without the symptoms of palpitations or tachycardia. Arrhythmia may present as syncope or an alteration of consciousness; long-term electrocardiographic monitoring may be required to delineate the specific disturbance of rhythm and permit appropriate therapy. First-degree atrioventricular block, premature atrial contractions, premature ventricular contractions, and atrial fibrillation are encountered with increased frequency in the elderly.

The aged are more sensitive to most cardiovascular drugs, including those used to manage cardiovascular arrhythmias. Patients with symptomatic complete heart block have attained a new lease on life with the advent of permanent pacemakers, which increase both survival and the quality of life. Prior to permanent pacing, 50% of patients who developed complete heart block survived less than two years. Now the majority of patients survive more than five years. The presentation of complete heart block may vary from profound weakness, to exacerbation of heart failure, to confusion, or syncope. Education regarding pacemaker surveillance is an important rehabilitative component.

ELECTROCARDIOGRAPHIC ABNORMALITIES

Electrocardiographic (EKG) abnormalities are common in the elderly but usually indicate cardiovascular disease. Indeed, there is little reason to change the EKG criteria for the aged (24); a significant proportion of apparently well older persons have entirely normal EKGs (5). Aged individuals have an increased incidence of heart disease and an increase in electrocardiographic abnormalities, which tend to parallel each other (8).

More commonly encountered in the elderly are first-degree atrioventricular block, bundle branch block, nonspecific ST segment and T wave changes, premature ventricular contractions, left anterior hemiblock, left ventricular hypertrophy, and atrial fibrillation. In one survey, left anterior hemiblock was far more common than either right or left bundle branch block and constituted the most common abnormality after ST-T changes and the pattern of left ventricular hypertrophy (14). In general, the presence of atrial fibrillation, left bundle branch block, or an intraventricular conduction delay correlate with organic heart disease.

The EKG abnormalities per se have little prognostic significance, in that the prognosis of EKG abnormalities in the elderly is equivalent to that of the underlying disease. EKG abnormalities common in the elderly, in the absence of appreciable heart disease, are a leftward deviation of the QRS axis, incomplete right bundle branch block, and first-degree atrioventricular block.

APPROACH TO AND MANAGEMENT OF THE PATIENT WITH CONGESTIVE HEART FAILURE

The initial approach to the problem of congestive heart failure in the elderly individual includes a search for precipitating features in patients known to have heart disease such as infection with fever and tachycardia, pulmonary embolism, anemia, and thyrotoxicosis. There may, in addition, be remediable heart disease, that due to hypertension or to valvular heart disease; pericardial disease rarely causes heart failure in the aged.

The cornerstones of therapy are physical and emotional rest, the relief of sodium and water retention, and the improvement of myocardial contractility.

The elderly patient with congestive heart failure is often restless and agitated; these symptoms respond better to control of the heart failure than to sedation (13). Digitalis (see discussion in subsequent section) and gradual diuresis are indicated, with particular attention to the avoidance of hypovolemia and hypokalemia; a transient elevation of the blood urea nitrogen (BUN) may be encountered early in the course of therapy. Dietary sodium restriction may be poorly accepted by elderly patients.

Initially the patient with heart failure may be more comfortable sitting in a chair than in bed. Early but gradual mobilization is indicated after control of the congestive heart failure; the patient should be carefully observed for weight gain, edema, fatigue, and breathlessness as activity is increased. Psychologic rehabilitation is important, with an optimistic attitude that the patient will not be a cardiac cripple. Indeed, the addition of vasodilator therapy has afforded an improved prognosis for patients with severe congestive heart failure.

Simplification of maintenance therapy is important, using as few drugs as possible and as limited a dosage schedule as feasible.

SELECTED PROBLEMS WITH DRUG THERAPY

Older patients often respond differently to cardiovascular medication because of their diminished hepatic, renal, gastrointestinal, and central nervous system function and diminished metabolism and cardiac output. The diminished glomerular filtration rate (even with a normal BUN) and decreased creatinine clearance prolong the half-life of digoxin, predisposing to digitalis toxicity, as does the often associated hypokalemia (13). On occasion, in addition to the standard presentation of digitalis toxicity, the patient may manifest this problem as lethargy or even psychosis.

Diuretics pose a particular problem as excessive diuresis with hypovolemia is poorly tolerated by the elderly individual and may result in hypotension, azotemia, and confusion. Even with the milder thiazide diuretics, in addition to checking for orthostatic complications, the patient should be watched for potassium depletion; this is especially prominent in the elderly whose dietary potassium intake may be limited. Digitalis toxicity and weakness may result from hypokalemia. In addition, the hyperglycemia encountered with thiazide therapy may aggravate preexisting diabetes mellitus.

Elderly patients have particular sensitivity to the effects of vasodilator therapy and beta adrenergic blocking agents, because of the predisposition with aging to orthostatic hypotension, compromised baroreceptor function, and frequently associated conduction system disease. Particularly in the hypovolemic patient, vasodilator therapy may produce unacceptable hypotension. Similarly, taking nitroglycerin while in the upright position may cause syncope.

Psychosocial factors assume a far greater importance in the elderly. Hearing or vision impairment may limit medication-taking ability, as may mental confusion. Elderly patients often have difficulty opening safety caps on medication bottles. Fixed incomes or limited insurance benefits may discourage medication purchase. Also, living alone, without reinforcement of medication-taking from family and friends, may limit drug adherence (17).

REFERENCES

1. Austen, W. G., DeSanctis, R. W., Buckley, M. D., Mundth, E. D., and Scannel, J. G. (1970): Surgical management of aortic valve disease in the elderly. *JAMA*, 211:624–626.
2. Bassey, E. G. (1978): Age, inactivity and some physiological responses to exercise. *Gerontology*, 24:66–77.
3. Bethel, C. S., and Crow, E. W. (1963): Heart sounds in the aged. *Am. J. Cardiol.*, 11:763–767.
4. Caird, F. I., and Kennedy, R. D. (1976): Epidemiology of heart disease in old age. In: *Cardiology in Old Age*, edited by F. I. Caird, J. L. C. Dall, and R. D. Kennedy, pp. 1–10. Plenum Press, New York.
5. Campbell, A., Caird, F. I., and Jackson, T. F. M. (1974): Prevalence of abnormalities of electrocardiogram in old people. *Br. Heart J.*, 36:1105–1111.
6. Chaturvedi, N. C., Shivalingappa, G., Shanks, B., McKay, A., Cumming, K., Walsh, M. J., Scaria, K., Lynas, P., Courtney, D., Barber, J. M., and Boyle, D. McC. (1972): Myocardial infarction in the elderly. *Lancet*, 1:280–282.
7. Finegan, R. E., Gianelly, R. E., and Harrison, D. C. (1969): Aortic stenosis in the elderly. *N. Engl. J. Med.*, 281:1261–1264.
8. Fisch, C., Genovese, P. D., Dyke, R. W., Laramore, W., and Marvel, R. (1957): The electrocardiogram in persons over 70. *Geriatrics*, 12:616–620.
9. Hamby, R. I., and Aintablian, A. (1976): Hypertrophic subaortic stenosis is not rare in the eighth decade. *Geriatrics*, 12:616–620.
10. Higgins, C. B., Reinke, R. T., Gosink, B. B., and Leopold, G. R. (1976): The significance of mitral valve prolapse in middle-aged and elderly men. *Am. Heart J.*, 91:292–296.
11. Hodgson, J. L., and Buskirk, E. R. (1977): Physical fitness and age, with emphasis on cardiovascular function in the elderly. *J. Am. Geriatric Soc.*, 25:385–392.
12. Kannell, W. B. (1976): Blood pressure and the development of cardiovascular disease in the aged. In: *Cardiology in Old Age*, edited by F. I. Caird, J. L. C. Dall, and R. D. Kennedy, pp. 143–175. Plenum Press, New York.
13. Kennedy, R. D. (1975): Drug therapy for cardiovascular disease in the aged. *J. Am. Geriatric Soc.*, 23:113–120.
14. Kitchin, A. H., Lowther, C. P., and Milne, J. S. (1973): Prevalence of clinical and electrocardiographic evidence of ischaemic heart disease in the older population. *Br. Heart J.*, 35:946–953.
15. Kolata, G. B. (1977): The aging heart: Changes in function and response to drugs. *Science*, 195:166–167.
16. Moser, M. (1979): Hypertension in the elderly. In: *Clinical Geriatrics*, edited by I. Rossman, pp. 606–617. Lippincott, Philadelphia.
17. National High Blood Pressure Education Program Coordinating Committee (1979): *Statement on Hypertension in the Elderly*. National Institutes of Health, Bethesda, Md.
18. Pathy, M. S. (1967): Clinical presentation of myocardial infarction in the elderly. *Br. Heart J.*, 29:190–199.
19. Pathy, M. S. (1976): Clinical features of ischemic heart disease. In: *Cardiology in Old Age*, edited by F. I. Caird, J. L. C. Dall, and R. D. Kennedy, pp. 193–208. Plenum Press, New York.

20. Perez, G. L., Jacob, M., Bhat, P. K., Rao, D. B., and Luisada, A. A. (1976): Incidence of murmurs in the aging heart. *J. Am. Geriatric Soc.,* 24:29–31.
21. Pomerance, A. (1972): Pathogenesis of aortic stenosis and its relation to age. *Br. Heart J.,* 34:569–574.
22. Saltin, B., Blomqvist, G., Mitchell, J. H., Johnson, R. L., Wildenthal, K., and Chapman, C. B. (1968): Response to exercise after bed rest and training. *Circulation,* 37–38(Suppl. 7):1–55.
23. Semple, T., and Williams, B. O. (1976): Coronary care for the elderly. In: *Cardiology in Old Age,* edited by F. I. Caird, J. L. C. Dall, and R. D. Kennedy, pp. 297–313. Plenum Press, New York.
24. Simonson, E. (1972): The effect of age on the electrocardiogram. *Am. J. Cardiol.,* 29:64–73.
25. Smith, J. M., Lindsay, W. G., Lillehei, R. C., and Nicoloff, D. M. (1976): Cardiac surgery in geriatric patients. *Surgery,* 80:443–448.
26. Stamler, J., Stamler, R., Reidlinger, W. F., Algera, G., and Roberts, R. H. (1976): Hypertension screening of one million Americans: Community Hypertension Evaluation Clinic (C.H.E.C.) Program, 1973–1975. *JAMA,* 235: 2299–2306.
27. Starr, A., and Lawson, R. (1976): Cardiac surgery in the elderly. In: *Cardiology in Old Age,* edited by F. I. Caird, J. L. C. Dall, and R. D. Kennedy, pp. 369–396. Plenum Press, New York.
28. Stephenson, L. W., MacVaugh, H., III, and Edmunds, L. H., Jr., (1978): Surgery using cardiopulmonary bypass in the elderly. *Circulation,* 58:250–254.
29. Thell, R., Martin, F. H., and Edwards, J. E. (1975): Bacterial endocarditis in subjects 60 years of age and older. *Circulation,* 51:174–182.
30. Whiting, R. B., Powell, W. J., Jr., Dinsmore, R. E., and Sanders, C. A. (1971): Idiopathic hypertrophic subaortic stenosis in the elderly. *N. Engl. J. Med.,* 285:196–200.
31. Williams, B. O., Begg, T. B., Semple, T., and McGuinness, J. B., (1976): The elderly in a coronary unit. *Br. Med. J.,* 2:451–453.

Rehabilitation in the Aging edited by
T. F. Williams. Raven Press, New York © 1984.

Rehabilitative Aspects of Peripheral Vascular Disorders in the Elderly

John A. Spittell, Jr.

Mayo Medical School, Mayo Clinic, Rochester, Minnesota 14603

The peripheral vascular disorders that affect the elderly and require rehabilitative measures are occlusive arterial disease, venous thrombosis, chronic venous insufficiency, and, on occasion, obstructive lymphedema of the lower extremities (1). Ulceration of the skin of the digits, feet, and ankles (due to ischemia, trophic changes, or venous stasis) may also be a problem that requires specific measures for successful long-term management and rehabilitation.

Before dealing with rehabilitative aspects of specific disorders, attention to some problems commonly seen in all types of painful conditions of the lower extremities are in order.

When bed rest is a necessary part of the management of a painful process in their lower extremity, patients commonly keep the knee and hip of the involved extremity flexed with the thigh externally rotated to provide a comfortable position for the limb. With longstanding problems such as ischemic rest pain or ulceration, the limb may be kept in this position for protracted periods of time and the unfortunate (and preventable) complication of flexion contracture of the knee may significantly delay ambulation once the underlying arterial insufficiency is corrected. Awareness of and attention to this problem, with regular passive and/or active extension of the knee, can prevent this complication. A similar type of problem can develop in the person with longstanding ulceration about the ankle who remains partially ambulatory walking on the toes of the foot of the affected limb and thereby over time developing a shortened Achille's tendon. This can also result from the continued use of high-heeled shoes. While dorsiflexion and plantar flexion of the foot on a regular basis is a simple thing, it is surprising how often it is overlooked. Soft woollen socks or stockings are less likely to traumatize the skin than hard synthetic materials. Shoes should be loose and comfortable, free from pressure points.

One additional point, basic to the management of chronic edema, is the need for the patient to not only use the proper elastic support whenever up, but to elevate the involved extremity whenever sitting or lying down and, if at all possible, to spend 30 to 60 min in the middle of the day with the elastic supports removed and the legs elevated. The converse in the patient with occlusive arterial disease should be evident, i.e., when in bed, the head of the bed should be elevated and elevation of the ischemic extremity should be avoided.

OCCLUSIVE ARTERIAL DISEASE

Peripheral arterial insufficiency in the older person is common and is most often due to arteriosclerosis obliterans. Other causes include embolic arterial occlusion (emboli arising from the heart or arterial aneurysms) and uncommonly from the involvement of extremity arteries by giant cell arteritis (2). For all persons with occlusive peripheral arterial disease, whatever the cause, measures to decrease or avoid vasoconstriction and care to protect the ischemic limb and digits from trauma of all types are indicated (3); for the person who is able to walk, a walking program is desirable in an effort to stimulate the development of collateral circulation (4). When the arterial insufficiency is causing disabling intermittent claudication or when there is ischemic ulceration, restoration of pulsatile flow by either reconstructive arterial surgery or percutaneous transluminal balloon angioplasty is indicated if it is feasible (3).

Minimizing Vasoconstriction

One of the most important but difficult things for patients with occlusive arterial disease (a large number of whom are smokers of long standing) is the interdiction of tobacco; an explanation by the physician of the basis for this recommendation and emphasis of its value is desirable to encourage compliance.

Keeping both the extremities and body warm are simple measures that avoid the cutaneous vasoconstriction that exposure to cold induces.

In the elderly patient with occlusive peripheral arterial disease, coronary artery disease, and hypertension are commonly associated conditions requiring therapy. Certain drugs used in their treatment may have an adverse effect on the circulation, particularly in the skin. Thus, we avoid the use of propranolol and clonidine in the patient with occlusive peripheral arterial disease if possible. For a patient with occlusive peripheral arterial disease and migraine headaches, we advise that ergot preparations not be used in treatment of the latter.

The many vasodilators available are not recommended for the treatment of intermittent claudication because these agents do not dilate the arterial circulation of the muscles of the extremity (5). Thus, the usefulness of these drugs is limited to those situations in which there is a need for cutaneous vasodilation and where restoration of pulsatile flow to the extremity is not possible.

Trauma

Since ischemic tissue withstands trauma poorly and heals slowly, it is not surprising that the majority of amputations of ischemic limbs are the result of some type of trauma (6). Trauma of all types should be avoided and, regrettably, unless the patient and therapists are carefully informed of the tremendous import, amputations of digits and limbs, otherwise preventable, result. The time spent in instructing elderly patients with occlusive arterial disease (a large number of whom are also diabetics) about proper foot care and protection of their feet from all types of trauma—mechanical, chemical, and thermal—will have a yield of secondary prevention, second to none.

Walking

Encouraging the patient with intermittent claudication due to occlusive arterial disease to walk to the point of symptoms several times each day has been shown to increase the walking distance of many, presumably because of the development of more collateral circulation. For the patient with ischemic rest pain and/or ulceration, such a walking program is not advised until the ischemia has been corrected. The patient with coronary artery disease may present a problem as far as a walking program is concerned if anginal pain occurs at a shorter walking distance than the intermittent claudication.

Care of the Feet

As important as protecting the ischemic limb from trauma is attention to care of the feet. Trimming of nails and the management of corns and calluses is more easily and properly accomplished by a podiatrist who is informed about the degree of ischemia present. The patient should be instructed in the use of a non-irritating lanolin containing ointment to prevent excessive drying and fissuring of the skin. The prompt treatment of dermatophytosis with one of the several effective topical antifungal agents may prevent the extensive ulceration and limb threatening infection that can develop without treatment. If the patient with occlusive arterial disease is bedridden for any reason, protecting the heels from abrasions by sheets with one of the several heel protection devices should always be requested.

Rehabilitation after amputation and the role of prostheses is covered in the chapter by Friedman and Capulong (*this volume*).

VENOUS THROMBOSIS

In the elderly patient, deep venous thrombosis is usually a complication of another medical problem necessitating immobilization. Awareness of this and the use of prophylactic measures can effectively reduce its incidence.

The rehabilitative aspects include informing the patient of the nature of venous thrombosis and the need for conscientious care to lessen the occurrence of long-term disability.

Reassurance regarding the resolution of the acute process is important to prevent the fear of clots (based on misinformation) that some patients have long after an episode of venous thrombosis has been properly treated and resolved. Time taken by physicians, nurses, and therapists to inform patients is undoubtedly the most effective way to avoid "postphlebitic neurosis" (7). A positive approach to ambulation once the acute process subsides is equally important.

The complications of postphlebitic venous insufficiency are likewise preventable by the instruction of the patient in the use of adequate elastic support for their postphlebitic limb. Not every patient will have significant postphlebitic deep venous insufficiency but early identification of those who will or will not have it is difficult and unreliable clinically. For this reason, we prefer to have every patient use elastic support in the form of Ace bandages up to the knee whenever they are ambulatory for at least a month after leaving the hospital. They then can try a day without the bandages and, if no dependent edema develops, can abandon their use. On the other hand, if dependent edema does develop by the end of the day without the elastic bandages, patients are advised to resume the use of elastic bandages when ambulatory for another month before trying a second day without support. If at the end of the second month there is still dependent edema, the long-term use of adequate elastic support with elastic bandages or elastic stockings (made-to-measure or fitted) is advised. The length of the stocking and its weight should be individualized according to the degree of venous insufficiency and the patient's desires. Ordinarily, no limitations of activity or ambulation are indicated as long as adequate elastic support is used whenever the patient is ambulatory. Prolonged sitting, as before a TV, with legs down to the floor should be avoided. An ottoman or suitable chair should be used to support the legs.

Chronic venous insufficiency due to varicose veins can usually be managed with adequate elastic support unless recurrent superficial thrombophlebitis or cosmetic problems warrant vein stripping (8).

LYMPHEDEMA

While uncommon, compared to chronic venous insufficiency, lymphedema warrants mention because of the diagnostic problems and implications it creates.

In the elderly, lymphedema is virtually always obstructive and usually secondary to a neoplasm of pelvic origin or lymphoma. Differentiating it from other causes of edema is not difficult since lymphedema is painless, progressive, and unaccompanied by venous stasis changes. The edema, once established, is firm and does not clear with elevation overnight.

From the rehabilitative standpoint, wearing heavy-duty elastic stockings made-to-measure (after maximum reduction of edema by elevation of the leg(s) for several days) is the basic approach. Often, the intermittent use of a diuretic—e.g., 3 or 4 times a week—and the avoidance of salt in the diet aids in control of the edema.

As long as the lymphedema does not interfere mechanically, no limitation of activity is advised.

Some patients with lymphedema experience recurring episodes of lymphangitis and/or cellulitis. These are usually caused by streptococci, which gain entrance through a break in the skin like that caused by trauma or dermatophytosis. Management of these patients should include attention to preventing the portals of infection and long-term prophylactic antibiotic therapy with penicillin—or erythromycin if the patient is allergic to penicillin. In our experience, an effective regimen has been benzathine penicillin G (Bicillin), 1,200,000 units administered intramuscularly once a month, or penicillin V, 250 mg orally four times per day for one week each month; for the patient who is allergic to penicillin, erythromycin, 250 mg four times per day for one week every month, has provided good prophylaxis (9).

ULCERATION OF THE LOWER EXTREMITY

Ulceration of the lower extremity is common in elderly persons. The etiology of the ulceration of the skin can be varied, but most of the ulcerations are one of four types—venous stasis ulcers, ischemic ulcers due to occlusive arterial disease, neurotrophic ulcers, and ischemic ulceration due to cutaneous arteriolar disease. Since each of these four common types of ulcers has a different pathophysiology, correct management and rehabilitation programs depend on accurate identification of the type of ulcer one is dealing with. In general, these four types are easily differentiated from each other by their rather typical clinical features, i.e., their location on the limb, whether painful or not, the appearance of the skin around the ulcer, the appearance of the edges and base of the ulcer, and the adequacy of the arterial and venous circulation in the limb.

Venous stasis ulcers typically occur on the medial distal leg. They are painful when infected but otherwise do not hurt. The skin about a venous stasis ulcer shows stasis (brownish) pigmentation because of the longstanding venous hypertension. The edges of the stasis ulcer are typically shaggy and the base is healthy in appearance. Patients with stasis ulcers often try to remain ambulatory and may walk on the toes of affected limb; if they persist in this for a long period the Achille's tendon may shorten and require special attention in the rehabilitation phase after the ulcer is healed. Needless to say, prevention is the easiest approach to the shortened Achille's tendon. Since venous hypertension in the extremity with chronic venous insufficiency is the basis of the stasis ulceration, the use of adequate elastic support on the limb, whenever the patient is ambulatory, is basic to successful prevention of future ulceration. To accomplish this it is often necessary to add an extra dimension of support to the area of the leg where stasis ulceration has occurred. A foam-rubber pad shaped to support the skin about the medial side of the ankle and held in place by two elastic bandages has been an inexpensive and effective type of support in our experience. The patient with chronic venous insufficiency should be advised of the need to use adequate elastic support indefinitely.

Ischemic ulcers due to occlusive arterial disease are most often the result of some type of trauma to the skin. Severe pain, particularly at night, is a hallmark of ischemic ulceration. Although they may occur anywhere on the ischemic limb, most often they are located on the toes or heel of the foot. The edges of an ischemic ulcer are discrete and the surrounding skin is normal unless there is infection present. These ulcers have a pale base and are often covered by an eschar. Absence or marked diminution of pulsation of peripheral arteries confirms the ischemic basis of the ulceration and is the problem that must be corrected before healing can occur. In general, once pulsatile flow has been reestablished to the limb, the severe pain will abate and the ulceration will develop a healthy base commensurate with healing or successful skin grafting; at this point, the patient can be ambulated with dressings on the ulcer. Since dependent edema is so often an early and transient development after arterial surgery, it is best for the patient not to sit with the limb dependent. The measures already outlined for occlusive arterial disease should be a part of every patient's long-term program, including a regular walking program.

Neurotrophic ulcers are most often seen in diabetic patients with neuropathy but can be seen in other neurologic disorders as well. Typically, neurotrophic ulcers are located on the sole of the foot over the heads of the metatarsals or on the heel over the calcaneus, since the trauma of weight bearing is a factor in their development. The other etiologic factor is impaired cutaneous sensation, so these ulcers are typically painless. Because chronic trauma is a factor in their development, neurotrophic ulcers usually develop in a callus or have a rim of callus about them. Healing of these ulcers requires control of any infection present, removal of the callus about the edge, and the absence of trauma. Once these ulcers are healed, it is necessary to protect the involved area of the foot by redistributing the weight on the foot; various means of adjusting the footwear to accomplish this are available, and the assistance of a podiatrist is invaluable in this aspect of rehabilitation. Any associated arterial insufficiency should be appropriately managed.

Ulceration due to cutaneous arteriolar disease is perhaps the least recognized of the common types of ulceration of the lower extremity. Although not as frequent as venous stasis ulcers, arteriolar ulcers are not rare. Most often, since arteriolar occlusive disease is their basis, they are seen in patients with longstanding hypertension (hypertensive ischemic ulcer) or with one of the connective tissue disorders (vasculitides). A distinctive feature of these ulcers is their predilection to occur on the posterior or lateral aspect of the distal leg. Since the basis of the ulceration is cutaneous infarction, these ulcers are quite painful. Occlusive disease of the major arteries may or may not be present. Once healing has been effected, the patient with this type of ulceration is best not ambulated fully until healing is complete. Careful instruction in care of the skin of the lower extremities is an important part of rehabilitation.

SUMMARY

The peripheral vascular disorders seen in the elderly can usually be controlled and their complications prevented by proper management. Basic to rehabilitation are measures appropriately designed to restore the circulation to as nearly normal as possible and to control the annoying symptoms and restriction of easy and comfortable ambulation that the peripheral vascular problems cause.

REFERENCES

1. Spittell, J. A., Jr. (1982): Peripheral vascular disorders. *Geriatrics,* 37:55.
2. Klein, R. G., Hunder, G. G., Stanson, A. W., and Sheps, S. S. (1975): Larger artery involvement in giant cell (temporal) arteritis. *Ann. Intern. Med.,* 83:806.
3. Spittell, J. A., Jr. (1981): Recognition and management of chronic atherosclerotic occlusive peripheral arterial disease. *Mod. Concepts Cardiovasc. Dis.,* 50:19.
4. Jonason, T., Jonzon, B., Ringquist, I., Öman-Rydberg, A. (1979): Effect of physical training on different categories of patients with intermittent claudication. *Acta Med. Scandinav.,* 206:253.
5. Coffman, J. D. (1979): Drug therapy: vasodilator drugs in peripheral vascular disease. *N. Engl. J. Med.,* 300:713.
6. Weis, A. J., and Fairbairn, J. F., II. (1968): Trauma, ischemic limbs and amputations. *Postgrad. Med.,* 43:111.
7. Kazmier, F. J., and Juergens, J. L. (1980): Venous thrombosis and obstructive diseases of the veins. In: *Peripheral Vascular Diseases,* Fifth edition, edited by J. L. Juergens, J. A. Spittell, Jr., and J. F. Fairbairn, II. W. B. Saunders, Philadelphia.
8. Lofgren, K. A. (1980): Varicose veins. In: *Peripheral Vascular Diseases,* Fifth edition, edited by J. L. Juergens, J. A. Spittell, Jr., and J. F. Fairbairn, II. W. B. Saunders, Philadelphia.
9. Schirger, A., and Peterson, L. F. A. Lymphedema. In: *Peripheral Vascular Diseases,* Fifth edition, edited by J. L. Juergens, J. A. Spittell, Jr., and J. F. Fairbairn, II. W. B. Saunders, Philadelphia.

Rehabilitation in the Aging edited by
T. F. Williams. Raven Press, New York © 1984.

Common Foot Problems in the Aged and Rehabilitative Management

Arthur E. Helfand

*Department of Community Health, Pennsylvania College of Podiatric Medicine, Narberth,
Pennsylvania 19072; Department of Podiatry, James C. Giuffre' Medical Center; and
Department of Medicine (Podiatry), Jefferson Medical College and Thomas Jefferson
University Hospital, Philadelphia, Pennsylvania 19107*

During a maturing lifetime and into the aging process, the human foot is subject to a significant amount of trauma, use, misuse, and neglect. The stress of today's society accompanied by the normal aging process and degenerative diseases that occur associated with aging, make painful feet a common source of discomfort in the elderly. It has been stated many times that when a person's foot hurts he or she hurts all over. The ability to ambulate freely and move about, to render care for oneself, and to remain an active and productive member of society is often lost when foot problems become painful and, in fact incapacitate the person from the normal activities of daily living. Ambulation is many times the key or the catalyst between an individual retaining dignity and remaining in a normal living environment or being institutionalized. Even in institutions the inability to ambulate and move about further removes an individual from normal activities. Motivation is one of the keys to health care in the elderly. Keeping people walking may be one of the most significant catalysts for that motivation. As we consider these concepts, it is clear that foot health programs and podiatric services must be an integral part of rehabilitative activities, and included in the overall team approach.

Foot problems in the elderly and disabled are basically chronic in nature and their early identification should be part of the initial patient evaluation. Their management must include attention to the primary complaint as well as the long-range planning for continued care and patient education.

There are a wide variety of clinically disabling conditions that have pedal manifestations. Some of these require continued care and continued management, the use of orthotic devices, continual review of patient care planning and programming, proper treatment, health education, and adequate planning to minimize future complications. Some of the conditions that provide significant foot problems in the elderly include the residuals of arthritis, elderly patients with cerebral palsy or mental illness, cerebral vascular accidents, the residuals of congenital deformities, degenerative spinal cord diseases, joint deformities, muscular contractures, paraplegia, peripheral nerve injuries, peripheral vascular disease, polyneuritis, the residuals of trauma such as fractured hips, stasis dermatitis, ulcers, diabetes mellitus, and other related degenerative and chronic diseases.

291

In many cases, the podiatrist can be one of the motivating factors in helping patients cooperate with others and accept other forms of therapy. The immediate comfort that podiatric care generally brings to patients with foot discomfort instills confidence in the professional who in turn can instill motivation in the patient. When any professional displays overt concern for the best care and needs of the patient, the patients themselves become motivated.

There are several factors that contribute to the development of foot problems in the elderly. Some of these include the degree of ambulation, the duration of institutionalization or prior hospitalization, previous types of foot care and management, the environment itself, emotional adjustments to disease, current medications and treatment programs with either local or systemic disease, and past foot conditions and the manifestations or residuals of these types of problems.

In identifying the most common foot problems in the elderly, it is important to look at people who have foot complaints or overt impairments and who seek foot care for what many consider to be minor problems, except that the patients generally consider them to be major problems. Many elderly patients are usually taking more than one drug at any given time and may in fact have more sensitivities to certain drugs than a younger population. They are usually more susceptible to some form of local infection. They often present more atrophy of tissue as a result of or associated with degenerative neuromuscular and skeletal diseases and the avascular status or neuropathic changes associated with other conditions such as diabetes mellitus or arteriosclerosis. In addition, the elderly patient may be more confused and have a lower threshold to physical and emotional stress. Their ambulatory status may be severely limited by their general physical deterioration, their environment, and their social isolation. The elderly patient often has one or more chronic systemic diseases and is more prone to injure his or her lower extremities than a younger individual. Falls in the aged are more common and are many times related to foot problems and/or inappropriate footwear for the activities that they are designed for. Finally, the elderly are more prone to immobility, impairment, disability, and major medical management following even minor foot infections. There is a greater risk involved in managing the elderly patient with foot problems that should not preclude definitive care but should temper the approach to the patient so that care reflects the functional needs of the individual and is based on medical necessity. The key to identifying foot care in the elderly lies in the ability of the practitioner to recognize the problem, look for abnormalities, and to listen to the complaints of the patient.

CHANGES IN THE FOOT WITH AGING AND DISEASE

To understand better the importance of foot health in a total geriatric rehabilitation program, it is important to have an overview of the wide variety of changes, caused by aging and disease, that take place in the human foot.

The skin is among the first structures to demonstrate change. The earliest signs generally include the loss of hair along the outer sides of the leg and on the dorsum of the foot. Brownish pigmentations follow with an associated increase in the presence of hyperkeratotic areas due to keratin dysfunction. The nails have a tendency to become thickened and brittle and onycomycosis seems to be more prevalent in this population group. There is a progressive decline in muscle mass and thinning of the subcutaneous tissues. All of these changes make the foot more susceptible to injury, and even minor injuries can result in limitations in activity. Peripheral vascular disease may lead to trophic changes, intermittent claudication, rest pain, coldness, and color variations. There may also be loss of sensation associated with diabetes and other causes of peripheral neuropathy. Any of these changes increases markedly the susceptibility to injury, infection, and gangrene. Various chronic diseases may also produce degenerative changes in the foot, as a result of complex gaits, reduced agility, and tremors.

The foot is a relatively rigid structure that, through the years into the aging process, must carry heavy physical work loads, both static (weight-bearing) and dynamic (walking). The foot bears weight in a triangular manner: the medial and lateral longitudinal arches form the long sides of the triangle and the metatarsal heads form the short base. Weight is generally transmitted from the striking force of the calcaneus along the fifth metatarsal head through the first metatarsal head. Lifelong experiences, in occupational as well as social activities, produce changes in morphology and in the physiologic functioning of the foot. A major problem is the fact that most walking in our current environment is on hard flat surfaces that do not absorb shock. Thus the foot itself is forced to absorb all of the shock, creating repeated microtrauma. In addition, the hard flat surfaces do not provide for appropriate weight distribution over the entire foot. This reduces the intrinsic muscular function of the foot and results in atrophy of the interossei and diminished toe function.

One of the primary effects of repeated tissue trauma is stress on one particular area. The inability of the foot to adjust or compensate for that stress may result in injury to the skin and in inflammatory changes in bone and soft tissue: osteitis, periostitis, synovitis, capsulitis, fasciitis, myositis, fibrositis, and arthritis.

Treatment is directed to eliminating the cause of the problem and to redistribute weight to nonpainful areas of the feet. This is approached through techniques of weight diffusion or weight dispersion and use of various types of orthoses to compensate for painful skin lesions or existing deformities.

MANAGING COMMON FOOT PROBLEMS IN THE ELDERLY

In managing common foot problems of the elderly in a rehabilitative sense, it is important for the practitioners to identify the etiologic considerations, the symptoms and complaints of the patient, the physical signs, and the clinical manifestations of both disease and degenerative changes. There are various diagnostic considerations, such as appropriate laboratory data and X-ray examinations, and pathology reports when indicated. The practitioner should note the presence of complications or sequelae, and identify relevant treatment programs, prognosis, and the overall management of the geriatric patient in relation to rehabilitative needs in a long-term sense.

Disorders of the Nails

There are many nail changes that can occur in the elderly patient as a result of long-term chronic disease. Onychia is an inflammatory condition involving the posterior nail wall, usually precipitated by local pressure (including that produced by support stockings). The inflammation is usually mild, producing a mild degree of erythema. Treatment is aimed at removing all pressure from the area and the use of tepid saline compresses for 15 min., three times daily. Lambs wool or polyurethane tube foam may also be used to provide additional protection for the area. When this condition is allowed to progress without adequate management, a paronychia may develop with significant infection and abscess of the posterior nail wall. Treatment consists of culture and sensitivity, X-ray examination to eliminate the possibility of osteomyelitis, and appropriate antibiotics and drainage if required.

Any foot infection in an elderly person, particularly if diabetes mellitus or other causes of peripheral vascular disease are present, carries the potential of leading to gangrene and amputation and calls for prompt, vigorous treatment.

Deformities of the toenails are common in elderly persons. Some are the result of continued trauma, and others are the result of degenerative changes. The nails of the elderly patient tend to become thickened, a condition known as onychauxis. Longitudinal striations may also appear. When the condition is permitted to progress, a ram's horn nail or onychogryphosis may develop. These become disabling because the person is unable to wear shoes in an appropriate manner. The nail tends to conform to the shape of a confined space and ultimately may reach lengths of over 3 inches and penetrate the skin. Treatment should be aimed at periodic débridement to provide as near normal a thickness as is feasible.

With the above condition, the nails tend to become free from the nail bed at the distal portion. This is termed onycholysis; when of significant degree, subungual debris and keratosis form. Treatment should be directed toward débridement and the use of emollients to minimize the keratotic areas.

Associated with these types of nail deformities are changes that occur as a result of a hereditary tendency known as involuted or incurvated toenails. In these cases the nails become "C" shaped and produce onychophosis, a callous formation of the nail grooves. This condition often mimics an ingrown toenail (onychocryptosis) and provides the same type of painful pressure. Treatment should be directed at removing the keratotic or offending area, thinning of the nail plate, and, where appropriate, surgical revision of the nail to reduce the total width of the nail thereby reducing the curvature. Matrix destruction is essential if recurrence is to be avoided.

An ingrown toenail is usually the result of the awkward growth of an incurved nail, ultimately penetrating the skin and giving rise to a periungual abscess; or from improper self care. Treatment consists of removing the offending portion of the nail to permit drainage of the abscess, along with saline or povidone-iodine (Betadine®) compresses. Systemic antibiotics may be needed if there appears to be any likelihood of serious foot infection.

When these conditions are left untreated they may become complicated by periungual ulcerated granulation tissue. This tissue tends to become organized and to epithelialize. Appropriate management consists of surgical removal of the nail and matrix area along with the ulcerative granulation tissue, followed by phenolization of the matrix area. Subungual and periungual abscesses, forming as a result of pressure or trauma, are managed in a similar manner with removal of much or all of the nail depending on the degree of extension of the abscess formation.

One of the most common nail problems in the elderly patient is onychomycosis or fungus infection of the nails. The nails tend to become brittle and thickened and granular in character. Onycholysis is generally present with a granular substance noted subungually. The nail discolors in a yellowish manner and provides an odor characteristic of the condition itself. Treatment should be aimed at management of the condition with the use of topical antifungals. Use of an antifungal in a solution permits the fungicide to penetrate around the nail in the onycholysed area. Adequate debridement is essential. For the most part, surgical avulsion of the nail is not necessary.

Subungual hemorrhage may be present as a result of direct trauma or may be associated with systemic diseases. Where trauma is involved, and pain is persistent, drilling a small hole through the nail plate may be required to remove the liquid hemorrhage. Where the condition is present for a period of time, the most appropriate management is to permit the nail to grow out with the hemorrhagic ecchymotic area, without drainage.

Elderly persons with significant pain involving the nail plate should be reviewed for the presence of subungual exostosis or spur or subungual heloma. The osseous diagnosis can easily be made by the use of a lateral radiograph of the digit. A heloma may be present as a result of shoe pressure or as a result of osseous projections. Treatment should be aimed at eliminating the cause. Where bony enlargement is present, surgery may be necessary for long-term relief.

Disorders of the Skin

One of the most common skin problems in the elderly patient is dryness or xerosis. The problem is a result of a lack of hydration and a lack of lubrication along with keratin dysfunction. Heel fissures may result. Appropriate management generally consists of the use of an emollient following hydration of the foot. A plastic or styrofoam heel cup may be needed to reduce pressure on the area.

Pruritus is common in the feet of aging patients. It may be due to dryness, scaliness, decreased glandular activity, keratin dysfunctions, environmental changes, or a defatting of the skin as a result of continuous hot foot baths. The effects of the resultant scratching must be differentiated from chronic tinea infection from various allergic neurogenic or emotional dermatoses, and any of the latter treated appropriately. Treatment of the skin itself should consist of the daily application of emollients preceded by the application of water to help hydrate and lubricate the skin. Topical steroids and antibiotics are of value where the scratching has produced a break in the skin.

Occasionally excessive sweating or hyperhidrosis is a problem. If it is localized to the feet and not due to any systemic disease (which would need its own appropriate treatment), it can be treated with careful attention to cleanliness and the use of appropriate foot powders. When there is inappropriate hygiene, the excessive sweat may decompose; this is known as bromhidrosis. Appropriate management consists of controlling the excessive moisture, the use of hydrogen peroxide swabs to clean the area, and the topical application of neomycin to eliminate bacterial contaminants.

Contact dermatitis may be present in elderly patients due to shoes or stockings, medications, or environmental factors. Typically there is a line of demarcation corresponding to the primary irritant. Appropriate skin testing can be utilized to confirm the diagnosis. Treatment consists of removing the irritant, then use of mild compresses and appropriate steroidal topical preparations.

Stasis dermatitis of the feet may be a problem in persons with venous insufficiency or systemic causes of dependent edema. In addition to treating the cause, the local treatment of the dermatitis on the feet may require elevation, cleansing compresses, and at times topical steroids and antibiotics.

Pyoderma or superficial bacterial infections should be cultured and treated with cleansing and appropriate antibiotics. They must be differentiated from fungal infections.

Fungal infections of the skin of the feet of older persons often prove to be an extension of mycotic toenails. They are generally caused by the *Trichophyton rubrum, Trichophyton mentagrophytes,* or *Monilia.* A Wood's light examination may be required to eliminate the possibility of an erythrasma infection. Wood's light is a useful diagnostic tool along with appropriate culture smear and identification. The clinical varieties of tinea caused by the *Trichophyton* group are vesicular, bullous, interdigital, or hyperkeratotic in character. The *Trichophyton rubrum* usually produces the hyperkeratotic variety. The possibility of secondary bacterial infection is present when the skin manifestations give rise to a break in the skin or produce an excessive amount of moisture, such as in the interdigital variety. Even with secondary bacterial infection, mild compresses of saline or povidone-iodine (Betadine®) solution along with topical fungicides are usually adequate to provide control. Most dermatologic manifestations can be controlled by the use of topical medications.

Other forms of dermatologic manifestations such as atopic dermatitis, nummular eczema, circumscribed neurodermatitis, psoriasis, or lichen planus may be found in the foot. Appropriate treatment involves the use of topical steroids and other supportive dermatologic measures. Other skin conditions include latent syphilis (with mal perforans) and neoplasms, which should be kept in mind during examination of the feet of elderly persons.

Simple bullae or hemorrhagic bullae occur frequently in patients in rehabilitation centers due to friction between the foot and footwear, particularly associated with soft athletic shoes prescribed as a part of the rehabilitation regimen. Often bullae can be drained and further trouble prevented by eliminating the pressure. One of the complicating factors involved in significant débridement is the resultant ulceration, which limits ambulation. Adequate supportive dressings should be in place and patients should be evaluated periodically to eliminate the cause and to minimize future complications.

A wide variety of ulcerations may be present in the elderly person. They may be the result of external etiologic factors such as trauma, trophic changes, decubitus, necrotic excoriations, and burns from thermal, electrical, or chemical factors. The use of heating pads and hot water bottles are significant sources of external ulcerations. An example of chemical ulcerations would be those created by the use of commercial corn cure products, high in salicylic acid concentration.

Management of ulcerations consists of supportive measures to reduce trauma and pressure, control the infection, and maintain a clean and healthy ulcerative base to permit gradual healing. Physical measures such as the use of whirlpool are of assistance in aiding healing. The use of low voltage therapy will also provide an increased localized vascular supply to the ulcerative area and, coupled with supportive measures, generally improves the healing time.

Ulcers on the feet may also be the result of systemic diseases, in particular peripheral vascular disease, diabetic or other neuropathy, and gout. Management consists of appropriate treatment for the underlying condition, examination for the possibility of osteomyelitis, the use of appropriate antibiotics, the use of appropriate supportive measures and dressings, and changes in weight-bearing. (See J. A. Spittell, Jr. *this volume.*)

Modifications in weight-bearing can be attained by the use of orthotics or changes in footwear, either newly fitted shoes or modifications such as padding, bars, and wedges. Increasing the sole thickness or the use of a softer material may also help. Where the ulceration is significant, a Plastazote or Aliplast sandal or a Plastazote boot would be most appropriate and can also provide additional support when used with or in addition to a modification of a surgical boot. This permits ambulation but decreases the pressure to the ulcerative area and provides a slowness of gait that aids in reducing trauma to the ulcerative site.

Elderly persons who have difficulty in bending to put on adequate footwear may tend to walk barefoot in their homes. In addition to the potential for major foot injury, tiny foreign bodies such as glass or slivers of wood or animal hair may be picked up and result in small cystic areas, a closed inflammatory tissue reaction that follows the initial puncture. These may appear to be hyperkeratotic plugs; appropriate evaluation and débridement relieves the problem.

One of the most significant problems and complaints of the elderly person may be classed as hyperkeratotic lesions. These include callous and corn formation as the various forms of tyloma and heloma such as hard, vascular, neurofibrous, soft, seed, and, as previously identified, subungual. Porokeratosis and eccrine poroma also present as initial complaints of hyperkeratotic lesions. Verruca are many times confused with a well-demarcated plantar heloma or intractable plantar keratosis. However, verruca are generally not common in the elderly patient, and many times are treated inappropriately.

There are many mechanical factors that cause hyperkeratosis to form, of which the most common are various types of stress: compressive, tensile, or shearing. In elderly persons such stresses are made more likely as a result of the loss of soft tissue, atrophy of the plantar fat pad, and changes associated with residuals of arthritis and deformity. A common contributing factor is incompatibility between foot type and shoe last.

Locations of hyperkeratoses may be anywhere on the foot but are most frequent on the dorsal surface of the digits, distal surface of the digits, plantar aspects of the digits and sole of the foot, and in the heel area. Marginal hyperkeratosis may be present on the heel associated with excessive friction, in particular when there is bony deformity such as may be present with an enlargement of the navicular medially or the dorsal aspect of the medial cuneiform and first metatarsal base. Deformities such as hammer toes, or digital rotational contractures, hallux valgus or bunions, bunionettes or Taylor's bunion are but precipitating factors when related to foot to shoe last incompatibility.

The treatment for these lesions varies based on the functional needs of the patient in relation to the activities of daily living. In general, initial treatment consists of débridement and the use of emollients to provide appropriate skin care. Secondary treatment consists of the removal of pressure by placed pads, removable pads, shoe modifications, or orthotics. Material to provide soft tissue replacement such as various densities of polyurethane foam, properly positioned and employed, will serve as an external form of soft tissue replacement. Shoe modification or change may be needed.

It is also important to be aware that the presence of hyperkeratosis for long periods of time represents a hyperplasia and may persist even with nonweight-bearing. Left untreated, the hyperkeratosis itself becomes a primary irritant creating local avascularity and residual ulceration. It is not uncommon to reduce a heloma and uncover a significant ulcer beneath the hyperkeratotic tissue.

Once débrided, and adequate local treatment provided, these lesions tend to heal rapidly, and there is a strong tendency to forget that the underlying causes may still be present and may lead to recurrence. A total understanding on the part of the patient, the patient's family, or those associated with patient care management is essential as the ultimate treatment for these conditions may prove to be periodic débridement and management. This concept is no different than the periodic monitoring of patients with cardiovascular disease, high blood pressure, or diabetes mellitus. They are chronic in nature by definition, and should not be viewed as routine elements of foot care. They represent specific diagnostic entities and require specific treatment and planning. If not adequately handled, the pain associated with them will interfere with ambulation, and the potential for spreading infection from underlying abscesses is present. These conditions can produce wards of society.

Nonspecific Symptoms

Elderly persons often present with vague foot complaints and symptoms that may or may not be identifiable with any specific disease entity. Examples include cramps, foot fatigue, and numbness, tingling, and pain on arising. Although overt disease may be unidentifiable at the onset and clinical manifestations not present, such symptoms should be thoroughly investigated for the presence of vascular insufficiency, arthritic changes, fibrositis, or neurologic deficiencies. These types of symptoms, left untreated, will generally reduce the patient's ability to ambulate, move about, or accept other forms of therapy.

Foot Deformities

There are a significant number of residual deformities that can present in a wide variety of combinations in elderly persons. These include hallux varus, hallux valgus, splay foot, hallux flexus, hammer toe deformities, digiti quintivarus, digiti quintiflexus, overlapping and underriding toes, and the residuals of mild forms of club foot, pes cavus, pes planus, pronation, hallux limitus, hallux rigidus, and numerous accessory bones. These deformities generally create functional problems in relation to adequate foot covering, ambulation, and the residual pain of localized inflammatory processes as a result of stress, microtrauma, pressure, and the residuals of arthritic processes.

Treatment consists of both surgical and nonsurgical approaches. Surgery should be utilized when conservative measures fail and when the deformity significantly limits ambulation or gives rise to additional problems such as ulcers. Age should not be a contraindication to remove a painful deformity from a patient. However, when surgery is considered, an adequate evaluation, particularly of the vascular status of the patient and the ability of the patient to adapt to whatever modifications are made, is essential. The activity needs of the patient should also be seriously considered in the total overall treatment program for these types of conditions.

For the most part, these deformities and residuals can be managed in a conservative manner. Analgesics can be employed to reduce pain. Physical modalities such as whirlpool, ultrasound, superficial heat, low voltage therapy, and exercise can reduce significantly the extent of pain and increase ambulation. Progressive resistive exercises can be employed in the elderly patient and can be significantly effective when appropriately programmed and taught.

Adequate footwear is a significant consideration in the conservative management of these types of deformities. The orthopedic shoe per se may or may not be needed, but shoes such as bunion lasts, high-toe box, or custom molded shoes may be needed, with or without adequate orthotics. These residual deformities may produce inflammatory changes including periarthritis, aseptic necrosis, sesamoiditis, and bursitis, and changes in the lateral segments, which produce similar metatarsalgic problems. Plantar fascial strain and heel pain are likewise common in the elderly patient. The subcalcaneal bursitis associated with calcaneal spurs, periostitis, and plantar fasciitis are the most common inflammatory problems.

Tenosynovitis is also a problem along with tendonitis in elderly persons. The dorsal extensor tendons may be significantly aggravated by inadequate shoe pressure. Synovitis, bursitis, and neuritis are also residuals of foot to shoe last incompatibility. The use of nonsteroid analgesics, injectable steroids, physical modalities, short-term steroid therapy, and supportive devices all have a place in the total overall management of these conditions in the geriatric patient.

Nerve entrapments should also be considered when pain persists in the intermetatarsal digital area. Where an entrapment is clearly defined, surgical excision is the treatment of choice. Where the entrapment is present in its early stages, local steroid injections may produce some resolution of the inflammation and provide some relief, together with mechanical therapy to provide positional changes in the metatarsal area.

Fractures

Fractures may occur in various bones of the foot in elderly persons. The stress type of fracture as the result of osteoporosis is often overlooked and left untreated. In general, most uncomplicated foot fractures in the elderly can be managed by the use of a surgical shoe and adequate dressing. Most elderly patients have difficulty with casts and learning to use crutches. Digital fractures can be easily managed by the use of moldable silicone compound that provides digital bracing. This mechanism for treatment is simple, inexpensive, and effective and provides the patient with the ability to maintain normal foot hygiene during the healing process.

Shoes and Orthoses

Shoe modifications that can be effectively employed in the management of foot deformities and gait changes in the elderly individual include: mild heel wedging, both medially and laterally to restrict sub talar motion or to provide some alteration in gait; metatarsal bars such as the Fay, Denver, or Hauser, to transfer weight over the metatarsal heads; the Thomas Heel to provide increased support on the medial aspect of the foot or the reverse Thomas Heel to provide similar support on the lateral aspect; the long counter to provide increased control to the medial longitudinal arch area; medial or lateral heel flares to provide increased stability for the ankle; shank fillers or wedgies to produce total weight-bearing on the plantar surface of the foot; and steel stiffeners in the management of hallux limitus and rocker bars to prevent flexion and extension of the shoe.

Some of the changes that can be employed internally in shoes are longitudinal arch pads, metatarsal pads, cut out pads, medial heel wedges, calcaneal bars, heel pads, heel lifts, and tongue or bite pads to prevent forward riding of the foot within the shoe.

Many types of foot orthoses are available for use in the elderly patient. They include both the rigid and flexible types of material. For the most part, a semi-flexible orthotic is generally more tolerable in the elderly patients. Various materials can be used. They include plastic, leather, laminates, polyurethane and sponge or foam rubber, Korex, felt, latex, and any combination of the above materials. Plastazote, Alimed, or other similar products are also adaptable to be molded to foot contours and shapes. Silicone, latex, or synthetic latex combinations can also be employed along with various removable densities of polyurethane to provide adequate support, the reduction of pressure, weight diffusion, or weight dispersion.

CHANGES IN THE FOOT RELATED TO CHRONIC DISEASES

The foot of an older person is likely to undergo degenerative changes related to chronic disease. It should be of primary concern to uncover the manifestation at its earliest onset, prior to the onset of symptoms or the presence of overt abnormalities.

Osteoarthritis in the foot of the aged patient is usually secondary to trauma, inflammation, metabolic changes, chronic microtrauma, strain, obesity, and osteoporosis. Deformities are present, with contracture and rigidity. Existing functional and mechanical problems such as pes planus, pes cavus, digital contractures, and hallux valgus tend to increase pain, limit motion, and reduce the ambulatory status of the patient.

The common pedal manifestations are plantar fasciitis, spur formation, periostitis, stress fractures, tendonitis, tenosynovitis, and deformity. The general principles of management include a proper diet, analgesics, muscle relaxants, and physical therapy in various forms including progressive resistive exercises and orthotics. Programs of activity should be utilized to a maximum degree to keep patients ambulatory.

Acute gouty arthritis as well as the chronic changes of tophaceous gout can occur in elderly persons. Systemic treatment for the disease is indicated with appropriate anti-inflammatory drugs, inhibitors of uric acid synthesis, and uricosuric agents. No local treatment is needed in most instances other than avoiding shoe pressure on the gouty joint. Steroids injected into the joint area may occasionally be needed for intractable pain. Ultrasound is also of use with this condition.

The chronic residual changes of rheumatoid arthritis are much more common in older persons than the acute manifestation of the disease. The fore part of the foot may exhibit any or all of the following entities: hallux rigidus, arthritis of the first metatarso-phalangeal joint, hallux valgus, cystic erosions, sesamoid erosions, metatarso-phalangeal dislocations, arthritis and residual hyperkeratosis, digiti flexus, fused interphalangeal joints, phalangeal reabsorption, talonavicular arthritis, extensor tenosynovitis, rheumatoid nodules, bow-stringing of the extensor hallucis longus tendon with hallux valgus, ulnar displacement of the extensor tendon, ganglion, and a rigid pronated foot. The hind part of the foot will demonstrate ankle arthritis, subtalar arthritis, tarsal arthritis, subachilles bursitis, retro-calcaneal bursitis, subcutaneous nodules, plantar fasciitis, spur formations, and achilles shortening. Therapy may include the use of analgesics, muscle relaxants, local injections of steroids, local anesthesia, orthotics and physical therapy.

The foot problems that may result from diabetic or other neuropathy and from peripheral vascular insufficiency have already been discussed.

CONCLUSION

Ability to ambulate depends on foot health. "Keep Them Walking"—the title of a special study of foot needs of elderly (19)—is a good motto for a comprehensive approach to foot care for elderly. This care requires both professional attention to the various problems discussed in this chapter and health education for the public and patients, to help them assume responsibility for their own foot health. The U.S. Public Health Service publishes a booklet entitled *Feet First* (34), which provides a well-documented foot health education program for patients and should be employed as a key tool both in institutions and for individual patients.

With the very high prevalence of foot problems in elderly persons, programs involved in rehabilitation of elderly patients should ensure that podiatric services are available to provide direct treatment and in-service education of patients and staff.

BIBLIOGRAPHY

1. Anderson, M. H. (1972): *A Manual of Lower Extremity Orthotics,* Charles C Thomas, Springfield, Ill.
2. Brachman, P. R. (1966): *Mechanical Foot Therapy,* Podiatry Books Co., Chicago, Ill.
3. Brachman, P. R. (1966): *Foot Orthopedics,* Podiatry Books Co., Chicago, Ill.
4. Bruno, J. (1967): Gross muscle evaluation by the podiatrist. *J. Am. Podiatry Assoc.,* 57:309–314.
5. Gamble, F. O. and Yale, I. (1975): *Clinical Foot Roentgenology.* R. E. Krieger Pub. Co., Huntington, N.Y.
6. Giannestras, N. J. (1973): *Foot Disorders, Medical and Surgical Management,* 2nd ed. Lea & Febiger, Philadelphia.
7. Gibbard, L. C. (1968): *Charlesworth's Chiropodical Orthopedics.* Balliere, Tindall & Cassell, London.
8. Gibbs, R. C. (1974): *Skin Diseases of the Feet,* W. H. Green, St. Louis.
9. Helfand, A. E. (1961): A study in podogeriatrics. *J. Am. Podiatry Assoc.,* 51:655.
10. Helfand, A. E. (1963): Podiatry—A basic long-term need for the chronically ill and the aged. *Nurs. Homes,* 12:9.
11. Helfand, A. E. (1964): Foot health education—A community health need for the aged and chronically ill. *J. Am. Podiatry Assoc.,* 54:178.

12. Helfand, A. E. (1965): Guidelines for podiatry service in nursing homes and related facilities. *Nurs. Homes,* 14:25.
13. Helfand, A. E. (1965): A survey of podiatric service in some Pennsylvania nursing homes. *J. Am. Podiatry Assoc.,* 55:440.
14. Helfand, A. E. (1966): Practice guide for podiatric programs in extended care facilities. *J. Am. Podiatry Assoc.,* 56:220.
15. Helfand, A. E. (1966): Foot impairment—An etiologic factor in falls in the aged. *J. Am. Podiatry Assoc.,* 56:326.
16. Helfand, A. E. (1966): Guidelines for podiatric programs in extended care facilities. *Hosp. Top.,* 44:26.
17. Helfand, A. E. (1967): Arthritis in older people as seen in podiatry practice. *J. Am. Podiatry Assoc.,* 57:82.
18. Helfand, A. E. (1967): Podiatry in a total geriatric health program—Common foot problems of the aged. *J. Am. Geriatric Soc.,* 15:593.
19. Helfand, A. E. (1968): Keep them walking. *J. Am. Podiatry Assoc.,* 58:117.
20. Helfand, A. E. (1968): Rules for foot health. *J. Pract. Nurs.,* 18:25.
21. Helfand, A. E. (1968): *The Need for Podiatric Service in Gerontology Programs and the Contributions Podiatry Can Make to a Total Geriatric Health Program; Working With Older People: A Guide to Practice, Vol. 3, Books 2 and 3.* PH-86-63-184, PH-108-65-205, PH-108-66-221, Gerontological Society, St. Louis.
22. Helfand, A. E. (1969): The principles and techniques of podogeriatric management. *J. Am. Podiatry Assoc.,* 59:295–299.
23. Helfand, A. E. (1971): Nursing homes: Podiatric considerations for the aged patient. *J. Am. Nurs. Home Assoc.,* 20:30–31.
24. Helfand, A. E. (1971): *Working with Older People, Vol. 4-Podiatry and the Elderly Patient.* PHSP No. 1459. Public Health Service, Department of Health, Education and Welfare.
25. Helfand, A. E. (1973): Podiatric services for the aged. *J. Am. Podiatry Assoc.,* 63:368–373.
26. Helfand, A. E. (1976): Consumer's guide to podiatric services. *J. Health Ed.,* 7:17–19.
27. Helfand, A. E. (1978): Foot health for the elderly patient. In: *Clinical Aspects of Aging,* edited by W. Reichel, pp. 303–314. Williams & Wilkins, Baltimore, Md.
28. Helfand, A. E. A positive approach to rehabilitation. *J. Am. Podiatry Assoc.,* 60:239–243.
29. Helfand, A. E., and Bruno, J. (1973): *Modern Therapeutic Approaches to Foot Problems: Some Physical Therapy Concepts in Managing the Podiatric Complications of Diabetes,* pp. 1–13. Futura Publishing Co., New York.
30. McGregor, R. R. (1968): Geriatric foot care. *Nurs. Clin. North Am.,* 3:687.
31. Riccitelli, M. L. (1966): Foot problems of the aged and infirm. *J. Am. Geriatric Soc.,* 14:1058.
32. Roberts, E. H. (1975): *On Your Feet.* Rodale Press, Emmanus, Pa.
33. Yale, I. (1980): *Podiatric Medicine.* 2nd ed. Williams & Wilkins, Baltimore.
34. U.S. Department of Health and Human Services, Public Health Services, National Institutes of Health (1970): *Feet First,* Document No. 0–388–126. Government Printing Office, Washington, D.C.
35. Helfand, A. E. (1981): *Clinical Podogeriatrics,* Williams & Wilkins, Baltimore.

Rehabilitation in the Aging edited by
T. F. Williams. Raven Press, New York © 1984.

Urologic Disorders in the Elderly

Robert S. Davis

Department of Urology, University of Rochester Medical Center, Rochester, New York 14642

The elderly person may suffer from any of the entire spectrum of urologic diseases and disorders. Infection, malignancy, bladder outflow obstruction, urinary incontinence, and sexual dysfunction are more common with the older person and are often in association with other disabling conditions for which restorative or maintenance therapy is needed. These urologic problems at times threaten longevity and frequently adversely affect the patient's social activities and quality of life. Fear of rejection, loss of independence, and a sense of inappropriateness by the older person will often keep many of these problems suppressed until they become advanced and obvious. Earlier detection will be prompted by health personnel who demonstrate a broad interest in the patient, encouraging trust, confidentiality, and communication. Thorough evaluation and treatment of these problems are essential components of any rehabilitation effort.

URINARY TRACT INFECTIONS

Urinary tract infections occur more frequently in the older individual of either sex. General factors accompanying aging that decrease resistance to infection include tissue atrophy, decreased blood flow, decreased immunologic response, poor nutrition, and other chronic illnesses. With age, the kidneys demonstrate a lower urine urea concentrating ability and an elevation of urinary pH which diminishes bacterial resistance. The postmenopausal woman will have a rise in the normally very acidic vaginal pH secretions, making the vaginal vestibule more susceptible to bacterial colonization with resultant ascending urinary tract infections (36). Older individuals may require bladder catheterization during the management of other illnesses resulting in an acquired infection, which appears to be associated with an increased mortality rate (13,39). Prostatic enlargement and resultant bladder outflow obstruction commonly occur in older men. Although obstruction does not usually lead to infection, treatment by catheterization may introduce an infection difficult to eradicate in the face of high residuals or acquired bacterial prostatitis (47).

The symptoms of urinary tract infections range from acute, toxic febrile illnesses, seen with acute pyelonephritis or prostatitis, to nearly asymptomatic reactions, seen in chronic pyelonephritis and prostatitis. Bladder irritative symptoms of frequency, suprapubic discomfort, and pain on voiding often accompany acute cystitis or prostatitis. Flank pain may be present in acute pyelonephritis; low back pain, perineal and upper inner thigh discomfort, and an acute slowing of the urinary stream may be seen with prostatitis. Urinary incontinence may be the predominant symptom of infection noted by other family members.

Diagnosis of a urinary tract infection is easily established by urinalysis and culture. Its localization may be further suggested by the symptoms and urinalysis findings. White blood cell casts and flank pain suggest pyelonephritis, but many white blood cells often in clumps from the expressed prostate secretions and a tender prostate point to prostatitis. In some cases, bladder wash-out tests or ureteral catheterization may be employed for infection localization (19,22).

Treatment of urinary tract infections varies with the location of the infection. Cystitis requires a short course of antibiotics of 3 to 5 days and may even respond well to a single large dose of antibiotic (1,15,45). Patients with acute pyelonephritis or prostatitis are frequently clinically very ill and benefit from parenteral antibiotic treatment of 7 to 14 days duration. Although urine cultures may not be obtained in all patients with cystitis, adequate culturing of urine and any other suspected site of infection is most important before commencing parenteral antibiotics. Although less symptomatic, chronic prostatitis and pyelonephritis require longer courses of antibiotic of 2 to 12 weeks (18,30). Many drugs are clinically effective in acute prostatitis; however, more careful selection of drugs achieving prostatic levels (trimethoprim, erythromycin, synthetic tetracycline) is required in chronic prostatitis (7,43,49).

Rapid return of the same bacterial infection (relapse) suggests a privileged and hard to eradicate focus of infection, such as prostatitis, chronic pyelonephritis, or infected calculi. Symptomatic or frequent relapses merit evaluation with intravenous urography (IVU) and cystoscopy. Patients who persist with asymptomatic bacteruria, despite protracted courses of adequate antibiotics or after removal of infected foci such as infected stones, may be left untreated, especially when chronic treatment cannot maintain urine sterility. Likewise, patients who have infections due to continuous catheterization are not given antibiotics unless symptomatic febrile infections occur (54). However, patients with frequent reinfections benefit from long-term, low-dose maintenance antibiotic therapy after treatment of their acute infection (50,51).

MALIGNANCIES

The common urologic malignancies affecting the older population are renal cell carcinoma, transitional cell carcinoma, and, in men, prostatic carcinoma. Early detection of carcinoma by evaluation of microhematuria, sterile pyuria, and changes in voiding habits is critical to early tumor detection, tumor control, and prolongation of longevity. In addition to appreciation of the importance of transient gross and microhematuria, a good physical exam including a thorough rectal exam is most important to the early detection of prostatic carcinoma.

Patients with hematuria are evaluated by IVU, cystoscopy, and possibly urinary cytology. When renal mass lesions are noted, they require additional evaluation by CT scan, ultrasound, and occasionally by fine needle aspiration or angiography (11,23). Filling defects in the renal pelvis, ureter, and bladder, which may be transitional tumor, clot, or stone, are further clarified by cystoscopy, CT scan, cytology, and occasionally repeat IVU examination after several weeks where clots will have lysed while tumor persists. Nodules and irregularities of the prostate may be further evaluated by transrectal ultrasound and needle biopsy of the prostate.

Renal cell carcinoma may be present in many ways in addition to the triad of flank pain, flank mass, and hematuria (8,52). Fever of unknown origin, anemia, polycythemia, and apparent hyperparathyroidism and Cushing's syndrome are other possible clinic presentations. Wide pulse pressure, hypertension, and high output cardiac failure may also occur due to the very vascular nature of the tumors which often have significant arteriovenous shunting.

When absence of metastatic disease is suggested by negative lung, bone, and liver evaluation, renal cell carcinoma is treated by radical nephrectomy (44). Radiation therapy and chemotherapy have not been effective, but early clinical trials with interferon and immunotherapy show some promise in patients with metastatic disease (29,32).

Transitional cell carcinoma can arise from the transitional epithelium of the renal calyx, pelvis, ureter, bladder, or urethra, though by far the most common location is the bladder. Bladder carcinoma may be totally asymptomatic except for episodes of painless hematuria; additionally, the patient may have bladder irritative symptoms of frequency and urgency. Patients with these symptoms must not be misdiagnosed as hemorrhagic cystitis, thus emphasizing the importance of further evaluation of refractory cystitis or apparent abacterial cystitis (53). Cystoscopy permits visual and biopsy confirmation of bladder and urethral lesions. Well-differentiated tumors confined to the bladder mucosa may be managed by endoscopic resection and regular follow-up endoscopic examinations. If the tumor shows invasion into the muscularis of the bladder, more aggressive treatment is imperative. Low-dose radiation followed by cystectomy and urinary diversion is the treatment of choice (41,46). Those patients with potentially curable invasive bladder tumors who are medically unable or unwilling to undergo combined radiation and surgical therapy may be managed by higher doses of radiation therapy alone.

Carcinoma of the prostate occurs with increasing frequency with age and has been reported in up to 50% of men over age 70 in autopsy series (3). After lung carcinoma, it is the second cause of cancer deaths in adult males (24). Although tumor markers for screening have been sought, the more specific immunoassays for prostatic acid phosphatase fail in that goal owing to significant numbers of false positive results (9,28). Rectal examination remains the most effective means of early detection of prostatic carcinoma; when abnormalities in consistency or contour of the gland are detected, biopsy is indicated.

Treatment of prostatic carcinoma is dependent on the stage and grade of the tumor. Metastatic disease is excluded by a normal bone scan, normal serum enzymatic prostatic acid phosphatase, and in some cases by absence of node metastasis on pelvic lymph node dissection. When the tumor is small, well differentiated, and localized to the prostate, radical prostatectomy offers the greatest survival (21,37). Higher grade tumors, tumors involving both lobes of the prostate, or tumors with suspected prostatic capsule extension but with absence of metastatic disease are better managed by radiation therapy (12,42).

Metastatic disease may be left untreated when asymptomatic. Estrogens, if administered early, will delay the progression of the disease but not increase longevity because of an increased number of cardiovascular deaths (24). Symptomatic metastatic disease should be treated by estrogens (DES 1–3 mg/day), bilateral orchiectomy, or antiandrogens. Pain from a localized metastatic deposit often responds well to radiation therapy. Chemotherapy shows some promise in hormonally refractory cases. Those tumors with extension into the bladder base with resultant azotemia can benefit from percutaneous nephrostomy drainage of the better functioning kidney.

BLADDER OUTFLOW OBSTRUCTION

Bladder outflow obstruction frequently results from benign prostatic hypertrophy (BPH) or prostatic carcinoma; both elongate and narrow the prostatic urethra. In men BPH occurs with advancing age and may in part be hormonally mediated. Symptoms of obstruction include hesitancy, decreased force of the urinary stream, incomplete bladder emptying, urinary frequency, and nocturia. Obstruction results in hypertrophy of the bladder wall manifested radiologically and endoscopically by thickening of the wall and trabeculation. Instability of the hypertrophied detrusor muscle often develops resulting in symptoms of urgency and precipitous voiding (40). The symptoms of obstruction often develop very slowly and may go unrecognized by the patient until urinary retention, overflow incontinence, or azotemia develops.

Patients presenting with chronic obstructive symptoms with retention and those with overflow incontinence should not undergo rapid bladder decompression, since this may result in severe bleeding or hypotension. A bladder that has chronically adapted to a high volume and pressure may bleed massively on rapid decompression. On catheter decompression, the azotemic patient will experience an osmotic diuresis. He may experience further obligatory fluid loss if there is associated hydronephrosis which may result in marked impairment of urine concentrating ability (25,33). This massive fluid loss in patients already significantly dehydrated by fluid restriction can result in severe hypotension. The bladder is gradually decompressed (600 ml followed by release of 200 ml hourly) and adequate i.v. fluid replacement instituted with close monitoring of vital signs, serum, and urinary electrolytes.

Once stabilized, cystoscopy is performed to evaluate prostate size and the presence or absence of other concomitant bladder pathology, such as large stones or diverticuli. Transurethral resection of the prostate, preferably under spinal anesthesia, is the operation of choice. Very large glands and severe associated bladder or urethral pathology will require an open prostatectomy via the suprapubic or retropubic approach. Patients should be reassured that though retrograde ejaculation may occur, loss of potency is the rare exception and not the rule of prostatectomy. An informed and reassured patient will not have the alarm of retrograde ejaculation or the fear of failure and hence sexual abstinence.

URINARY INCONTINENCE

Urinary incontinence is a common problem among older people which unfortunately can have as great a negative social as medical impact (16,34). Loss of satisfactory urine control can lead to withdrawal or depression, or result in transfer from a family to an institutional environment. It is a frequent concomitant of other disabling conditions, such as stroke or dementia, and may represent the most pressing social problem. Improved understanding of incontinence and better treatment methods have improved the previous, very negative prognosis for patients with incontinence (35,56). The patient with incontinence deserves a full evaluation, even though this problem is not always correctable.

Stress incontinence (SI) is leakage of urine from a sudden rise in abdominal pressure often brought on by coughing, laughing, or standing up. It is more commonly seen both in the multigravida with loss of urethral support and in the obese where higher abdominal pressures are generated by coughing and positional changes. A history of leakage occurring at times of transient elevation of abdominal pressure without associated urgency suggests the diagnosis. Further confirmation can easily be obtained by observation of urine leakage with a full bladder by coughing or straining, and its correction by urethral suspension without compression. Urodynamic testing in complex cases can be useful. Provocative cystometrics can help exclude leakage from active bladder contractions brought on by similar stimulating events (coughing, laughing, jumping, etc.) owing to detrusor instability. Some cases may benefit from simultaneous midurethral and bladder pressure measurements where poor transmission of the transient abdominal pressure rise to the mid urethra will be documented as the cause of SI (17).

Treatment of SI is normally surgical by urethral suspension and repositioning to ensure transmission of transient pressure rises to it. In mild cases of SI, improvement may be achieved by α-adrenergic drugs, such as phenylpranolamine or ephedrine, though their potential vasoconstrictive and excitatory side effects must be considered. Pelvic floor exercises may also help cases of mild SI. Newer surgical procedures, such as Pereyra and Stamey urethral suspensions, are very effective, rapidly performed, and amenable to shorter and lower risk anesthetics, permitting surgical correction on older and higher risk patients (38,48).

Overflow incontinence (OC) results in the frequent dribbling of small amounts of urine from a very overdistended bladder. Poor bladder emptying can result from obstructive causes, such as BPH, or from poor bladder detrusor function from diabetic neuropathy or lower spinal cord or cauda equina lesions. Initial slow bladder decompression should be employed and management performed as discussed above under the topic of outflow obstruction. Such obstructive causes as BPH, carcinoma of the prostate, urethral stricture, urethral carcinoma, and uterine procedencia are then corrected with resultant correction of the overflow incontinence. In those with poor detrusor function, bladder management by clean self-intermittent catheterization is a most helpful method (26). The older patient may show reluctance to learn this technique, but by repeated reassurance and instruction many can master it. Occasionally, when surgical intervention is too great a risk or when severe dementia or disability predicts failure, long-term catheter drainage may prove necessary.

Detrusor instability (DI) represents the most common cause of urinary incontinence among the elderly (56). Bladder contractions that the patient cannot inhibit and that are often immediately preceded by a sense of urgency result in the incontinence. Voiding is integrated at the midbrain level, and there are both facilitory and inhibitory cortical pathways to this center. As the predominant cortical outflow is inhibitory, injury to cortical pathways to the midbrain voiding center by stroke, Parkinson's disease, multiple sclerosis, low pressure hydrocephalus, and Alzheimer's dementia may result in bladder instability. Excessive peripheral stimulation of the micturition center by such processes as cystitis, perivesical inflammation, vesical calculus, and malignancy of or into the bladder may also trigger bladder instability. Bladder instability can also result from deranged voiding habits, which may vary from negative conditioning when medical personnel insist on toileting the incontinent patient immediately after an episode of incontinence or by excessive volitional efforts of the patient to void at very frequent intervals to avoid the embarrassment of incontinence.

Detrusor instability is suggested by a history of urgency, precipitous voiding, frequency, and nocturia. Coughing, laughing, jumping, and so forth, may trigger uninhibited bladder contractions, and a careful history may be required to differentiate DI from SI (6). Provocative cystometrics looking for bladder contractions of greater than 15 cm of water pressure which the patient cannot inhibit under the stress of rapid bladder filling, coughing, upright positioning, and jumping will confirm the diagnosis.

Treatment of bladder instability may be as simple as providing a bedside commode or urinal to provide easier access to an acceptable collecting device, or can be as complicated as surgical procedures for bladder denervation (10,20). Trials of such drugs as oxybutynin, propantheline, or imipramine are often very helpful, although side effects of constipation, obtundation, dry mouth, or glaucoma may weigh against their use (2,5). Correction of an irritable focus in the pelvis such as cystitis, when present, is clearly indicated. Patients suspected of having some deconditioning of voiding reflexes may well benefit from a regular toileting program that reinforces retaining urine but does not penalize episodes of incontinence should they occur (14). Encouraging socialization, avoiding emphasis on accidents, and reinforcing the patient's sense of self-worth can greatly help in improving continence. Use of combined toileting program and drug therapy, most notably with imipramine, can be very helpful in improving incontinence from DI.

UROLOGIC RELATIONSHIPS TO SEXUALITY IN THE AGING

Sexuality of the geriatric population is a suppressed, ignored, and nearly taboo topic for the present younger, liberated generation. Unfortunately, the affected older generation often were reared with more restrictive sexual attitudes, further inhibiting communication when problems arise. An active sexual life can continue for both sexes throughout its duration to very old age. Many problems may develop that can result in impairment or loss of sexual function. Lack of information and fear may cause patients to stop sexual activity following recovery from a myocardial infarction or stroke despite the very remote risk with an established sexual partner. Others may terminate sexual activity following an illness to their partner, not wanting to place undue stress or demands on them. Patients may expect impotency following some operations, such as prostatectomy, and terminate sexual initiative as a form of performance anxiety. Chronic pain from arthritis may cause unnecessary sexual abstinence which can be avoided by better physician counseling and improved communication between patients and their partners. Those caring for the elderly should be aware of how the seemingly nonsexual problem they are treating may affect sexuality. A concern for the maintenance of sexuality and a discussion on its resumption following an illness should be part of the discharge instructions.

Impotence may develop from neurological, vascular, surgical, or pharmacological causes (27,31). Occasionally it may be the presenting symptom of diabetes mellitus. Antihypertensive drugs may bring on impotency, and male patients placed on them should be warned of the possible side effects that the patient might otherwise regard as part of aging (31). This lack of communication can result in impotency which might have been altered by drug changes. Radical pelvic surgery, such as radical cystectomy, abdominoperineal resection, radical prostatectomy, and some vascular surgery, such as aortic iliac bypass grafts, have a high incidence of postoperative impotency. The new procedure of transluminal angioplasty and nerve-sparing, open surgical procedures can decrease the incidence of impotency from therapy of aortoiliac occlusive disease (55). Patients facing surgical intervention with a high risk of impotency should have this discussed preoperatively and be reassured that penile prostheses are available for implantation if impotency should occur.

Organic impotency can be differentiated from psychogenic impotency by history, nocturnal penile tumescence monitoring, penile blood flow and pressure studies, and, where revascularization is considered, pelvic angiography (4,57).

These studies demonstrate that psychogenic impotency occurs in only a minority of patients. (See Bray, *this volume.*)

Recognition of the importance of sexuality in the older individual, coupled with expanding capabilities of counseling those with functional disorders and providing a variety of penile prostheses, should substantially improve the outlook for the impotent. Future refinements with penile revascularization may provide normal erections without the use of a penile prosthesis in selected patients (31,58).

REFERENCES

1. Allan, R., Boutros, P., and Mourtada, H. (1976): Bacteriuria localization and response to single-dose therapy in women. *J.A.M.A.,* 235:1854–1856.
2. Applebaum, S. M. (1980): Pharmacologic agents in micturitional disorders. *Urology,* 16:555–568.
3. Ashley, D. J. B. (1965): On the incidence of carcinoma of the prostate. *J. Pathol. Bacteriol.,* 90:217–224.
4. Bennett, A. H. (1982): *Management of Male Impotence.* Charles C. Thomas, Springfield, Ill.
5. Blaivas, J. G., et al (1980): Cystometric response to propantheline in detrusor hyperretlexia: theraputic implications. *J. Urol.,* 124:259–262.
6. Booth, C. M., Whiteside, C. G., and Turner-Warwick, R. T. (1981): A long term study of the persistance of the urodynamic characteristics of the unstable bladder. *Br. J. Urol.,* 53:310–314.
7. Brannan, W. (1975): Treatment of prostatitis. *Urology,* 5:626–631.
8. Brereton, H. D., et al (1974): Indomethacin-responsive hypercalcemia in a patient with renal-cell adenocarcinoma. *N. Engl. J. Med.,* 291:83–85.
9. Bruce, A. W., et al (1981): The significance of prostatic acid phosphatase in adenocarcinoma of the prostate. *J. Urol.,* 125:357–360.
10. Clarke, S. T., Forster, D. M., and Thomas, D. G. (1979): Selective sacral neurectomy in the management of urinary incontinence due to detrusor instability. *Br. J. Urol.,* 51:510–514.
11. Clayman, R. V., Williams, R. D., and Fraley, E. E. (1979): Current concepts in cancer- The pursuit of the renal mass. *N. Engl. J. Med.,* 300:72–74.
12. Cupps, R. E., et al (1980): Definitive radiation therapy for prostatic carcinoma. *J. Urol.,* 128:502–504.
13. Dontas, A. S., et al. (1981): Bacteriuria and survival in old age. *N. Engl. J. Med.,* 304:939–943.
14. Elder, D. D., and Stephenson, T. P. (1980): An assessment of the Frewen regime in the treatment of detrusor dysfunction in females. *Br. J. Urol.,* 52:467–471.
15. Fang, L. S., Tolkoff-Rubin, N., and Rubin, R. H. (1978): Efficacy of single-dose and conventional amoxicillin therapy in urinary-tract infection localization by the antibody-coated bacteria technique. *N. Engl. J. Med.,* 298:413–416.
16. Fenely, R. C. L., et al (1979): Urinary incontinence; prevalence and needs. *Br. J. Urol.,* 51:493–496.
17. Gaudenz, R., and Weil, A. (1980): Motor urge incontinence: Diagnosis and treatment. *Urol. Int.,* 35:1–12.
18. Gleckman, R., Crowley, M., and Natsios, G. (1979): Therapy of recurrent invasive urinary tract infections of men. *N. Engl. J. Med.,* 301:876–880.
19. Harding, G. R., et al. (1978): Urinary tract infection localization in women. *J.A.M.A.,* 240:1147–1150.
20. Jannegt, R. A., et al (1979): Transection of the bladder as a method of treatment in adult enuresis nocturna. *Br. J. Urol.,* 51:275–277.
21. Jewett, H. J. (1980): Radical perineal prostatectomy for palpable, clinically localized, non obstructive cancer. *J. Urol.,* 124:492–494.
22. Jones, S. R., Smith, J. W., and Sanford, J. P. (1974): Localization of urinary-tract infections by detection of antibody-coated bacteria in urine sediment. *N. Engl. J. Med.,* 290:591–593.
23. Kam, J., Sandler, C. M., and Benson, G. S. (1981): Angiography in the diagnosis of renal tumors. *Urology,* 18:100–106.

24. Klein, L. A. (1979): Prostatic carcinoma. *N. Engl. J. Med.,* 300:824–833.
25. Landsberg, L. (1970): Hypernatremia complicating partial urinary tract obstruction. *N. Engl. J. Med.,* 283:746–748.
26. Lapides, J., et al (1972): Clean intermittent self-catheterization in the treatment of urinary tract disease. *J. Urol.,* 107:458–461.
27. Levine, S. B. (1976): Marital sexual dysfunction: erectile dysfunction. *Ann. Intern. Med.,* 85:342–350.
28. Lindholm, G. R., et al (1980): Prostatic acid phosphatase radioimmunoassay. *J.A.M.A.,* 244:2071–2073.
29. Mc Cune, C. S., et al (1981): Specific immunotherapy of advanced renal cell carcinoma. *Cancer,* 47:1984–1987.
30. Meares, E. M., and Stamey, T. A. (1972): The diagnosis and management of bacterial prostatitis. *Br. J. Urol.,* 44:175–179.
31. Miles, J. R., Miles, D. G., and Johnson, G. (1982): Aortoiliac operations and sexual dysfunction. *Arch. Surg.,* 117:1177–1181.
32. Montie, J. E., et al (1982): A critical review of immunotherapy of disseminated renal adenocarcinoma. *J. Surg. Oncol.,* 21:5–8.
33. Muldowney, F. P., et al (1966): Sodium diuresis after relief of obstructive uropathy. *N. Engl. J. Med.,* 274:1294–1298.
34. Ouslander, J. G., Kane, R. L., and Abrass, I. B. (1982): Urinary incontinence in elderly nursing home patients. *J.A.M.A.,* 248:1194–1198.
35. Overstall, P. W., Rounce, K., and Palmer, J. H. (1980): Experience with an incontinence clinic. *J. Am. Geriatr. Soc.,* 28:535–538.
36. Parsons, C. L., and Schmidt, J. D. (1982): Control of recurrent lower urinary tract infection in the postmenopausal woman. *J. Urol.,* 128:1224–1226.
37. Paulson, D. F., et al (1982): Radical surgery versus radiotherapy for adenocarcinoma of the prostate. *J. Urol.,* 128:855–859.
38. Pereyra, A. J., and Lebherz, T. B. (1967): Combined urethrovesical suspension and vaginourethroplasty for correction of urinary stress incontinence. *Obst. Gynecol.,* 30:537.
39. Platt, R., Polk, B. F., Murdock, B., and Rosner, B. (1982): Mortality associated with nosocomial urinary tract infection. *N. Engl. J. Med.,* 304:939–943.
40. Price, D. A., Ramsden, P. D., and Stobbart, D. (1980): The unstable bladder and prostatectomy. *Br. J. Urol.,* 52:529–531.
41. Prout, G. R. (1971): Preoperative irradiation as an adjuvant in the surgical management of invasive bladder cancer. *J. Urol.,* 104:116.
42. Ray, G. R., Cassady, R., and Bagshaw, M. A. (1973): Definitive radiation therapy of carcinoma of the prostate. *Ther. Radiol.,* 106:407–418.
43. Ristuccia, A. M., and Cunha, B. A. (1982): Current concepts in antimicrobial therapy of prostatitis. *Urology,* 20:338–345.
44. Robson, C. J., Churchill, B. M., and Anderson, W. (1969): The results of radical nephrectomy for renal cell carcinoma. *J. Urol.,* 101:297–301.
45. Rubin, R. H., et al (1980): Single-dose amoxicillin therapy for urinary tract infection. *J.A.M.A.,* 244:561–564.
46. Skinner, D. G. (1980): Current perspectives in the management of high grade invasive bladder cancer. *Cancer,* 45:1866–1874.
47. Smith, J. W., et al. (1979): Recurrent urinary tract infections in men. *Ann. Intern. Med.,* 91:544–548.
48. Stamey, T. A. (1980): Endoscopic suspension of the vesical neck for urinary incontinence in females. *Ann. Surg.,* 192:465–471.
49. Stamey, T. A. (1980): *Pathogenesis and Treatment of Urinary Tract Infections.* Williams & Wilkins, Baltimore.
50. Stamey, T. A., Condy, M., and Mihara, G. (1977): Prophylactic efficacy of nitrofurantoin macrocrystals and Trimethoprim-Sulfamethozazole in urinary tract infections. *N. Engl. J. Med.,* 296:780–787.
51. Stamm, W. E., et al (1980): Antimicrobial prophylaxis of recurrent urinary tract infections. *Ann. Int. Med.,* 92:770–775.
52. Tveter, K. J. (1973): Unusual manifestations of renal carcinoma. *Acta. Chir. Scand.,* 139:401–409.
53. Utz, D. C., and Zincke, H. (1974): The masquerade of bladder cancer in situ as interstitial cystitis. *J. Urol.,* 111:160–161.

54. Warren, J. W., et al. (1982): Cephalexin for susceptible bacteriuria in afebrile, long term catheterized patients. *J.A.M.A.,* 248:454–458.
55. Wasserman, M. D., et al (1980): The differential diagnosis of impotence—The measurement of nocturnal tumescence. *J.A.M.A.,* 243:2038–2042.
56. Williams, M. E., and Pannill, F. C. (1982): Urinary incontinence in the elderly. *Ann. Intern. Med.,* 97:895–907.
57. Zorgniotti, A. W., and Rossi, G. (1980): Diagnosis and therapy of vasculogenic impotence. *J. Urol.,* 123:674–677.
58. Zorgniotti, A. W., and Rossi, G. (1980): *Vasculogenic Impotence.* Charles C Thomas, Springfield, Ill.

Rehabilitation in the Aging edited by
T. F. Williams. Raven Press, New York © 1984.

Specific Assistive Aids

*†Lawrence W. Friedmann and *Ernesto S. Capulong

*Department of Physical Medicine and Rehabilitation, Nassau County Medical Center,
East Meadow, New York 11554; and †Department of Rehabilitation Medicine, State
University of New York, Stony Brook, New York 11790

In the care of the aging person, assistive devices are used primarily to relieve pain and to maintain or restore function. Aging implies a deterioration of functional capacity with the onset of acute and chronic disorders that limit physical, mental, emotional, and social function. There may be acute episodes that leave chronic residue or chronic progressive disorders that diminish the patient's ability to deal with the world.

In the first category there are, for example, the acute episodes of chronic occlusive arterial disease. These episodes may be in the form of a myocardial infarction, reducing the patient's cardiac reserve, or a cerebrovascular accident, giving a permanent hemiparesis and possibly some disturbance in speech, with or without balance difficulties or amputation.

The joints may be involved by the wear and tear of degenerative arthritis or have the damage of acute inflammatory rheumatoid arthritis. The patient may have the complications of various neurologic disorders or just the gradual onset of dementia and debility. Various environmental and work exposures, or diseases, may have given rise to chronic pulmonary disease, impairing the patient's ability to do heavy work or to work for a prolonged period due to a diminished breathing capacity. The general slowing down of physical activities in the aging individual predisposes to disuse muscular weakness. This muscular weakness decreases the patient's desire to be physically active, which further increases the tendency to back pain due to muscular insufficiency, decreases the cardiac work capacity, and places the patient on the downhill spiral that we see too often. The deterioration is usually unnecessarily early and rapid. The limitations of function may be systemic or confined to one or more extremities.

The specific disorders are dealt with in other chapters of this book. Here we outline some of the wide variety of measures that may assist the elderly in improving their comfort, their general physical status, and, most of all, their ability to function as independently as they can. It is important for the individual's self-respect to be as independent as the physical and mental conditions allow. It is the deprivation of the dignity of independence that is most damaging as people grow older. Relying on an assistive device to help one to function is nowhere near as demeaning as the need to ask for someone else to help with a formerly simple task. This is especially true when help is required to perform the activities of daily living, some of which are intimate in the highest degree (Figs. 1 and 2).

PAIN

The first thing that limits independence in individuals is pain. Pain has many detrimental biologic effects. It certainly restricts the individual's ability to perform activities.

The first effort toward relief of pain is, of course, directed at correcting its cause. However, it is often also necessary to treat the pain itself. There are many measures for the relief of pain. They may be classified as chemical, physical, psychologic, and surgical. In appropriate cases, all of these may need to be used. The most common method of treatment of pain is pharmacologic. Often this is the only pain-relieving measure that is considered. The various analgesics have side effects and these adverse effects are most common in the elderly. They tend to obtund the individual's already diminished alertness and may make the patient confused and disoriented, especially at night, when sensory deprivation is most severe. The simple analgesics such as aspirin may have side effects such as diminished coagulation with bleeding and blood dyscrasias. Sedative drugs are also too often prescribed to relieve discomforts. The elderly person's inability to sleep may have a psychologic basis or may be due to discomfort because of such a simple thing as a wrinkle in the bed sheet. Often the first thing that is thought of by medical personnel is to give the patient a sleeping pill or tranquilizer. These further diminish the sensory feedback in an individual whose sensory acuity, hearing, seeing, and touch may already be diminished.

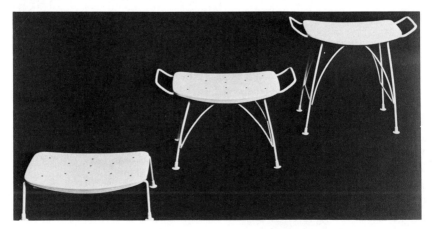

FIG. 1. Bathtub elevated seats to allow self-transfer in tub bathing. (From Everest and Jennings Corporation, with permission.)

The elderly individual may, under these circumstances, become agitated because of disorientation when out of familiar surroundings and, say, in the hospital or nursing home in the evening when the lights are out and the room is quiet. The simplest and most effective measure is to use a simple assistive device—a night light. This allows the person who awakens in the middle of the night with, perhaps, a bad dream, to see the surroundings. This visual stimulation is usually more effective than any amount of sedatives. Sensory deprivation is known for its ability to cause disorientation.

HEAT

A large component of most painful conditions is muscle spasm. Muscle spasm and many other forms of pain are relieved by physical measures that have few side effects when used appropriately. The most effective of these is the use of heat. Heat may be classified as either superficial or deep and either wet or dry. There is as yet no proof that one is definitely superior to the other. For any one individual, a trial of the various types may be used if the first type that one tries is ineffective. Heat is effective in relief of pain not only of muscles but also of other conditions. It is effective in relieving the pain of inflamed joints and spasmodic episodes in the gastrointestinal, urogenital, and gynecological tracts. It relieves stiffness and allows the patient to have an improved range of motion, allowing the patient to function better. It is important that everyone understands that any heat treatment for muscle spasm should always be followed by appropriate exercise of the involved muscles.

Superficial heat may be conductive, as with paraffin or water, either free

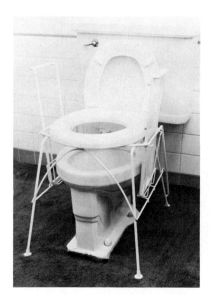
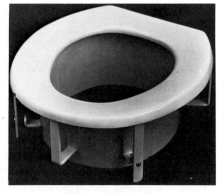

FIG. 2. Elevated toilet seats. **Left:** Elevated seat on frame. **Right:** Elevated seat to attach to bowl. (From Everest and Jennings Corporation, with permission.)

flowing or in hot packs or mud; radiant, as with a heat lamp or the use of the sun; inductive, as with the electromagnetic flux of short wave or microwave diathermy; or by ultrasonic movement.

The radiant and conductive applications give superficial heat, whereas the inductive and ultrasonic types of heating give deeper heating. Short wave diathermy heats the least deeply of the inductive heating types, with microwave giving somewhat more deep heat and ultrasound giving the deepest heat. It has not yet been determined by controlled clinical studies whether deeper heat is actually more beneficial for the treatment of deep conditions than superficial heat. Although we do not know exactly how heat exerts its beneficial effects, millennia of experience indicate that these effects do exist.

WATER

One of the most common and ancient ways of providing superficial heat is the use of warm water. That this method is efficacious can be testified to by its ancient history. Warm spa baths have been used throughout the world in every known culture. Warring American Indian tribes would allow an enemy soldier to go through their lines, even during the midst of a battle, if he were going for treatment to a warm water spring.

Warm water baths, with or without dissolved salts and with or without agitation, as in a natural spring or in a whirlpool bath, are excellent methods of applying heat to the entire hand, leg, and/or trunk. The temperature of the water can easily be regulated, according to the tolerance of the individual (Fig. 3).

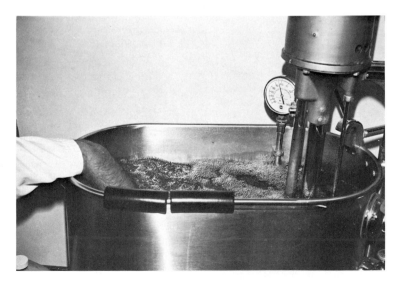

FIG. 3. Whirlpool bath.

Water is cheap, clean, easily available, and requires no special equipment. Although there is disagreement on whether added or natural salts are beneficial, spa treatments, although not much used in America, are extremely popular overseas. Certainly, the ambience of the spa is helpful for conditions worsened by emotional and muscular tension. Water agitation increases the heat transfer.

PARAFFIN

Paraffin is a method of applying superficial heat by conduction. It is a very good method for combating stiffness and pain, especially in the hands of persons with arthritis. It is inexpensive and relatively easy to use, both in the physical therapy department and, more importantly, for the patient at home (Fig. 4). The heat is transferred from the paraffin to the skin by conduction after the hands, for example, are dipped into the melted paraffin-mineral oil mixture. The precise temperature at which the paraffin will be melted is determined by the amount of mineral oil relative to the amount of paraffin. The more mineral oil, the lower the heat at which the paraffin melts. This may be adjusted to meet patient comfort. It is important that the circulation and sensation in the hands be normal and that there be no open wounds.

A great advantage of paraffin treatment is that the extremity may be elevated during the treatment. The hand, for example, is dipped into the paraffin and withdrawn repeatedly until a "paraffin glove" is formed. The joints are not moved. Multiple layers, usually 10 or 15, are applied in this way. The hand is then wrapped in a Turkish towel to retain the heat. The extremity may then be elevated during the rest of the treatment, allowing the edema to diminish. This is in contrast to the use of the whirlpool bath in which the limb must be kept in the dependent position for the entire treatment. Paraffin is more useful when the heat treatment is followed by centripetal massage. Another advantage is that it softens the skin and makes it pliable. It does not dry out the skin as

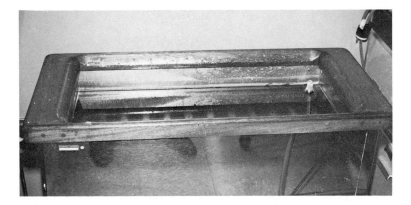

FIG. 4. Therapeutic paraffin bath.

does the whirlpool bath. The whirlpool, however, may be modified to decrease the drying capacity by using a small amount of olive or mineral oil in it.

A disadvantage of paraffin treatment is the difficulty in melting it at home and in finding the exact proportion of paraffin to oil to attain the most efficacious and comfortable temperature for the individual. A good place to start is a mixture of four parts of paraffin to one of oil. If a cooler temperature is desired, more mineral oil should be added. If a warmer temperature is felt desirable, more paraffin should be added. The patient should be aware that it takes a long time to melt the paraffin and if it is to be used a number of times a day it may be advisable to keep the container on the stove on the lowest heat. The patient should be cautioned that there should always be a slight "skin" on the top of the paraffin, even when it is completely melted on a stove. If the "skin" is not there the bath may be too hot. This does not apply to a therapeutic temperature controlled unit.

DEEP HEAT

Short wave and microwave diathermy are excellent methods for electrically induced moderately deep heating. Short wave is safer, as the patient can feel overheating. Microwave is quicker, but the dosage is more exacting (Fig. 5).

Ultrasound is a form of deep movement-induced heat that is often successful in the treatment of arthritis, bursitis, capsulitis, periarthritis, trigger points, and painful neuromas. As with all forms of heat, it is to be used in conjunction with exercise. The use of heat alone, without the exercise required, is analogous

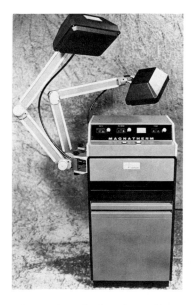

FIG. 5. Microwave diathermy for moderately deep heat. (Courtesy of International Medical Electronics, LTD.)

to treating a patient with appendicitis by giving him anesthesia and not doing the surgery required to alleviate his condition. Heat is a symptomatic treatment to relieve pain and muscle spasm and to increase blood flow, but it is rarely therapeutic by itself. It is the exercise, which increases the range of motion, maintains the pain-free state, and improves the physiologic condition of the muscles, that is therapeutic. The improvement of function, which is the ultimate goal of therapy, is primarily determined by the subsequent exercise and not by the heat.

ELECTRICAL STIMULATION

Electrical stimulation has been used for many years for the reduction of pain. It is most successful in the pain due to muscle spasm. Muscle spasm is the body's defense against painful movement and is, therefore, associated with almost all types of painful conditions, both internal and external. This reflex, painful spasm is used diagnostically but the patient can be markedly relieved of pain by the use of heat or electrical stimulation. Electrical stimulation may also be used for the relief of muscle spasm in back and neck pain and is extremely successful for that purpose. Usually, continuous tetanizing stimulation is used and often followed by surging sinusoidal electrical stimulation, generally in that sequence (Fig. 6).

A newer way of giving electrical stimulation which has been highly successful in some acute and chronic pains is the TENS (transcutaneous electrical nerve stimulator unit). Electrical frequency is far higher than for muscle stimulation and the pulse width narrower. Pain of almost any etiology can be diminished by some of these units. Much of the work that has been done indicates that it is more helpful for chronic pain than for acute pain. There is some indication that the pain of Sudeck's atrophy, neuromata and arthritic joints and some cases of postfracture pain, responds well to transcutaneous electrical stimulation. In more chronic conditions, nerve stimulation seems to become less efficacious with time. Intraspinal and intracerebral stimulators have also been attempted

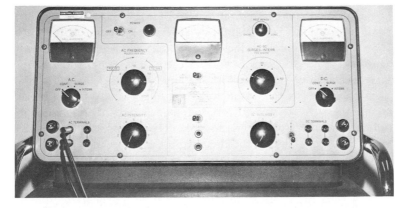

FIG. 6. Therapeutic electrical stimulator for galvanic and faradic stimulation.

with varying degrees of success. In our experience, the success rate of the implanted stimulator is approximately the same as with that of the transcutaneous nerve stimulator. If the transcutaneous nerve stimulator and all else fails, the implanted stimulator may be worth a try as a last resort before denervating surgical procedures.

EDEMA CORRECTION

Edema inhibits function by preventing joint motion and by causing pain. It may be a consequence of (a) trauma, either mechanical or thermal; (b) lack of motion with dependency, which we term dependent edema, as occurs with lower limb dependency when the patient sits for long periods of time without walking; (c) hand dysfunction, as in the shoulder-hand syndrome after myocardial infarction, bursitis or stroke; (d) obstruction of the lymphatic or venous drainage, including cardiac failure; or (e) hypoalbuminemia, as in nephrosis and malnutrition and liver failure. The treatment of edema due to these nonmechanical causes is not considered here.

The correction of edema is obtained by elevation to drain the part. The elevation must be above heart level to counteract dependency. Exercise is used to improve the "muscular pump," which forces venous blood and lymphatic fluid toward the heart. Edema is also corrected by centripetal massage, which improves the lymphatic and venous return. Compression of the exterior part of a limb helps to prevent or reverse swelling by decreasing the available volume of the limb. It inhibits the accumulation of fluids that we call edema. This external compression may be by means of elastic stockings or gloves. These give mild compression, decreasing the edema, which helps in the restoration of the motion of the joints and in pain reduction. For the hand, an inexpensive elastic glove called an Isotoner® glove is available. It is a brand of elastic glove that comes in one size and has as its main advantage being inexpensive. As with most gloves, it is made of a blend of fibers—in this case of nylon, Lycra, and Spandex. They are readily available in most department stores. Custom-made stockings and gloves are better.

Edema may be reversed by intermittent or constant compression. Intermittent compression therapy has been helpful in reducing swelling of the limbs. It is helpful to get the limb to a smaller size. It must be used in conjunction with compression stockings or gloves to prevent the recurrence of edema. The hand, for example, is placed in the sleeve with the fingers in either flexion or extension. The pressure machine is placed on for a varying period of time, say 5 min, and then the pressure is released for the same period of time. All of this is done with the part elevated, where possible. The compression time can be increased as the patient tolerates the therapy.

SPLINTING

Splinting is used for many conditions. The basic purposes of splinting are (a) to prevent or correct deformity; (b) to enhance or substitute for function;

(c) to support the weight of a body part; and (d) to protect a fragile body member or structure.

Orthoses or splints are prescribed for specific purposes. Each part of the orthosis must have a well-planned design to accomplish a particular purpose for the individual. Some splints assist in holding a patient's foot perpendicular to the lower leg so that, for example, in the case of paralysis due to a stroke, the patient would not develop a foot drop and trip over a toe. In this case, usually a nonmovable or static splint is used to prevent the foot drop. In other cases, a dynamic splint, which performs a movement function or gives therapy, will be used. Such a type of splint may be used after hand injury or burns, where there are contractures. Elastic rubber bands will move the fingers in such a way that the contractures that have developed will be reversed. Not only must the splint itself be prescribed, but the material of which it is to be made should also be specified. The time that the patient should wear the splint and the time it should be off also need prescription. Any splint or brace is only a part of an overall patient management program, of which assistive aids are a small but vital feature.

Static Splints

Static splints may be protective, supportive, and/or corrective in their design, with no movable parts. The joints are the means by which the power of the muscles move the bones to bring about useful function. Where these joints are stiffened by fibrosis, destroyed by disease, or deformed by dislocation or fracture, the function of the body part is impaired or destroyed. A static splint may be indicated to protect a weak muscle from being overly stretched by the contraction of the stronger opposing muscle. The splint can support the joints, as in the arthritides. The splint may act as a substitute for the weak muscles by supporting joints, as in the case of peripheral nerve palsies. Static splints whenever possible should hold the involved part in the most functional position for that individual's needs.

The so-called functional position of the hand for most people is with the wrist in 30° of dorsiflexion with the distal metacarpal arch maintained and with the thumb in abduction and opposition, lined up with the pads of the second and third digits, in a three-jaw chuck arrangement. The metacarpal, phalangeal, and proximal interphalangeal joints are in approximately 45° of flexion and the distal interphalangeal joints are in approximately 20° of flexion.

Dynamic Splints

Dynamic splinting is the application of a force to a moving part that ideally remains nearly constant as the body part moves. This means that the force should be applied as near as possible at 90° to the body part that one wants to move.

The movement of joints decreases the formation of adhesions around the joints. This keeps the integrity of the joints intact. It nourishes the joint cartilage. It prevents the contracture of soft tissues that always contract on the concave side of a flexed joint and stretch on the convex side of that joint. By moving the joint, this contraction, which can come on very rapidly, is avoided. In addition, if there is already a contracture of the joint with tight soft tissues, dynamic splinting along with the active and active-assistive motion tends to stretch out these tissues and restore joint range of motion and, therefore, function. Even if the range is not restored entirely to normal, the range can be at least made more functional. Rehabilitation is, of course, the restoration of function for the patient, which is usually more important to the individual than anything else. Older people are usually more concerned with their lack of function than with their appearance.

Dynamic splints may be required for the following.

1. Skeletal substitution: to support bones and joints with intrinsic pathology.
2. Muscle balance: to counteract the deforming forces of paralyzed muscles when opposing forces are present and to hold in position previously divided tendons or muscles.
3. Joint motion: to preserve existing joint motion where a deforming potential cause of contracture is present and to increase joint motion where it is restricted.

A dynamic splint must be designed and constructed carefully to provide specific forces to achieve the goal intended. It must be made so that the patient can continue to wear the splint without discomfort. All new devices are somewhat uncomfortable, including new shoes, so absolute comfort cannot be attained at the beginning but should be attainable after the patient has worn the splint for some time. The forces applied must be the minimal that will do the job. The attempt to give a great deal of correction quickly makes a splint or brace uncomfortable, and the device may then be discarded by the patient. Only very small forces are needed to counteract the forces applied by the muscles. The muscles fatigue quickly and light weights are adequate. The direction of force application is very important. Outriggers, which are attachment points for the traction devices (usually rubber bands or spring steel), must be placed accurately and securely onto the body of the splint.

Medical Principles in Splinting

The forces acting on a joint must be balanced. If they are not, a constant deforming force will exist, eventually causing contractures and diminished function. Where the forces are not equal, a splint must be given to counterbalance the stronger of the forces. This maintains the periarticular soft tissues, the elastic tissues in the muscle, and the nutrition of the muscles, joints, and bone in optimal condition.

Joints should not be immobilized needlessly.

Where there is injury on one surface of the limb, the body parts should be so placed as to not stress the recently repaired subcutaneous structure such as the tendon or muscle. By contrast, if the skin is involved and tends to contract, the body part must be placed so that the maximally stretched position is maintained.

Specific assistive devices are needed for specific problems. In a short chapter, only a few can be mentioned. To prevent stiffness in the shoulder, common in the elderly due to bursitis, tendonitis, and arthritis (see J. Baum, *this volume*), various maneuvers may be used in addition to standard exercises. These are important to prevent the so-called shoulder-hand syndrome, which is a consequence of the "frozen shoulder" (adhesive capsulitis of the shoulder). The simplest technique is to have the patient "walk" the fingers up a wall. A more formal way of doing that is to have a "shoulder ladder," which is a small series of steps in which the patient uses the fingers to slowly abduct and elevate the hand and shoulder. Active motion of the shoulder is, of course, most important.

A simple device that may be used at home as well as in a formal therapy setting is the over-the-door pulley. This may be adapted from the home cervical traction set. The patient has a pulley over the door and pulls down with the good hand while the other hand holds a loop and is pulled up over the head. This may be used for forward flexion, abduction, or extension. This is useful in patients with hemiplegia, paralysis, shoulder contractures, mastectomy, burns, and fractures.

The patient may also use various circumduction devices such as troughs with ball bearings that roll on tables, to assist in moving the shoulder. These are also useful for elbow flexion. Another device useful for the upper limb is the "hand gym." This is an exercise unit originally designed for patients with hand involvement of rheumatoid arthritis. It exercises the intrinsic and extrinsic muscles of the hand, for patients who have lost finger dexterity and strength. Theraplast is a Silicon, moldable dough that can be pulled, squeezed, and twisted to improve range of motion, strength, and endurance of the hand.

Assistive devices may also be needed for the spine. Various types of assistive devices are frequently needed to maintain the neck, especially after injury in this area. Soft tissue injuries may be held by cervical collars, either soft or rigid. They may be made of cloth, plastic, or metal. They may be easily bendable or may be rigid. Various designs holding the chin and occiput in relation to the chest are available, e.g., the soft foam, plastic, two poster, four poster, rigid occipital, sternal, mandibular immobilizing devices, and the most rigid device, which contours to the chest and holds the head rigidly in a halo-shaped ring through which four metal pegs are inserted into the bones of the outer table of the skull. The latter is used only for fractures of the neck with danger of severance of the spinal cord.

To hold the shoulders back in a patient who has a kyphosis of the upper thoracic spine with drooped shoulders, there are various devices that loop in front of the delto-pectoral groove and in the axilla and remind the patient to hold the shoulders back. It should be remembered in this context that spinal devices are rarely strong enough to support the spine physically but, instead, tend to remind the patient to move in the proper directions and to hold body posture properly.

For the dorsal spine, the Taylor brace is helpful to maintain the erect posture and to prevent excessive motion. There are many modifications of all these devices, literally numbering in the hundreds. The Taylor brace modifications may include not only axillary straps to prevent forward and sideward flexion but also "cow horns," which are metal devices that press on the anterior chest, making the patient uncomfortable if the patient forward flexes. Still better devices are the modifications of the Jewett hyperextension brace. These braces work on the three-point pressure principle more directly than do most other braces. The middle point of the brace is in the upper lumbar spine while the other two points are at the manubrium of the sternum and the pubic symphysis. If an attempt is made to forward flex, the patient gets pain in the manubrium and in the pubis and does not continue to flex. These devices are generally used for compression fractures of the bodies of the vertebrae to inhibit the patient from flexing and increasing the collapse of the vertebrae, and other situations where spinal flexion is contraindicated.

For the lumbar spine, devices inhibit motion in various directions, depending on where their rigid structures are. Most of them have rigid structures posteriorly, but these are less effective than those that have rigid structures anteriorly to prevent forward flexion. For the most part, the devices are immobilizing. Those for back pain have a tight front to support the abdominal organs to replace the function of weak abdominal musculature. The simplest devices are corsets, which may be made in many styles. They are lightweight, comfortable, and more cosmetic, especially for women. Simple devices such as groin belts and athletic supports are useful. As the patient needs more support for the abdominal muscles, more rigid devices, including those with firm pads, are sometimes required. It is the abdominal compression that is the most important feature and not the rigid steels. For that reason, we prefer corsets to the more complex braces, in most cases. One exception is the use of the Williams flexion brace, which induces a posture-correcting reaction on the part of the body by causing a pelvic tilt that, in turn, induces a reflex contraction of the hip extensors in order for the patient to stay erect.

Devices to correct scoliosis are many. The most efficient ones are those based on the principle of inductive bracing, in which the body self-corrects because of slight discomfort. Pads are placed over the apex of the curve by pressing on the rib, which goes to the apex of the curve. The patient stands in this brace and, after a period of time, becomes slightly uncomfortable because of pressure over the rib. The patient then actively uses the musculature to curve around that pad and to self-correct. Active use of exercise is required in the brace and the patient must wear the brace all the time. Daytime use of the brace is said to help support the trunk during the erect posture but probably gives little or no correction. Most of the correction probably occurs at night when the patients sleep, as the pad is rolled over. The body is relaxed and curves around the pad, which acts as a fulcrum with the body weight helping to correct the curve. The original principle of the Milwaukee brace, which included traction to straighten the spine, has been abandoned for the obvious reason that traction alone can only partially straighten the curve and is not really the best way of doing so. The reader may prove that by attempting to straighten a paper clip by pulling on its ends. It should be remembered in this context that spinal devices are rarely strong enough to support the spine physically but, instead, induce the patient to move in the proper directions and to hold the body posture properly.

All of the above assistive devices must be used in an integrated plan of total patient care, including exercises to prevent the inevitable disuse atrophy caused by a device whose prime function is to decrease the work demand on the back and abdominal muscles.

ASSISTIVE DEVICES FOR THE LOWER LIMBS

Orthoses

Elderly people have a lifetime of walking behind them. They have much wear and tear in the lower limbs, frequently with osteoarthritis of the hips or knees. They may have rheumatoid arthritis, bunions, and other foot deformities. These foot deformities affect their entire lives. If they have painful feet their mobility and comfort are diminished and they put excessive strain on other parts of their bodies, especially their backs. For this reason, comfortable, appropriate footwear is crucial.

The podiatrist is the logical therapist to consult in the care of the feet (see A. Helfand, *this volume*). The following principles are essential in preventive foot care.

1. Wash the feet nightly with tepid, not hot, water. Use a mild, nonmedicated soap. Dry the feet carefully by patting, particularly between the toes, then apply a thin coat of lanolin to all unbroken skin. Leave for 5 min and then gently pat off, especially between toes. Dust the feet in the morning with light, nonmedicated talc (baby powder), particularly between the toes.
2. Inspect the feet daily for blisters, cuts, or scratches. Any break in the skin is a potential area of infection and should be treated with great care.
3. Avoid wet feet, wet shoes, or wet socks, especially in winter months.
4. Wear wool bed socks if the feet are cold at night. Do not use heating pad or hot water bottle.
5. Cut nails short in the center and never below the juncture of the nail and the flesh at the corners. Never cut the corners of the nail out.

6. Inspect the insides of shoes frequently for foreign objects, nail points, and torn linings. Any object that creates pressure or a break in the skin is dangerous since they are potential sites for ulcers or infection.
7. Wear properly fitted stockings of cotton or wool. Make sure that they are large enough to allow considerable toe motion. Change the stockings daily. Do not wear mended stockings and avoid seams and stretch or tube socks.
8. Do not wear garters or any other support garment that causes localized constrictions.

Special last shoes may be required such as bunion lasts, modified lasts, or even custom-made shoes. Special inserts are often required to transfer body weight to foot locations on which the patient can walk without pain or skin damage. When the patient has cocked toes a high, soft toe box is required. The leather should usually be kid leather, deerskin, or antelope. Crepe soles are sometimes required to give cushioning. With the use of specially designed orthoses for inside the shoes, patients may frequently be made much more mobile and free to enjoy their lives.

After certain conditions, such as a stroke, a foot drop may occur. At this point, support for the weight of the foot and shoe may be required. A simple elastic tip strap may be used in therapy but this is inappropriate for permanent use. In this case, an ankle-foot orthosis is required. Many types are available. They may be attached to the shoe by means of metal stirrup or caliper attachments, single or double bar devices. Double bar devices are more stable and control rotation better. In heavy individuals a single bar device may be bent out of shape by the weight of the patient but this is not usually the case unless the patient is obese. Metal braces are slightly less expensive than the plastic braces. In addition, the metal joints allow elastic control of dorsiflexion and allow some plantar flexion at heel strike that is adjustable and easily controllable. These may vary from a posterior leaf spring brace to the single and double bar braces mentioned.

Since the development of resilient plastic materials, a number of braces in which there is a plastic footplate are used for the lower limb to prevent foot drop. The use of a plastic footplate usually means that a larger shoe size is required for that foot and the patient must buy split size shoes or two pairs. If this is a problem, a larger size shoe can be obtained for both sides and an insole placed in the opposite shoe to take up the extra room. Appropriate modifications will be built into the shoe and brace as required. The elasticity and resilience of the plastic allow some plantar flexion at heel strike and recoil to lift the foot during swing phase. The elasticity at heel strike may be somewhat adjustable by modifying the amount of plastic left on the medial and lateral sides of the brace. If more resistance is required, more plastic may be added to decrease the flexibility. These devices are somewhat more costly than the metal braces and less adjustable. Their appearance is much better and they are much lighter in weight.

Metal, plastic, and combination braces are available for patients who need control over the knee. Various types of knee joints are available, free or locking in case the patient has no muscle strength or, where strength is diminished, eccentric posteriorly placed knee joints. Knee locks may be of the drop lock variety, either assisted or unassisted by means of springs. The French, Swiss, or bail lock allows the patient to unlock the brace without reaching down. This should not be used in crowded areas or where there are children as they may accidentally hit the bail and unlock the brace, causing the patient to fall.

The knee-ankle-foot or knee orthosis is often used to compensate and prevent the further progression of mediolateral instability or anteroposterior instability. A double bar brace is required for this. Plastic braces may also be used to decrease the weight in these types of braces. Recurvatum is also inhibited by this brace.

For patients who do not need a long leg brace but who need some help with mediolateral instability or anteroposterior instability because of internal derangement of the knee joint, a number of braces have been used. In my experience, most of the lightweight braces are ineffective. Probably the most effective is the Lenox Hill derotation brace which, if properly made, assists the patient to be active. This is usually used by athletes but may be used by the elderly as well. The complexity of putting it on may be a little difficult for those who are not as alert as they once were. A number of modifications are available but are no better. Also available are braces to control the hip joint with a long leg brace and pelvic band but these are rarely used for the elderly because they are very heavy.

Another type of orthosis used by the elderly is for patients with ununited fractures of the lower limb or peripheral neuropathy. When peripheral neuropathy is present, with neuropathic ulcers on the bottom of the feet, often the patient cannot be managed by the use of modified footwear alone. The patient may also be unable to use crutches. The patient must then be kept at bedrest or use a walker, which is extremely difficult if not impossible to use on steps. For this reason the patient may become a prisoner at home. One device that can be used is a patellar tendon bypass orthosis, in which the patient doesn't bear weight on the foot at all but bears weight basically on the patellar tendon and the medial tibial flare. The ulcer then has time to heal and the patient can still be mobile, at home and outside, without a problem.

A similar type of bypass orthosis may be used to enable the patient to walk in case of a fracture of the tibia. It is a form of fracture bracing, of which there are a number of modifications.

If the patient has a fracture of the femur, a similar type of bypass may be used except that a quadrilateral ischial and gluteal bearing socket is used and the body weight is transferred from the ischium around the fracture site and around the knee, down to the floor. This type of device may also be used for patients with severe arthritic or otherwise painful knee joints.

If weight-bearing is bypassed in the gluteal ischial orthosis, the knee joint must be fully extended and locked and the shoe must have a rocker bar on it in order to transfer weight from the floor to the ischium.

There are a number of categories of technical aids that are important for elderly people and especially for the disabled. These may be classified into mobility aids, manipulation and control of the environment aids, patient handling devices, and communication devices.

Mobility Aids

Transportation is a great problem for the elderly, particularly to allow them to shop independently and to socialize, to remove the very frequent isolation from peers, friends, and family. Social isolation is one of the greatest dangers and fears of the elderly and transportation is a very important means of avoiding this.

Among the mobility aids available are conventional crutches, canes, artificial limbs, orthoses, and walkers. There are also wheelchairs and licensed motor vehicles of various types.

The most common device for the lower extremity is the cane (Fig. 7). It is frequently used by elderly people. The basic purpose is to enhance balance, which may be impaired due to generalized weakness and loss of coordination. A common gait in elderly people is a shuffling type of gait with a wide base. The cane increases the width of the base of support and gives some sensory feedback through the handle of the cane, which may compensate for the dimin-

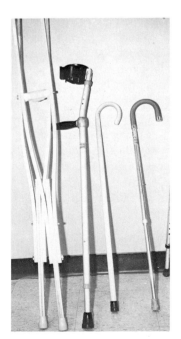

FIG. 7. Canes and crutches, *left-to-right,* standard adjustable wooden crutch, lofstrand crutch, wooden standard cane, and adjustable aluminum cane.

ished sensation of the lower extremies, which may be a part of aging or peripheral neuropathy due to diabetes mellitus. A cane is useful for taking the pressure off arthritic joints by decreasing weight-bearing on the legs and providing some weight-bearing through the arms. This is useful after fractures, amputations, and strokes.

The length of a cane is important. The cane should be of such height that when its tip is on the ground (15 cm to the front and to the side of the tip of the shoe) and the hand is resting on the handle, the elbow should be flexed about 30°. This gives maximum support. Canes, of course, are used not only for support but, in the visually impaired, as a searching instrument to find out where objects are. The cane is usually felt to be most comfortable and most useful for body support when it is held in the hand contralateral to the painful or diseased limb. Some patients find that this is not the case. They prefer to hold it in the ipsilateral hand. The patient should be allowed to do whatever is comfortable. The physician, however, is well advised to examine both lower extremities because if the patient really prefers to use the cane in the ipsilateral hand it may be determined that there is a problem with the contralateral limb as well as with the ipsilateral limb.

The patient should be trained to ascend steps and ramps with the good limb first, followed by the cane and the disabled limb. Descending steps should be the reverse—that is, the cane and the disabled limb should descend first, followed by the good limb. Usually the patient would not go down or up steps in a step-over-step fashion but will take one step at a time, using the procedure mentioned.

The tip of the cane and the crutch should be of the type that has a relatively flat surface with concentric rings that grip the ground. The minimum cross-sectional diameter should be 3 cm; this helps prevent slipping. Special crutch tips for ice are available, which are useful for canes as well. The patient should be taught to use the cane for ascending and descending steps and ramps, not only on level surfaces, but on slippery surfaces and irregular terrain. Various sizes and shapes and material grip surfaces are available on canes and should be chosen by the patient to suit the patient's own convenience. There are also specialized canes. Examples of these are the tripod and quadruped canes, which give additional support (Fig. 8).

If the patient needs more support than a cane provides, crutches may be used. Some elderly people are afraid to use crutches, and for them a walker can be used. For those who are not afraid to use crutches, a number of types are available. The standard adjustable wooden type is the most common. The measurement for a crutch should be as described for the cane—that is, the crutch tip should be as described for the cane, and the handle of the crutch should be such that the patient has a 30° flexion of the elbow when the crutch is placed as described for the cane.

The axillary piece should be low and the patient should push up on the cane so as not to rest the axillary bar in the axilla at all during walking. At

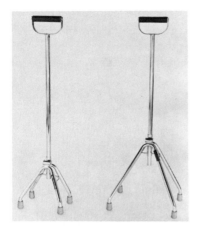

FIG. 8. Quadruped canes with varying bases of support. (From Everest and Jennings Corporation, with permission.)

most, the elderly patient should rest while standing still, with pressure in the axilla. If excessive pressure occurs in the axilla, it may cause a paralysis of some of the muscles in the hand. Such crutch palsy is not uncommon. Some patients, however, need support in the axilla, and in that case the axilla top, which is generally of wood, can be made more comfortable where resting is required by placing a rubber pad over it. For long-term users, the top may be replaced by a leather sling to diminish pressure further.

If the patient can use it, the Lofstrand or forearm crutch is desirable. It has many advantages. It is light in weight and there is no way the patient can get an axillary palsy. In addition, the main advantage is that one can let go of the cane and open a doorknob or carry something without having the cane drop to the ground. This is especially true when, instead of the standard forearm piece that opens in the front, the side-opening Lofstrand is prescribed. It is the same price as the standard Lofstrand but is much better in northern climates where topcoats are used and the patient needs a cane both inside and outside the house.

One or two crutches may be used, depending on the needs of the patient. They act in a similar fashion to canes but can take more of the body weight. They transfer much of the body weight from the lower limbs to the upper limbs and reduce pressure on the painful joints, allowing ambulation even with markedly weak muscles or total paralysis. They increase stability by markedly increasing the area of support of the body. One must accurately evaluate the patient's ability to use these devices. The patient must be trained in their use to get the maximum benefit. Strengthening of the patient's lower extremities, upper extremities, and trunk is required.

For patients who need crutches or a walker but who have severe hand deformities from rheumatoid arthritis, forearm crutches that bear weight on the forearm and elbow rather than through the hand and wrist may be desirable (Fig. 9).

Various crutch gaits can be taught. Each patient should be taught one fast

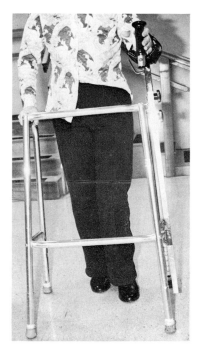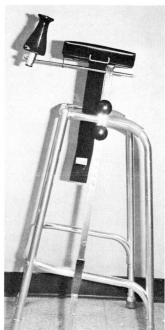

FIG. 9. Walker with forearm crutch. **Left:** Front view. **Right:** Side view.

gait and one slow gait. The four-point gait, in which each crutch and each limb is moved individually, allows for maximum balance and stability. It is a very slow gait. A slightly faster gait is the two-point gait, in which alternate crutches and lower limbs are moved simultaneously. The three-point gait is most rapid. Both crutches and both lower limbs are moved alternately. The two lower limbs are moved simultaneously, as are the two crutches. This may be a drag-to gait when the lower limbs are entirely paralyzed or a swing-through gait where a rapid gait is feasible.

If the patient is not stable and cannot use crutches, the use of a walker is desirable. This is a four-point device that the patient holds with both hands (Fig. 10). The patient lifts the device, which is very light in weight, usually of aluminum, and places it in front, leaning the body forward. The patient then takes a step or two into the walker and lifts up the device again and then places it in front. This gives an extreme amount of stability but, because of its mode of use, obviously does not allow a reciprocating natural walking pattern. This is particularly useful for the aged. It is sometimes used as the first walking device outside the parallel bars when retraining a patient to walk. Wheeled variants are less safe (Fig. 11). As there is improvement, the patient then proceeds to crutches, canes, and then no assistive device, if possible. Original training usually starts in the parallel bars.

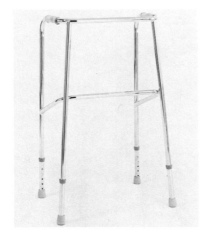

FIG. 10. Adjustable aluminum walker. (From Everest and Jennings Corporation, with permission.)

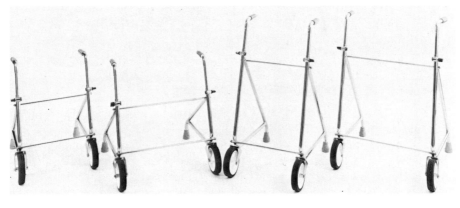

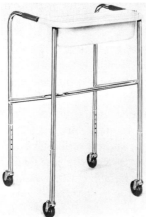

FIG. 11. Wheeled walkers. **Top:** Wheels on the front allow rolling, while crutch tips in the back can be placed on the ground for stability. **Bottom:** Walker with wheels on all four legs with no provision for stopping rolling. (From Everest and Jennings Corporation, with permission.)

Walkers are used when neither canes nor crutches suffice but full-time wheel-chair use is not required. They are helpful so that a patient can get out of the wheelchair and walk into the bathroom, for example, especially when the bath-room door is narrow. They are used almost entirely at home or in the hospital for ambulating short distances.

A walker should be used only for physiologic and early ambulation or for permanent ambulation. The gait pattern is much different from the normal gait. If a patient can walk with a normal gait it is preferable to teach walking in the parallel bars using a more normal gait pattern, for a longer period of time, and then graduate directly to crutches or canes. In certain patients, how-ever, who are afraid of crutches and yet in whom it is psychologically important to take them out of the parallel bars, a reciprocating walker is less detrimental than a standard walker because you do not want to develop a poor walking pattern. The use of the walker will require exercises for strengthening.

A reciprocating walker is basically constructed like a regular walker except that the two sides are attached by hinges to the front bars. This construction allows each side to move forward in conjunction with the leg and arm of that side and still provide the support of a regular walker.

If the patient cannot ambulate at all on foot, then one of the various types of wheelchairs should be used. Wheelchair prescription is a very complex subject and cannot be gone into completely here. There are standard wheelchairs that are used in the hospital pushed by someone else, with or without commodes (Figs. 12 and 13). There are folding wheelchairs that the patient can move without assistance with a large front wheel for indoor use only. Many attach-ments and sizes are available. Folding wheelchairs are generally most useful for patient use at home and outside. If the wheelchair is to be used inside, a solid thin rubber tire is best (Fig. 14). If there is occasional use of it outdoors, a semipneumatic tire is useful (Fig. 15). If soft, irregular terrain is frequently traversed, a balloon tire is required. Elevating leg rests may be needed if the patient has edema of the lower limbs. Foot rests are usually standard. Desk-type arms are available for patients who want to wheel under a standard table or desk. The arm rest may be solid or padded. Removable side arms are available for those who wish to transfer from the wheelchair to the bed and vice versa and to the toilet from the side of the wheelchair rather than from the front. There are crutch holders and back modifications.

The wheelchair is primarily a vehicle of transportation. It does, however, help the patient stimulate activity somewhat, getting the patient to use the upper extremities and, if used actively, gives some mild exercise. It reduces cardiac work in patients since the energy used in propelling a wheelchair is minimal and it thus can be used for patients with severe cardiorespiratory defi-ciency who find crutch walking too strenuous. Wheelchairs may make the elderly patient much more functional, particularly for performing various homemaking chores in which the use of both hands is required and standing is not necessary.

A wheelchair must be prescribed, as any other assistive aid, after a thorough

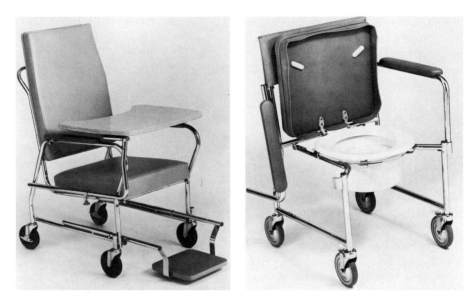

FIG. 12. Left: Hospital attendant wheeled wheelchair with lap board to hold such items as food, occupational therapy projects, or books. **Right:** Hospital commode wheelchair where patient cannot self-propel chair. (From Everest and Jennings Corporation, with permission.)

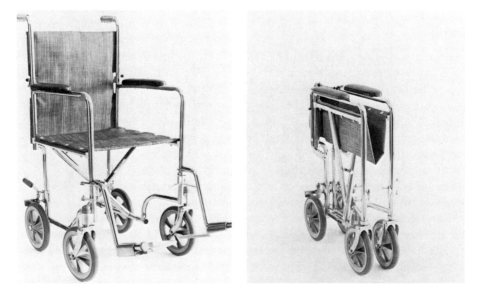

FIG. 13. Hospital folding wheelchair where patient cannot self-propel chair. **Left:** Open. **Right:** Folded. (From Everest and Jennings Corporation, with permission.)

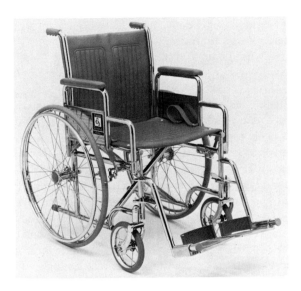

FIG. 14. Folding adult wheelchair with desk arms, foot rests with heel loops, and thin, solid, rubber tires for indoor use; note large front wheels for rolling over surface irregularities. (From Everest and Jennings Corporation, with permission.)

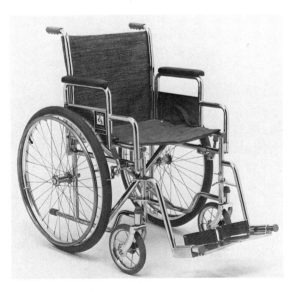

FIG. 15. Folding adult wheelchair with removable desk arms for getting close to table, with semi-pneumatic wheels for going over surface irregularities and moderately soft terrain. (From Everest and Jennings Corporation, with permission.)

evaluation. Unnecessary dependence on the wheelchair should be avoided.

For the bilateral lower limb amputee, especially when a prosthesis is not worn, an amputee wheelchair is available with the axle 5 cm posterior to the standard axle, to provide a more appropriate fulcrum for balancing the body weight.

For most patients, the standard wheelchair is desirable. This has a 24- or 26-inch rear wheel and 8-inch front casters for stability in going over doorsills. Smaller front wheels are generally inadvisable as the wheelchair may tip in going over the edge of a rug or doorsill (Fig. 16).

Wheelchairs may be manually propelled. In addition, there are externally powered wheelchairs, usually electrically powered, with many variations in control mechanisms and function. Some are useful only indoors whereas others can go over uneven outdoor terrain and some can even climb curbs and steps. They may have a variation in speed and can be controlled by movement of many parts of the body such as by movement of legs, hands, arms, head attitude, breath, and even eye motion, voice and acoustic controls.

There may be licensed vehicles such as automobiles with various types of hand or foot controls, power augmentation devices to lift the person and/or a wheelchair into the car (Fig. 17), vans with or without ramps or lifts to lift the patient into the van either to have the person transported or to lift the patient, with wheelchair, into the vehicle and enable the person to drive the vehicle.

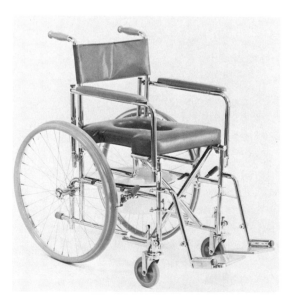

FIG. 16. Commode self-propelled wheelchair with small front wheels, which may be unsafe going over doorsills or carpet edges. (From Everest and Jennings Corporation, with permission.)

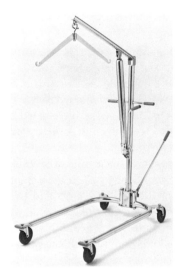

FIG. 17. Pneumatic lift, to lift patients from bed to wheelchair, tub, car, and vice versa. (From Everest and Jennings Corporation, with permission.)

Equipment is available to help a person to transfer from the wheelchair to a vehicle if this is a problem. Hand controls are available for those who cannot use their legs. An automatic transmission vehicle with power steering and power brakes is almost invariably required but can be obtained from the car manufacturer. Providing mobility so that the person is not trapped in the house is psychologically very important, particularly to the aged. Any type of mobility is important psychologically, socially, and sometimes vocationally. Many people work well into advanced years and we have many patients who continue to work at remunerative employment, either in their own businesses or elsewhere, well into their eighties. This gives them a feeling of accomplishment and self-respect.

In all vehicles, chairs, and wheelchairs, seating is a very important factor. For persons with coccygodynia, a cut-out donut may be required. Frequently, a seat board is required in wheelchairs with a cut-out to avoid continual pressure over the ischial tuberosities. The use of a 3- or 4-inch foam cushion is helpful. There are special devices with water, air, or gel cushioning, but these generally are not required for the aged person in a wheelchair but for those who have had seating problems and decubitus ulcers over the ischial tuberosities.

Elderly persons may need a back brace to support their spines in vehicles and may use special car seats to provide comfort.

Another type of mobility aid is an unlicensed vehicle, such as a golf cart or tricycle, either for the nondisabled but weak who are elderly and cannot walk long distances, or for those with balance problems. These may be leg powered or hand powered. The vehicles may have three or four wheels. There are also wheelchairs that function as stretchers, standing devices, and therapeutic aids, and some that can serve as shower chairs and commode seats.

Prostheses

The elderly need safe mobility most of all. The characteristics needed in a prosthesis, therefore, are stability for safety, lightweight, ease of donning and use, and appearance. The prosthesis should be inexpensive to buy and maintain. Complex, sophisticated devices are unwise, especially for the elderly.

For patients who have partial foot amputations, shoe fillers are generally all that is required. Prostheses are available for patients with Syme amputations through the ankle. Below-knee amputation patients generally use the patellar tendon weight-bearing prosthesis with varying suspension means, with varying amounts of minimal to total contact, and with different interfaces between the skin of the residual limb and the prosthesis. For elderly people, suspension is generally by means of a soft suprapatellar cuff suspension, although an occasional patient with knee instability or great demands needs a thigh corset. For the above-knee amputee, elderly people can only infrequently use a prosthesis. Some patients may use lightweight endoskeletal devices, which have knee locks for stability. In general, elderly people with above-knee amputations do much better with single axis joints, rather than the solid ankle cushion heel (SACH) feet used for the below-knee amputee. Elderly below-knee amputee patients sometimes do not do well with SACH feet because they are less stable than single axis ankles and feet.

Elderly patients with amputations at the hip are generally confined to the use of a wheelchair. Prosthetic fitting for these patients is extremely infrequent. A soft insert liner used with thick stump socks is usual for padding and absorption of perspiration.

Patients with an upper limb amputation rarely use a prosthesis because they can do almost everything with one hand. The cosmetic prosthesis is rarely desired by the amputee of advanced age. However, a prosthesis should certainly be prescribed for a person who wishes to have one.

An accurate evaluation of the patient's cardiorespiratory, neuromotor, and muscular strengths, vision, and ability to learn is required prior to prescribing a prosthesis. It is most important that the patient's true desire to have a prosthesis be evaluated. A temporary limb is always required to help evaluate the patient and his needs for special components and to have the patient evaluate whether it is worth the time and effort to learn to use a limb, prior to prescribing a permanent and expensive artificial limb. The patient must understand that hygiene and gait training are required, and this requires general conditioning exercises and exercises of the trunk, upper limbs, both lower limbs, and so on. The patient must have the mental ability to learn to use a prosthesis, to put it on, to take it off, and to use it in the home. This is all taught in both occupational and physical therapy and includes care of the stump and of the prosthesis.

Prosthetic training should be undertaken and during that time the patient's ability to be independent will be evaluated. Where possible, preprosthetic training and even preamputation training are desirable. The training flows naturally as part of one ongoing process the patient generally understands. For all persons, but for the elderly most of all, the importance of below-the-knee amputation must be stressed. It takes at least three or four times as much energy to walk with an above-the-knee prosthesis as with a below-the-knee prosthesis. In addition, the patient who retains the knee joint always knows where the prosthetic foot is, if the prosthetic knee is bent. A locked prosthetic knee gives a poor gait and only then does the patient know that the prosthetic foot is in a direct line with the thigh. The physical and mental work is much less and, therefore, the locked knee should be used, if required.

The saving of the knee joint often makes the difference between an elderly patient who can walk and an elderly patient who is confined to a wheelchair. This may make the difference between the family's ability to take the patient home and the need for institutionalization in a nursing home. The psychological, social, and economic costs of this difference are crucial.

Elderly people with weak muscles, who have difficulty in strengthening them because of cardiac or respiratory difficulties, may need special support for their abdominal and back muscles. Corsets, braces, and other labor-saving devices can be crucial for this population.

Communication Devices

Communication is very important to all individuals. The elderly who have hearing problems may be able to use hearing aids, and those with visual problems may be able to use eyeglasses. For the deaf and the blind, very special devices are important for transmission of information. The inability to communicate by either speaking or writing is catastrophic for the individual. Some speech disorders in which cerebral involvement is not a factor can be helped by technical aids. The simplest are the various symbol, picture, or alphabet boards that can convey information. The patient points to the various symbols, either with a digit or with a device. Some more sophisticated aids have voice outputs.

One communication problem that occurs is that the patient cannot read, simply because the patient cannot turn pages. Page-turning devices are available. Other aids, such as overhead projectors and those that project a photographic image, such as microfilm, can be used. (See also A. L. Kornzweig, *this volume.*)

Sensory aids for the blind include the long and white canes, and ultrasonic and laser devices to probe surroundings. They can give either an audible or tactile feedback to the person. The use of the seeing-eye dog is the use of another living creature to help the disabled. The use of other animals to perform various functions for the elderly and the disabled is just being started; primates are being researched.

Of course blind persons can be taught Braille, but there are some people who have sensory loss in the fingers for whom Braille is inappropriate. One may have the input and/or the output in Braille, depending on what is needed for a particular individual. The magnetic tape cassette player brings the written word to the blind, free of charge, through the Library of Congress. It also may be used in place of writing. A speech output calculator is available and may be used at the workplace. For the deaf, there are hearing aids and writing.

The electric typewriter has been a boon to the elderly. The typewriter may be activated by the fingers, with or without special guides for the keys where coordination is a problem; used with a mouth stick or head stick; or can be an automatic device. This type is activated by a light-sensing board (which the patient activates by pointing a light attached to a movable and controllable body part onto the receiving board). This is a special narrow-beam flashlight attached, for example, to a head band. Voice-activated typewriters are available, usually as part of a total environment control system. Information regarding such equipment can be obtained from any established rehabilitation center.

Environment Manipulation

The average person uses many controls for the environment. These are especially helpful for the elderly. Examples include air conditioning, and the automatic door openers used in supermarkets and department stores. The removal of the door sills and the provision of ramps all are a help to the elderly, so that they do not have to raise their legs to go up curbs, steps, or other obstacles. The provision of wide doors in all rooms, including the bathroom, is important for many elderly so that they may walk with their canes and walkers as well as use wheelchairs.

The arm amputee will have artificial arms to grasp and to manipulate the environment. People must be able to grasp, manipulate, transport, and release objects. The prostheses are inadequate replacements for what the individual has lost, but they certainly assist function and dignity.

For those who are bedridden or wheelchair-bound, many household chores still need to be done. There are devices that are activated by voice, puff and suck pneumatic controls, head controls, or switch controls. The patient can open and close doors and windows, control air conditioners, radios, television sets, toasters, ovens, and so on. Multiple channel systems are available for individual needs, such as raising and lowering a bed or the head of the bed. Typewriters are often part of such a system.

Manipulation devices are an outgrowth of manipulators for the atomic industry. To move radioactive materials, manipulators that amplify the reach and grasp of the individual had to be developed. Some remote manipulators can be used by the severely disabled. Simpler manipulators are used as braces and orthoses for grasping, holding, and manipulating for those with hand function loss, such as after a nerve injury or stroke.

Patient-handling devices may be lifting devices, which may be pneumatic, hydraulic, electrical, or manual. This may assist in moving the patient from one side to the other or allow the patient to be stood upright or put into a bathtub or bed.

Various types of beds are available, from the standard bed with a different mattress, bed boards, water mattresses, hospital beds, alternating pressure pad mattresses, mobile beds, and air fluidized beds. There are also electrically operated tilting and turning beds for those with decubitus ulcers, rotary beds, and flotation mattresses and bed.

The list of available assistive devices is almost endless. Ingenuity must be exercised to choose the best for and with the patient, to maximize function and self-respect at minimal cost in money and gadgetry.

The sense of self-worth is aided if the older person can participate in some of the sports and activities that were earlier enjoyed. Special assistive aids are of help in this regard.

Rehabilitation in the Aging edited by
T. F. Williams. Raven Press, New York © 1984.

Self-Help Devices for the Elderly Population Living in the Community

*Masayoshi Itoh, *Mathew Lee, and **Joyce Shapiro

*Department of Rehabilitation Medicine and **Occupational Therapy Service, Goldwater Memorial Hospital, New York University Medical Center, F. D. Roosevelt Island, New York, N.Y. 10044*

In this chapter the words *elderly* or *aged* are used generically and do not refer to any particular age group. The aging process is a continuous one throughout life.

The now well-recognized overall increase in life expectancy and in numbers of old (and very old) people in our society present problems our society is not yet prepared to solve. Financial support for many elderly is inadequate. Physical environment such as housing, household services, personal protection, and transportation do not meet their needs, and psychologically and socially a large segment of this population is isolated and lonely. Although the medical community can be credited for its remarkable achievement in the increase in life expectancy, it must take a measure of responsibility for the lagging development of geriatric medicine.

The degenerative processes that appear with aging do not occur evenly in particular organ systems or evenly in all organ systems, but rather are observed in various systems in varying degrees. These changes are very slow in their progression and may or may not have clinical significance until the resultants interfere with normal activities of daily living (ADL).

Elderly persons may not recognize the decline of their functional ability and endurance in ADL (1) from the peak functional level of younger days. Thus, they typically try to perform these tasks without modification. They undoubtedly possess sufficient skills and experiences to perform a variety of other activities. This is no assurance, however, that physical endurance, dexterity, and mental capacity remain the same as it was a few decades earlier. The elderly population must learn or recondition themselves to adjust their performance according to their present physical and mental capacities.

It is difficult and frustrating for the elderly to accept a new pace and a modified method of performing their accustomed activities. However, it is the responsibility of medical practitioners to emphasize to elderly people the importance of "moderation and modification" of life style. It must be noted that moderation and sedentary are not synonymous. Rather, elderly persons should be as active physically and mentally as possible. It is to assist them in maintaining the best feasible levels of activity that self-help devices have their role.

Self-help devices are gadgets, materials, articles, or equipment that assist persons in various physical activities. Some of them may be used for ADL and others aid vocational or recreational activities. The primary purpose of the self-help device is to provide a particular body function that was lost or diminished due to a trauma or disease.

This group of devices should not be confused with orthotic and prosthetic devices. Orthotic devices are also substitutes for lost functions. But this group of devices provides gross functions such as the long leg brace for standing and ambulation or the spinal brace used to maintain posture. Prosthetic devices fill a void wherein a part of body is missing and they may or may not be functional. A prosthesis for an extremity amputation or a dental prosthesis are functional whereas a prosthesis for an enucleated eye is strictly cosmetic. On the other hand, self-help devices are intended for more specific functions such as feeding and grooming.

There are many studies on self-help devices for the physically handicapped. Our approach, which promotes self-help devices for the aged who are not overtly disabled, is new. This concept does not imply that the aged are considered disabled. Many elderly people have various underlying conditions that are often degenerative, progressive, and chronic. These conditions may not limit their overall function to any great degree. A careful observation of their physical performance and a thorough assessment of their physical and mental conditions, therapeutic regime, and living environment provide a base that determines what self-help devices will make life safer, easier, and more enjoyable for them.

Many self-help devices for the physically disabled are custom made in order to meet the patient's specific needs. These are often called adaptive devices. For the purpose of economy and easy availability, many devices that will be described below have been selected because they can be purchased in regular retail or discount stores. Some items can be fabricated very easily and economically. Many items can be found under different brand names but are equally good and serve the same purpose. The important considerations are meeting the needs of each individual, soundness of construction, and durability. The various items described here were not originally intended to be self-help devices and creative and imaginative thinking will find many other commercial items that are useful for the elderly.

CONSERVATION OF ENERGY EXPENDITURE

In general, the aged have less cardiovascular reserve and fatigue easily. Thus, even those who do not have overt cardiac conditions should avoid stressful physical activities. In kitchen activities, standing for a long period is stressful and tiring. An "admiral's chair" or bar stool is high enough for one to work comfortably on a counter top in a sitting position. The feet can rest on the foot rail section of the chair. If a bar stool is used, select one with a backrest to provide better support for the trunk.

A regular gas or electric range usually has the oven section under the range top. Thus, to operate the oven one must bend, stoop, or kneel on the floor. Returning to the upright position from these positions consumes extra energy and the sudden change in posture may cause dizziness. This can be avoided by using a table top electric broiler-oven, which is often combined with a toaster. They come in many sizes that accommodate small or large quantities of food.

A rolling cart is a convenient device to transport various items such as food, plates, and serving and eating utensils from the kitchen to the dining room table. This will eliminate the necessity of making several trips between these two areas. The rolling cart comes in a stationary construction or folding type. If the living space is limited, the folding type may be more useful. Obviously, this cart can be utilized to carry many items in the home that are either heavy or cumbersome.

To eliminate several trips to various electric appliances, there is a device to which several appliances can be connected and it can be switched on and off by means of remote control. There are different types on the market that serve the same purpose and their prices depend on the degree of sophistication in the design of the mechanism.

Many housekeeping activities can be made easier. A long-handled dustpan can be operated in a standing position and there is no need to stoop to collect dust after sweeping. To minimize the necessity of stooping or climbing, which is always hazardous for the elderly, a reacher (Fig. 1) may be used to pick up items from the floor or a high shelf. Similarly, long-handled pullers and pruners eliminate stooping and climbing in the garden or yard.

The basic concept for utilizing specific equipment and devices by the aged is to eliminate stressful and hazardous movement while promoting maximum ADL. With this concept in mind, one can find many gadgets on the market that are relatively inexpensive and serve to promote safety or activity without unnecessary energy expenditure.

PREVENTION OF FALLING ACCIDENT

Some of the general characteristics of the aged are decreased muscle tone, strength, joint motion, coordination, vision, memory, slower body motion, and reflex time. Each of these characteristics can be contributory factors in a falling accident. The osteoporosis that is common among the elderly adds greatly to the likelihood of a fracture with a fall. The resulting immobilization and physical inactivity produce loss of muscular strength that is often not regained; the traumatic experiences of hospitalization and surgery often hasten mental deterioration.

There are many correctable environmental hazards—throw rugs that slip, obstacles left in walkways, poorly lit halls or stairways, lack of handrails. However, the place where the most serious falling accidents happen is in the bathroom.

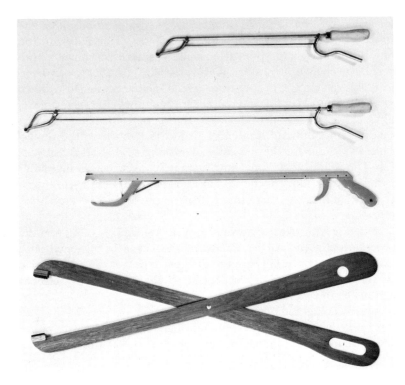

FIG. 1. Reacher. (Reprinted by permission. Copyright © J. A. Preston Corporation.)

A grab-bar installed on the wall (Fig. 2) or on the rim of the bathtub (Fig. 3) should be mandatory in the homes of all elderly persons. The expenditure for nationwide installation is miniscule compared to the annual costs of medical and nursing home care for elderly victims of bathroom accidents. There is

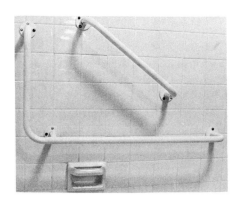

FIG. 2. Grab-bar installed on the bathroom wall.

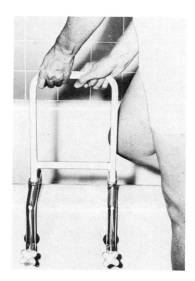

FIG. 3. Grab-bar attached on the rim of bathtub. (Reprinted by permission. Copyright © J. A. Preston Corporation.)

also a guard-rail designed for toilets (Fig. 4), which can be purchased from medical and surgical supply stores.

Another dangerous area in the bathroom is the floor of the shower and bottom of the bathtub. There is nonskid tape especially made for these fixtures that comes in various colors and designs. This tape has its own adhesive backing and merely pressing it to the dry surface completes installation. It provides sufficient friction even when the tub or shower is wet and soapy. As with the grab bar, all elderly should have the nonskid tapes. A shower chair may be

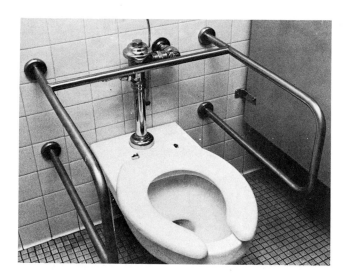

FIG. 4. Guard rails for toilet.

used when the person is prone to dizziness for any reason. A shower chair can be purchased from surgical supply stores and some bath shops. The same result may be obtained by placing a metal chair under the shower if the legs of the chair have rubber tips. Rubber tips are common items in hardware, discount, and home decorating stores.

INCOORDINATION

Incoordination is a common finding in the elderly. This often makes their physical performance clumsy and shaky. Incoordination can also cause slow body movement and delayed reflex time. These functional deficiencies not only cause falling accidents but make performance of ADL difficult and result in other injuries such as bruises, cuts, and burns.

A hand-held shower head connected to the regular shower outlet (Fig. 5) may be easier for some elderly persons to use, particularly if they must shower

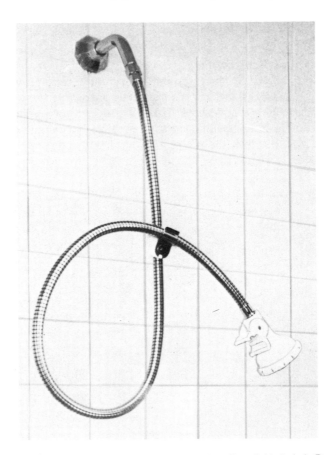

FIG. 5. Hand-held shower head. (Reprinted by permission. Copyright © J. A. Preston Corporation.)

while sitting down. The incoordinated hand may drop a cake of soap. Soap-on-a-rope, which hangs from the neck of the bather, is convenient and secure. Less costly but equally effective is a bar of soap in a bag made of a loosely woven string or mesh dishcloth with a loop of soft cord attached. It is large enough to hold a bar of soap and has the added advantage of reuse with a favorite soap.

A shower caddy (Fig. 6) can store such items as brushes and shampoos within easy reach in the shower or bathtub. When one wishes to take a bath, a child's pool raft, a small air mattress, can be floated on water and various items needed for bathing may be placed on it.

Shaving by both elderly men and women for cosmetic reasons should be encouraged but incoordinated persons can cut themselves even with a safety razor. Electric razors for men and specially designed ones for women to use under the arms or on the legs are available. However, these should not be used in the bathroom by any elderly person since it is possible that the cord or razor could touch a wet surface.

Household and kitchen activities also present problems. If a gas range is not equipped with an automatic lighter, one must use matches to light the oven. It is safer for the elderly to use the long fireplace matches to prevent burns. They should always use padded mitts or pot holders when carrying hot pots or dishes. A mop pail with caddy is a pail with casters and easily rolls from one place to the other. It may not be easy to reach the bottom of a clothes hamper but a reacher (Fig. 1) can do it. Laundry baskets can be carried on a rolling cart. There is an ironing board with an electric outlet. This ironing board may prevent tripping on the iron cord.

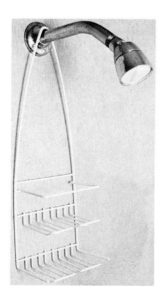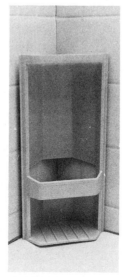

FIG. 6. Left: Shower caddy on the shower pipe. **Right:** Shower caddy on the bathtub.

Incoordinated hands may drop articles on the floor. Melamac dishes (plastic) are unbreakable. Plastic colanders and other utensils are much lighter in weight than the metal ones and are easier to handle.

Those who have difficulty negotiating door knobs may find levers (Fig. 7) or pulls are handier. Some who find it difficult to get up from an armchair may use a so-called cushion lifting chair, which can assist one to stand up by pressing a button.

LOSS OF MANUAL DEXTERITY

Many old people lose hand dexterity and become somewhat clumsy. This decline in hand function may be caused by various factors, e.g., incoordination, weakened muscle power, limitation in joint movement, or tremor. In addition, decreased tactile sensation may contribute to difficulty in performing fine manual work.

If the hand is weak, it is hard to open a can or jar. An electric can opener or jar opener (Fig. 8) may be extremely useful. If one finds various cooking utensils or mixing bowls too heavy to handle, similar utensils or bowls made of plastic materials may suffice. Those who have a poor grip may be afraid of dropping a glass on the floor. A stretch knit coaster slipped onto the bottom of a glass provides additional friction and secures the grasping area. For leisure activity, a playing card holder (Fig. 9) eliminates the need to hold cards in the hand.

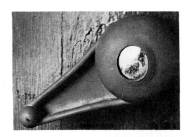

FIG. 7. Door lever. Made of rubber and slips on the door knob.

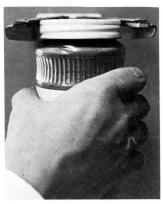

FIG. 8. Jar opener.

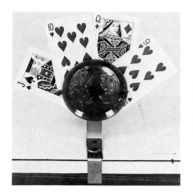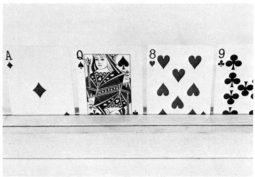

FIG. 9. Playing card holder. **Left:** Commercial style. **Right:** A piece of wood approximately 1 × 1.5 × 16 inches with two parallel grooves. One groove is ⅛ inch wide and ½ inch deep and the other is ⅛ inch wide and ¾ inch deep.

LIMITATION IN RANGE OF JOINT MOTION

Limitation of movement in various major joints can interfere with ADL. These limitations may be caused by some forms of arthritis or pathological changes in tendons or other soft tissues (see J. Baum, *this volume*). When these limitations are combined with limitation of motion in the hands, performance of ADL is even more difficult. These changes are again common findings among the elderly.

In general, limitations in motion of major joints make reaching activity difficult. One approach to overcome these obstacles is to extend the handles of objects so that the individual can perform the intended task with the limited range of motion. A long-handled shoehorn, hair brush, or bath sponge and long-handled weed puller and pruner are some examples that can be found in many stores. If it is so indicated, an extension handle attached to a comb or other items can be constructed without too much difficulty.

A long-reach zipper pull (Fig. 10) is simply a cord approximately 18 inches long with metal hook attached to its end. A stocking put-on device (Fig. 11) is a stick with a looped wire and hook on one end. A stick with a girdle garter attached at one end is another type of device that serves the same purpose. Other items helpful to those who cannot reach their feet are the shoe and boot jack (remover) (Fig. 12) and elastic shoe laces.

Other aids to dressing include the dressing stick, cuff and collar extenders, and button hooks. More information of these items can be obtained from specialized surgical supply stores or any occupational therapy department of a hospital or rehabilitation center.

A hoop apron is an apron with a resilient elastic band on the top instead of apron strings. The person just hooks the band at the side of the waist instead of having to tie a sash (strings) in the back. Front closure bras are available for those women who have limitations in the shoulder joints.

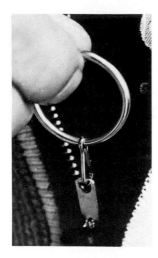

FIG. 10. Zipper pull. A ring is attached to the zipper. If necessary a string may be attached to the zipper or to the ring.

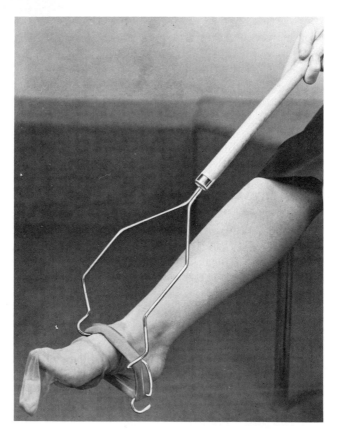

FIG. 11. Stocking put-on device. (Reprinted by permission. Copyright © J. A. Preston Corporation.)

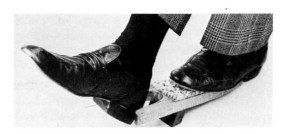

FIG. 12. Bootjack.

Some modification may be needed in the home. For example, a person who has limitation of hip and knee joints may need a raised toilet seat (Fig. 13). The toilet paper holder may have to be moved to a location that is easier to reach. Storage of daily necessities should not be placed too high or too low because such locations make ADL more difficult. The installation of a peg board, shelves, or counters at a convenient height or the use of a lazy susan may make a person more independent and more functional.

DECREASED TACTILE SENSATION

Tactile sensation is somewhat diminished in many elderly people and this can present problems. If there is a severe loss of this sensation, there must be some neurological condition that should be investigated. Elderly persons with

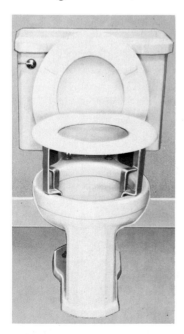
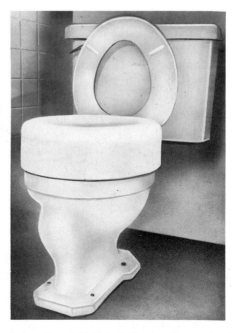

FIG. 13. Raised toilet seats. (Reprinted by permission. Copyright © J. A. Preston Corporation.)

such conditions are not within the scope of this chapter. There is concern, however, for those with slight loss of this sensation because they are often not aware of the loss.

The elderly must be careful to prevent burns. Padded pot holders or mitts should be used to handle pots and pans on a stove. It is preferable to have pots and pans and other cooking utensils that have nonheat conducting handles. Insulated rubber gloves can be used for dishwashing. The hot water temperature should be set low enough (no more than 130 to 140°F) that it will be unlikely to cause burns. If the hot water is running for a long time, the metal faucet handle may become dangerously hot. Thus the handle of the faucet should be covered with nonheat conducting tape.

LOW VISION

Low vision is a common condition that the elderly encounter. Various magnifying glasses are available to enhance vision. Some may have stands or may hang on the neck of the user (Fig. 14) so as to free the user's hands. Magnifying make-up mirrors can be purchased with or without light fixtures. Other magnifying glasses are available for specific purposes, e.g., rectangular ones sized to fit book pages or newspaper columns, and large ones in stands for sewing or handicrafts. The soap-on-a-rope referred to earlier is also useful for the person with low vision. (See also A. L. Kornzweig, *this volume*.)

The needle threader for sewing has been used by many, both young and old, and can be found in any sewing center or dime store. A measuring cup with large print is manufactured by Westland Plastics. This can be purchased in a hardware store or by mail order. Sometimes an elderly person may find it difficult to read the temperature control knob of the oven. In reality, every

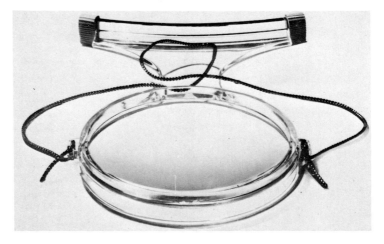

FIG. 14. Neck magnifier. (The photograph is the courtesy of Hoffritz for Cutlery Inc., 515 West 24 Street, New York City.)

nd he made other moves, | refused

recall of the Ame

from Moscow, in

Soviet military inte **Clues Found**

nistan.

ition officials, who

Continued From Page C1

cision to delay actic virgin female American roaches, identified the scent chemical, or sex phero-
eaty, also said tha mone, used to attract males. Last year,
Columbia University chemists an-
; had dropped its pl nounced the successful synthesis of the
substance, for possible use in trapping
an issue to the Unite males. But, after all this work, it is
doubtful that the chemical could be
l Assembly and in: used to control this pest because
American roach females can repro-
a proposal by Euro duce parthenogenetically — without
the services of males.
ld nations to put the ¶Japanese researchers showed that
the small German roach, most com-
: Security Council, v mon of the household varieties, ex-
cretes an aggregation pheromone, a
ain Soviet veto. chemical scent that attracts others of
the species to the same area. Thus, just

FIG. 15. Comparison of regular and large-type newspaper.

temperature registered on the knob is not used by the average person. Certain temperatures are used more often than the others. For example, baking a cake is done at 350°F. Thus, if the commonly used temperatures are marked with colored tapes, there is no need to read the knob.

The elderly person often has difficulty reading a newspaper with regular-type print. *The New York Times,* for example, issues a weekly large-type newspaper (Fig. 15). G. K. Hall Company of Boston, Massachusetts, is one of the publishers of large-print books on various subjects. There are even large-print cookbooks as well.*

POOR MEMORY

One of the very early signs of the common dementia of the elderly (usually Alzheimer's type) is forgetfulness. The onset of this syndrome is insidious and

---

* *Campbell Cookbook: Easy Way to Delicious Meals.* Large-type edition published by Volunteers Service of the Blind. *Large-Type Cookbook of General Mills, Inc.* Published by Betty Crocker Kitchens, Minneapolis, Minnesota. *The New York Times Large Type Cookbook.* Published by Golden Press, Inc., New York.

those who are close to an individual must observe very carefully to detect this change. Distant past memory is well preserved but the recent past memory becomes poor. Immediate recall may or may not be disturbed at this stage. During this period the elderly may need reminding by audio and/or visual means. A timer may be useful as a reminder for taking medication or during cooking. Electric appliances for the elderly should have a red reminder light to show that the appliance is on. Tea kettles that whistle should be used to boil water, as an open pan may boil dry. It is often useful to color code burners and switches on the stove with color tapes.

DISCUSSION

In 1975, 51% of the elderly in the United States were living in the community with their spouse, whereas 27% lived alone and 5% were cared for in institutions (3). Many of the elderly living in the community have various physical limitations, each of which may be minor and separately may not interfere greatly with their ADL. However, the cumulative effects of numerous minor limitations may, in aggregate, be detrimental to their well-being and to their ability to continue to live independently. Self-help devices can make the life of the elderly in the community more comfortable, enjoyable, and functional; through helping to prevent the need to enter institutions they reduce the costs of health care. For all of these reasons it seems justified to seek to include reimbursement for such devices in health insurance coverage, including Medicare and Medicaid.

There is a general lack of knowledge and understanding of self-help devices among medical practitioners (2). Occupational therapists specialize in these devices in addition to giving functional therapy, and can give expert guidance. Community-based occupational therapists should be a part of the health care delivery system.

All health professionals—physicians, nurses, social workers, as well as occupational and physical therapists—need to learn to assess the environment, the home, of elderly clients, to be sensitive to early signs of functional limitations, and to know what self-help devices may not only prolong elderly peoples' independence but also ease and enhance their daily lives.

REFERENCES

1. Deaver, G. D., and Brown, M. E. (1945): *Physical Demands of Daily Life.* Institute for Crippled and Disabled, New York.
2. Itoh, M., and Lee, M. H. M. (1971): The epidemiology of disability as related to rehabilitation medicine. In: *Handbook of Physical Medicine and Rehabilitation,* edited by F. H. Krusen, F. J. Kottke, and P. M. Ellwood. Saunders, Philadelphia.
3. Reichel, W. (ed.) (1978): *The Geriatric Patient.* HP Publishing Company, New York.

Subject Index